ASIAN PARENTING

Asian Parenting provides a comprehensive and scholarly discussion of the distinct features, meanings, and implications for human development of contemporary Asian parenting, beyond Western theoretical frameworks. It explores how cultural beliefs and values shape socialization goals and practices and guide Asian parent-child interactions. Edited by Xinyin Chen, contributions from leading scholars discuss key topics including conceptual and methodological issues in the study of Asian parenting; the role of social circumstances and cultural values in shaping Asian parenting; culturally prescribed socialization processes; the influence of Asian parenting on children's socioemotional functioning, learning and academic achievement, and psychological wellbeing; and the impact of social, economic, and cultural changes in Asian societies on parenting beliefs, attitudes, and behaviors.

Asian Parenting is an essential text for students and scholars of psychology, sociology, cultural anthropology, education, and family studies who are interested in culture and human development. It will also guide interventions on the parts of governmental and nongovernmental organizations operating in Asian societies.

Xinyin Chen is Professor of Psychology at the Graduate School of Education, University of Pennsylvania. His research interest is mainly in children's and adolescents' socioemotional functioning (e.g., shyness-inhibition, social competence, depression), social relationships, and family processes from a cultural-contextual perspective. With international collaborators, he has conducted a series of large-scale, longitudinal projects in Brazil, Canada, China, Italy, South Korea, and the United States. His recent work has tapped the implications of macro-level societal changes for human development in Asian societies.

Studies in Parenting Series

Marc H. Bornstein, Series Editor

The chief aim of this series of volumes is to provide a forum for extended and integrated treatments of fundamental and challenging contemporary topics in parenting. Each volume treats a different perspective on parenting and is self-contained, yet the series as a whole endeavors to enhance and interrelate studies in parenting by bringing shared perspectives to bear on a variety of concerns prominent in parenting theory, research, practice, and application. Reflecting the nature and intent of this series, contributing authors are drawn from a broad spectrum of the humanities and sciences—anthropology to zoology—with representational emphasis placed on active contributing authorities to the contemporary literature in parenting.

Parenting Across Cultures Across Development: Parenting from Childhood to Adolescence in Nine Countries
Edited by Jennifer E. Lansford, W. Andrew Rothenberg, and Marc H. Bornstein

Parenting, Infancy, Culture: Specificity and Commonality in Argentina, Belgium, Israel, Italy, and the United States
Edited by Marc H. Bornstein

Parenting and Child Development in Low- and Middle-Income Countries
Marc H. Bornstein, W. Andrew Rothenberg, Andrea Bizzego, Robert H. Bradley, Kirby Deater-Deckard, Gianluca Esposito, Jennifer E. Lansford, Diane L. Putnick, and Susannah Zietz

Asian Parenting: Meanings, Characteristics, and Implications
Edited by Xinyin Chen

ASIAN PARENTING

Meanings, Characteristics, and Implications

Edited by
Xinyin Chen

Routledge
Taylor & Francis Group
NEW YORK AND LONDON

Designed cover image: Winnie Vinzence via Getty Images

First published 2025
by Routledge
605 Third Avenue, New York, NY 10158

and by Routledge
4 Park Square, Milton Park, Abingdon, Oxon, OX14 4RN

Routledge is an imprint of the Taylor & Francis Group, an informa business

ISBN: 978-1-032-46950-8 (hbk)
ISBN: 978-1-032-46955-3 (pbk)
ISBN: 978-1-003-38394-9 (ebk)

DOI: 10.4324/9781003383949

Typeset in Optima
by codeMantra

CONTENTS

SERIES FOREWORD

Parenting is fundamental to the survival and success of the human species. Everyone who has ever lived has had parents, and the vast majority of adults in the world become parents. Opinions about parenting abound, but still surprisingly too little solid scientific information or considered reflection exist about parenting. *Studies in Parenting* redresses this imbalance. The chief aim of this series of books is to provide a forum for extended and integrated treatments of fundamental and challenging contemporary topics in parenting. Each book treats a different perspective on parenting and is self-contained, yet the series as a whole endeavors to enhance and interrelate studies in parenting by bringing shared perspectives to bear on a variety of concerns prominent in parenting theory, research, practice, and application. As a consequence of its structure and scope, *Studies in Parenting* will appeal individually or as a series to professionals and parents alike. Reflecting the nature and intent of this series, contributing authors are drawn from a broad spectrum of the humanities and sciences—anthropology to zoology—with representational emphasis placed on active contributing authorities to the contemporary literature in parenting.

Parenting is a job whose primary object of attention and action is the child—human children do not and cannot grow up as solitary individuals—but parenting is also a vital status in the life course with consequences for parents themselves. In this forum, parenting is defined by all of children's principal caregivers and their many modes of caregiving. *Studies in Parenting* encompasses five central themes in parenting.

Who Parents?

Biological and adoptive mothers, fathers, single parents, and divorced and remarried parents can be children's principal caregivers, but when siblings, grandparents, and nonfamilial caregivers as well as mentors mind children, their parenting is also pertinent.

Whom Parents Parent?

Parents parent infants, toddlers, children in middle childhood, and adolescents as well as special populations of children including multiple births, preterm, ill, developmentally delayed or talented, and aggressive or withdrawn children.

The Scope of Parenting

Parenting's direct effects include parents' genetic endowment as well as the experiences they provide children that are instantiated in parents' cognitions and practices; parenting's indirect influences take place through parents' relationships with each other and their connections to community and culture. Parenting's direct and indirect effects on children can be both positive and negative.

The Determinants and Consequences of Parenting

Evolution and history; biology and ethology; family configuration; formal and informal support systems, community ties, and work; circumstances, tasks, and demands; social, educational, legal, medical, and governmental institutions; socioeconomic class, designed and natural ecology, and culture—as well as children themselves—each shapes parenting.

The Nature, Structure, and Meaning of Parenting

Parenting's pleasures, privileges, and profits as well as frustrations, fears, and failures are all explored in *Studies in Parenting*. Contemporary parenting studies are diversified, pluralistic, and specialized. This fragmented state needs counterforce in an arena that allows the extended in-depth exploration of cardinal topics in parenting. *Studies in Parenting* vigorously pursues that goal.

Marc H. Bornstein
Series Editor

CONTRIBUTORS

Liane Peña Alampay is a Professor of Psychology at the Ateneo de Manila University, Philippines, where she has been teaching for over 20 years. She obtained her BA and MA Psychology degrees from the University of the Philippines, and her PhD in Human Development and Family Studies from the Pennsylvania State University. Her research focuses on parenting and child and adolescent development in cultural contexts, and interventions for youth and families at risk. She is a co-Investigator in the Parenting Across Cultures study, and Principal Investigator of Parenting for Lifelong Health-Philippines, wherein she contextually adapts, tests, and scales evidence-based parent support interventions to prevent child maltreatment among vulnerable Filipino families. Her research and policy contributions in the area of child protection have earned her the recognition of Outstanding Young Scientist from the Philippines' National Academy of Science and Technology in 2013, and Outstanding Psychologist from the Psychological Association of the Philippines in 2023.

Marc H. Bornstein holds a B.A. from Columbia College, M.S. and Ph.D. degrees from Yale University, honorary doctorates from the University of Padua and University of Trento, and an Honorary Professorship at the University of Heidelberg. Bornstein is President Emeritus of the Society for Research in Child Development, and he has held faculty positions at Princeton University and New York University as well as visiting academic appointments in Bamenda (Cameroon), Bristol, London, Munich, New York, Oxford, Paris, Santiago (Chile), Seoul, Tokyo. Trento, and the Institute for Fiscal Studies (London). Bornstein is Editor Emeritus of *Child*

Development and founding Editor of *Parenting: Science and Practice*. He has administered both Federal and Foundation grants, sits on the editorial boards of several professional journals, is a member of scholarly societies in a variety of disciplines, and consults for governments, foundations, universities, publishers, the media, and UNICEF. Bornstein has published widely in experimental, methodological, comparative, developmental, and cultural science as well as neuroscience, pediatrics, and aesthetics.

María Paula Yávar Calderón is a Research Associate in the Department of Psychology at the University of Texas at Austin. She received her BA in Psychology with a minor in English from the University of Texas at Austin. Yávar Calderón is a member of the American Psychological Association and was the recipient of the SUPER Fellowship from the American Psychological Association. Yávar Calderón's research interests include the study of the influence of discrimination on Hispanic/Latinx populations, the impact of environmental and societal factors on physical and mental health, and higher education.

Megan Chan was a Ph.D. student in psychology at University of California Berkeley. She received both a BA and a MA from University of California Berkeley. She was a National Science Foundation Graduate Research Fellow. Her research interests include emotion socialization and cultural influences on parenting and family dynamics. She has published in developmental and educational journals.

Lei Chang, PhD from University of Southern California, is Chair Professor of Psychology and Head of Department of Psychology, University of Macau. He conducts research in the areas of developmental psychology focusing on parenting and child and adolescent social and cognitive development and evolutionary psychology, including cultural evolution and social learning, life history and childhood environmental impact, and sociosexuality and human mating behavior. He has published eight books and over 300 refereed journal papers, with close to 27,000 citations and h-Index = 75 (by Google Scholar).

Ginger C. C. Chau is a Research Associate in the Department of Applied Social Sciences at The Hong Kong Polytechnic University. She obtained a BA from the Shanghai University of Finance and Economics and a MSW from the University of Hong Kong. Prior to joining The Hong Kong Polytechnic University, she worked as a social worker in Hong Kong for seven years, with a specific focus on older people and their families. She is a certified InterRAI Home Care assessor in the Hong Kong Social Welfare Department. When she worked as an Instructor at The Hong Kong Polytechnic University, she taught subjects on leadership and service-learning. Ginger's research interests involve positive youth development, qualitative and quantitative evaluations of the Tin Ka Ping P.A.T.H.S. Project in Mainland China, and service-learning. She has published research articles in different peer-reviewed journals and presented some research at various international conferences. She is committed to providing a learning environment that fosters positive and independent learning for adolescents.

Xinyin Chen is Professor of Psychology at the Graduate School of Education, University of Pennsylvania. He received a BA at East China Normal University, a MA from Shanghai Normal University, and a MA and a PhD from University of Waterloo. His research interest is mainly in children's and adolescents' socioemotional functioning, social relationships, and family socialization processes from a cultural-contextual perspective. He has been conducting, with his international collaborators, a series of large-scale, longitudinal projects in Brazil, Canada, China, Italy, and the United States. His recent work has tapped the implications of macro-level societal changes for human development. His articles have been published mostly in developmental journals, such as *Child Development, Developmental Psychology, Annual Review of Psychology, Child Development Perspectives,* and *Developmental Review*. He has served as the president of the International Society for the Study of Behavioural Development (ISSBD) and an Associate Editor of *Child Development*. He has received a Scholars Award from the William T. Grant Foundation, a Distinguished Scientific Contribution Award from ISSBD, and several other awards for his scientific work.

Yoonsun Choi is the Mose J. and Sylvia Firestone Professor in the Crown Family School of Social Work, Policy, and Practice and the College at the University of Chicago. Choi is the Director of the Doctoral Program at Crown and a fellow of the American Academy of Social Work and Social Welfare. She served as the Vice President of the Society for Social Work and Research and as the Chair of the Asian Caucus of the Society for Research on Child Development. Choi received a BA from Ewha Womans University in South Korea, an MSSW from the University of Texas, Austin, and a PhD from the University of Washington, Seattle. Choi is a PI of the Midwest Longitudinal Study of Asian American Families (MLSAAF), a longitudinal survey research following about 800 Filipino- and Korean-American families since 2014 to identify multiple developmental trajectories of young

Asian Americans. Choi's scholarship is particularly interested in the role of culture in family, racial prejudice and discrimination, ethnic/racial identity, culture change and formation, and the intersection of culture and socioeconomic class. Choi has published in the *Journal of Youth and Adolescence*, *Family Process*, and *Child Development* and co-edited *Asian American Parenting: Family Process and Intervention*.

Pamela Cole is the Liberal Arts Professor of Psychology and Human Development and Family Studies at The Pennsylvania State University—University Park. Pamela received a BA from Mercy College, an MA from The College of William and Mary and a PhD from The Pennsylvania State University. Pamela first taught at University of Houston, then was a Senior Staff Fellow in the Laboratory of Developmental Psychology at the National Institute of Mental Health. Since 1994, she has been a professor in the child clinical doctoral program at Penn State. She is a Fellow of Division 7 (Developmental Psychology) of the American Psychological Association and was twice awarded Fulbright Research Scholarships for her work in Nepal. She has also received several mentoring awards, including one from the Society for Research in Child Development. Pamela's main research interests include the early childhood development of emotion regulation and its implications for both children's mental health and risk for psychopathology. She co-edited *Emotion Regulation: A Matter of Time*.

Ziarat Hossain is A professor of Family and Child Studies and Regents' Lecturer in the College of Education and Human Sciences (COEHS) at the University of New Mexico. He received a PhD in Child and Family Studies from Syracuse University and did post-doctoral research training at the University of Miami Medical School in Florida. He was awarded a year-long Fulbright Fellowship at the University Putra Malaysia, Malaysia. He also taught in the Department of Psychology at Fort Lewis College in Colorado. He also served as interim associate dean, department chair, and program coordinator for several years. His research focuses on parenting, child development, globalization, and gender roles across cultural communities. In particular, he examines the levels of fathers' involvement in childcare and household labor and the influence of fathers' involvement on children's school and social outcomes in U.S. ethnic minority and international families. His co-edited book titled *Grandparents in Cultural Context* was published by Routledge. He is a past president of the Society for Cross-Cultural Research (SCCR).

Kihyun Kim is a Professor in the Department of Social Work at the Sungkyunkwan University in Seoul, Korea. She received a BA from Ewha Womans

University (Seoul, Korea), an MA from the University of Chicago, and a PhD from the University of Southern California. Kim is a current President of the Korean Society of Child Welfare and a member of the Society for Social Work Research and the International Society for Prevention of Child Abuse and Neglect. Kim's main research interests include the study of parenting, family process, and child maltreatment. She has led several large-scale longitudinal, interdisciplinary studies following families where child abuse occurs and published papers in international journals. She has published in *Journal of Youth and Adolescence, Interpersonal Violence*, and *Child Abuse and Neglect.*

Su Yeong Kim is a Professor in the Department of Human Development and Family Sciences at the University of Texas at Austin. She received her B.A. in Psychology and B.S. in Business Administration from the University of Southern California, and a Ph.D. in Human Development from the University of California, Davis. Kim is Editor of Journal of Research on Adolescence and former Editor of Cultural Diversity and Ethnic Minority Psychology. Kim is also a fellow of the Association for Psychological Science, American Psychological Association, and Asian American Psychological Association. Kim is a recipient of the American Psychological Association's Division 45 Distinguished Career Contributions to Research Award. Kim's main research interests include the role of cultural and family contexts that shape the development of adolescents in immigrant and minoritized families in the U.S.

Yeon-Jin Kim is Affiliated Researcher in the School of Social Work at Lund University, where she received a Ph.D. Yeon-Jin Kim's research focuses on Korean fatherhood in policy and practice and her current work is situated at the intersection of culture, fatherhood, and social policy. She has written on topics such as parental leave policies in Korea and Sweden, policy transfer, Confucianism, work norms, sense of entitlement, fathers' community, and parenting strategies in Korea and beyond.

Yeunjoo Kim is a doctoral candidate in the child clinical program at The Pennsylvania State University—University Park. She received her BA from Yonsei University in Korea and completed post-baccalaureate research training at University of California—Berkeley. She is a member of the Society for Research in Child Development and the Society of Clinical Child and Adolescent Psychology (APA Division 53). She received the Strumpf Scholar Award from Penn State's Child Study Center for her research. Like Dr Cole, Yeunjoo also spent time in Nepal, working with school children. Yeunjoo's interests include the early development of emotion regulation, the role of language development in children's coping with frustration, and the dynamics of fear regulation in preschool age children.

Jennifer E. Lansford is the S. Malcolm Gillis Distinguished Research Professor of Public Policy at the Sanford School of Public Policy and Director of the Center for Child and Family Policy at Duke University, USA. She earned her PhD in Developmental Psychology from the University of Michigan. She is Editor-in-Chief of the *International Journal of Behavioral Development* and President-Elect of the Society for Research in Child Development. She is a Fellow of the American Psychological Association, the Association for Psychological Science, the International Society for the Study of Behavioral Development, and the International Science Council. She is a recipient of the American Psychological Association Mary Ainsworth Award for Excellence in Developmental Science. Dr. Lansford leads the Parenting Across Cultures Project, a longitudinal study of children, mothers, and fathers from nine countries. She has consulted for UNICEF on evaluations of parenting programs and on the development of a set of international standards for parenting programs.

Moon Y. M. Law is a Lecturer at the Department of Social Work at The Chinese University of Hong Kong. She received her BSW degree at the Hong Kong Baptist University, MSW degree at The Chinese University of Hong Kong, and DSW degree at The Hong Kong Polytechnic University. Dr. Law is a registered social worker in Hong Kong and has extensive frontline social work experiences in youth work, school social work, and families. She also has rich experiences in curriculum development and initiating innovative programs and projects for adolescents and families. Her research interests include parenting, youth development, and school social work. She has received several research and teaching grants. Currently, she is working on a research project about family factors and youth indecisiveness, and a project about the use of immersive technologies in social work education. Dr. Law's work has been published in *International Journal of Child and Adolescent Health* and *Journal of Environment Research and Public Health*. Additionally, she performs journal reviews for different journals, including *Applied Research in Quality of Life, Youth, Asia Pacific Journal of Social Work and Development, Sustainability,* and *International Journal of Environmental Research and Public Health.*

Janet T. Y. Leung is Professor in the Department of Applied Social Sciences at The Hong Kong Polytechnic University. She received her BSSc at The Chinese University of Hong Kong, MA at University of Sussex in the U.K., and PhD at The Hong Kong Polytechnic University. She is a registered social worker and was a service supervisor in a social service organization supervising a wide range of social services. Leung is currently the Chairperson of Social Work Panel in the Department. Her areas of interest include poverty, family processes and adolescent development. Leung obtained different research grants from the Research Grant Council and various charitable/trust funds. Particularly, she received the sponsorship of HK$41.69 million (US$5.34 million) from the Hong Kong Jockey Club Charities Trust to conduct a large-scale "The Promoting Family Resilience Project." Furthermore, Janet received the Research Fellow Award from the International Society of Quality-of-Life Studies in 2019, recognizing her substantial contributions to quality-of-life research. Her work appears in *Journal of Youth and Adolescence, Family Process, Applied Research in Quality of Life* and *Journal of Research on Adolescence*. Leung is currently the Associate Editor of *Applied Research in Quality of Life* and *China Journal of Social Work*.

Dan Li is a professor at the School of Psychology and the Director of the Center for Child Development and Family Studies at Shanghai Normal University. She received a BA and PhD from East China Normal University and a MA from Shanghai Normal University in China. She has served as a Council Member of The Chinese Psychological Society and the Deputy Director of the Development Psychology Professional Committee, a Council Member of the Chinese Family Education Society, the Vice Chairman of the Shanghai Psychological Society and Vice Chairman of the Shanghai Psychological Health Society, as well as an editorial board member for journals such as *Journal of Youth and Adolescence*. Her main research interests are in children's moral and social development, including the development of values, social emotions, and social competence and behavior, and family and school environmental factors.

Xuan Li is Associate Professor in the Department of Psychology in the Faculty of Social Sciences at the University of Copenhagen. She received a BA in German language and literature and a double-degree BSc in Psychology from Peking University and both an MPhil and a PhD from the University of Cambridge. Xuan Li previously taught at New York University Shanghai and researched at the German Youth Institute. Xuan Li is a member of the Society for Research in Child Development and the International Society for the Study of Behavioral Development. Xuan Li is recipient of John & Beatrice Whiting Memorial Award for Outstanding Student in Cross-Cultural Studies, Society for Cross-Cultural Research. Her main research interests include fatherhood, parent-child interactions and relationships, and children and adolescents' socioemotional and gender development.

Yan Li is a professor in the Shanghai Institute of Early Childhood Education at Shanghai Normal University. She received a BA from East Normal University, a MA from Shanghai Normal University, and a PhD from Northeast Normal University. Yan Li is the Associate Dean in the Shanghai Institute of Early Childhood Education. Her main research interests include the study of family interactions and children's social and emotional adjustment. She has published in *Family Education, Young Children's Play, Young Children's Socio-emotional Learning,* and *Child Development.*

Yan Li is a PhD candidate in the Department of Educational Psychology at the Chinese University of Hong Kong. She received her BA in Education and MA in Psychology from Beijing Normal University. Yan's main research interests include parenting as well as children's social and academic adjustment. Her current research focuses on parents' child-based worth and its implications for both parents and children.

Albert Y. H. Lo is an Instructor in Psychology in the Department of Psychiatry at Harvard Medical School, an Outpatient Child Psychologist/Clinical Research Associate at Cambridge Health Alliance, and a Research Scientist at Boston Medical Center. Dr. Lo received a B.S. from the University of Delaware as well as an MS and PhD in Clinical Psychology from the University of Massachusetts Amherst. He completed his clinical internship at the Virginia Treatment Center for Children/Virginia Commonwealth University Medical Center and his fellowship at the Center for Multicultural Training in Psychology at the Chobanian & Avedisian School of Medicine. His research interests include parenting processes and child development in families from marginalized backgrounds and the intersection of mental health, culture, and health care use.

Florrie Fei-Yin Ng is Professor and Chair of the Department of Educational Psychology at the Chinese University of Hong Kong. She received her B.S. in Psychology as well as M.A. and Ph.D. in Developmental Psychology from the University of Illinois at Urbana-Champaign. She was a postdoctoral fellow at New York University and the Graduate Center of the City University of New York. Ng was an Associate Editor of *Child Development* and currently serves as an Associate Editor of the *Journal of Pacific Rim Psychology*. She co-organized the 2019 regional workshop of the International Society for the Study of Behavioral Development titled "Parenting Among Asians," with the aim of nurturing the next generation of parenting researchers in Asia. Ng's research focuses on understanding the role of parents in children's development and the factors that shape parenting. She has conducted a number of studies to examine parenting in the academic domain among Chinese families. She is particularly interested in how cultural and socioeconomic contexts may shape parents' beliefs and practices and thereby contribute to children's academic and socioemotional functioning over time.

Sumie Okazaki is Professor Emerita in the Department of Applied Psychology in the New York University Steinhardt School of Culture, Education, and Human Development. She received a B.S. in psychology from the University of Michigan and MA and PhD in clinical psychology from the University of California, Los Angeles. Okazaki previously taught at the University of Wisconsin-Madison and the University of Illinois at Urbana-Champaign. Okazaki is past President of the Asian American Psychological Association and is a fellow of the American Psychological Association Division 45 (Society for the Psychological Study of Culture, Ethnicity, and Race). Okazaki's main research interests include the study of the impact of immigration, social and cultural change, and race on Asian and Asian American adolescents, emerging adults, and parents within local and transnational contexts. Her most recent co-authored book, with Nancy Abelmann, is *Korean American Families in Immigrant America: How Teens and Parents Navigate Race*.

Xiaolin Ou is a current student in Columbia University pursuing a MA degree in Developmental Psychology. She received a B.S. in Applied Psychology from New York University. Ou is currently working as a research assistant in the Science of Human Connection Lab. Ou also previously worked as a research assistant in the Baby's First Years Lab studying Language Functions in Mother's Verbal Interactions with Their Infants. She has presented Patterns of Resistance and Adherence to Norms of Masculinity in a Sample of Urban Adolescents in China in Society for Research on Adolescence, and Influences of Multicultural Background: Crisis of Connection among Chinese Boys in America in L. Starling Reid Undergraduate Psychology Research Conference. Ou's main research interests include the study of adolescent development, parenting styles and gender norms within a changing social context in China.

Michael Park is an Assistant Professor at the School of Social Work and the Chancellor's Scholar for Inclusive Excellence in Racial Minority Health at Rutgers, The State University of New Jersey. Before joining Rutgers, Park completed a NIMH postdoctoral fellowship at the Center for Mental Health Services Research at Washington University in St. Louis. He earned his PhD in Social Work and his master's degrees in Social Work and Biostatistics from the University of Chicago, and his BA in History from the University of Georgia. His research centers on investigating how social positionality within the intersection of race/ethnicity, and immigration explains health disparities among racial/ethnic minorities in the United States. Specifically, his current research focuses on understanding how racial stereotypes contribute to disparities in mental health and mental health service utilization among Asian American immigrant youth and identifying protective factors that can mitigate the harmful effects of discrimination. He has published in *Child Development, Journal of Youth and Adolescence, Emerging Adulthood*, and *Journal of Racial and Ethnic Health Disparities*.

W. Andrew Rothenberg is a Research Scientist at the Duke University Center for Child and Family Policy. He holds a BA from North Carolina State University and MS and PhD degrees in child clinical psychology from the University of North Carolina at Chapel Hill. He is interested in preventing and treating the intergenerational transmission of deleterious parenting and child mental health problems. He has collaborated with UNICEF, is a member of the UNICEF Inclusive Policy Lab, and has taught and trained scientists and clinicians in Kenya, Italy, Sweden, and Thailand among other places. He is a winner of the United States' National Institutes of Health's Matilda White Riley Early Stage Investigator Award, is a practicing child clinical psychologist, and is the author or co-author of 100 scientific publications, including two books, *Parenting and Child Development in Low- and Middle-Income Countries* and *Parenting Across Cultures from Childhood to Adolescence: Development in Nine Countries.*

Daniel Shek is Chair Professor of Applied Social Sciences, Li and Fung Professor in Service Leadership Education, and Associate Vice-President at the Hong Kong Polytechnic University. He is also Advisory Professor of East China Normal University, Honorary Professor of Guangdong University of Technology, and Changjiang Scholar. He received a BSSc and a PhD from the University of Hong Kong. Daniel previously taught at the Chinese University of Hong Kong. Daniel has received several QS Reimagine Education Awards: Bronze Award (Ethical Leadership), Bronze Award (Social Enterprise), Silver Award (Ethical Leadership), Gold Award (Sustainability), and Gold Award (Nurturing Well-Being and Purpose). He has also received the University Grants Committee Teaching Award. He is Editor-in-Chief of *Applied Research in Quality of Life* and a Series Editor of *Quality of Life in Asia* published by Springer. He is Editorial Board member of several international journals, including *Children and Youth Services Review* and *Journal of Adolescent Health*. He is a volume editor of *Encyclopedia of Child and Adolescent Development*. Daniel is a Board member of International Society for Quality for Life Studies and International Positive Psychology Association.

Yishan Shen is an Associate Professor of the Human Development and Family Sciences Program in the School of Family and Consumer Sciences at Texas State University. She received a B.S. in Space Physics and another B.S. in Psychology from Peking University in China. She then received an MA and a PhD in Psychology from the University of Texas at Austin in the United States. Shen previously served as the Chair for the International Scholars Network subcommittee of the Asian Caucus of the Society for Research in Child Development and is a current member of the Society for Research on Adolescence and the American Psychological Association. Shen has received awards from the Society for Research in Child Development, the American Psychological Association, and the National Science Foundation for her research and teaching/mentoring. Shen's main research interests include parent-adolescent relationships and adolescents' psychosocial and academic development in immigrant and racial/ethnic minority families. She has published peer-reviewed articles in journals such as *American Psychologist, Child Development, Journal of Youth and Adolescence*, and *Cultural Diversity and Ethnic Minority Psychology*.

Jingyao Wang is a doctoral student at the Shanghai Institute of Early Childhood Education, Shanghai Normal University. Her main research interests include the study of children's social-emotional learning, family education and parent-child relationships and children's development. She served as the deputy editor-in-chief for the publication *Curriculum of Social and Emotional Learning for Young Children* and co-wrote *Instructional Design and Guidance of Social and Emotional Learning for Young Children, both of which were published by East China Normal University Press*.

Qi Wang is Joan K. and Irwin M. Jacobs Professor of Human Development, Psychology, and Cognitive Science at Cornell University. She holds a BSc in Psychology from Peking University, China, and a PhD in Psychology from Harvard University. Her research examines the mechanisms underlying the development of a variety of cognitive and social-cognitive skills in the context of culture, focusing particularly on autobiographical memory. She has undertaken extensive studies to examine how cultural variables sustain autobiographical memory by affecting information processing at the level of the individual and by shaping social practices of remembering between individuals (e.g., sharing memory narratives between parents and children). Wang has also pioneered research to examine the impact of the Internet and social media as a cultural force on autobiographical memory reconstruction and the consequences for psychosocial functioning. Her research has been supported by grants from the National Science Foundation, National Institutes of Health, United States Department of

Agriculture, and National Natural Science Foundation of China. Wang frequently publishes in scientific journals and in volumes of collected works. Her single-authored book *The autobiographical self in time and culture* (Oxford University Press, 2013) is regarded as the definitive work on culture and autobiographical memory. Wang is Editor-in-Chief of the *Journal of Applied Research in Memory and Cognition*.

Niobe Way is Professor of Developmental Psychology at New York University (NYU), the founder of the Project for the Advancement of Our Common Humanity (PACH), co-founder of agapi.kids, and the PI on the Listening Project. She received her B.A. from the University of California, Berkeley, and completed her doctoral degree at Harvard University. Dr. Way was also a NIMH postdoctoral fellow at Yale University. Dr. Way's research, developed over three decades, examines the social and emotional development of children and adolescents, the impact of ideologies on families in the U.S. and China, and strategies for building a just and humane democracy. Her work integrates her theoretical, empirical, and applied work on the intersections of culture, context, human development, and wellbeing. Dr. Way teaches the "The Science of Human Connection," "Transformative Interviewing," and "Culture, Context, and Psychology" courses. Her major publications include *Deep Secrets: Boys' Friendships and the Crisis of Connection* (Harvard University Press), which inspired the acclaimed film *Close*. Her latest books are *Rebels with a Cause: Reimagining Boys, Ourselves, and Our Culture* (Dutton/Penguin/Random House), and *The Science of Human Connection and Disconnection: A Five-Part Story* (Harvard University Press).

Wen Wen is a postdoctoral scholar in the Crown Family School of Social Work, Policy, and Practice at the University of Chicago. She received her BA from the Psychology Department at Remin University of China and her MA and PhD from the Department of Human Development and Family Sciences at the University of Texas at Austin. Wen is a member of the Society of Research on Adolescence and the Society for Research in Child Development. She is a recipient of the University Graduate Continuing Fellowship from the University of Texas at Austin and an APS Student Grant from the Association for Psychological Science. Wen's main research interests include understanding the adaptive/maladaptive parent-child relationships for youth from disadvantaged families and empowering youth from marginalized populations by revealing how they can develop psychological resilience and physiological adaptation in the face of contextual stress. Wen has published *Parent-child Relationships* in *Encyclopedia of Adolescence*.

Min Wu is Professor at Gannan Medical University. She received a PhD at Beijing Normal University. She is a member of the Student Development and Education Committee of the Educational Society of China and a member of the Family and Education Society of China. Her research focuses on positive development of children and adolescents. She has received grants from the Humanities and Social Sciences Council of the Ministry of Education of China. She has published many articles in important academic journals.

Yoko Yamamoto is a Visiting Associate Professor in the Department of Education at Brown University. She has also served as an invited consulting scholar at Osaka University's Graduate School of Human Sciences in Japan since 2013. Yoko earned her B.A. and M.A. from Kobe College in Japan and a Ph.D. from the University of California, Berkeley. She is a former Abe Fellow and a recipient of an Erin Phelps Award from the Society for the Study of Human Development. Yoko's research focuses on family engagement in education and parental support for children's learning, particularly at the intersections of culture, socioeconomic status, and immigration. Integrating psychological and sociological theories, she leads several research projects that examine parental beliefs and practices among Asian families and family-school relationships in Japan and the United States. She is deeply committed to community-engaged teaching and research, collaborating closely with schools and nonprofit organizations that support families, children, and educational initiatives.

Jinjin Yan is a postdoctoral fellow in the Psychology Department at Fordham University. She received a B.S. from Shaanxi Normal University and MA and PhD from University of Texas at Austin. Her research interests broadly center on understanding ethnically-racially minoritized families' well-being through the lens of culture and family context. Her work aims to inform culturally sensitive interventions and educational programs that promote developmental and educational equity for parents and adolescents from underrepresented families, helping them thrive despite challenges related to cultural adaptation and low socioeconomic status. Her primary research line is to identify risk factors (e.g., discrimination) and resilience factors (e.g., heritage cultural values) that shape the development of ethnic-racial minoritized youth and parents, and to investigate the potential family-related mechanism (e.g., parenting) between these associations. Her second research line is to investigate how acculturation and enculturation experiences influence positive psychosocial adjustment among immigrant-origin families. She has also published a chapter in the book *Close Relationships and Happiness across Cultures*.

Yang Yang is an Education Research Scientist at the Centre for Research in Child Development in National Institute of Education, Nanyang Technological University, Singapore. Yang received her Bachelor of Medicine and Bachelor of Science in psychology from Peking University in China, her Master of Education from Harvard University, and her PhD in developmental psychology from Cornell University. Prior to joining NIE, she worked as a Postdoctoral Research Associate at Rutgers University. Yang is a recipient of ISSBD Jacobs Foundation Mentored Fellowship for Early Career Scholars. Her research has focused on 1) the development of emotion recognition, emotion knowledge, and emotion regulation from infancy to middle childhood in different cultural contexts; 2) the factors that affect children's socioemotional development, such as cultural backgrounds, parenting behaviors, parent-child interactions, and child temperament; 3) how children's emotional development relates to their later psychological wellbeing and academic achievement. Yang has published her work in distinguished journals, such as *Child Development, Psychological Science, and Social Development*. She also co-edited a special issue in Culture and Emotional Development for *Culture and Brain*.

Kuang-Hui Yeh is a research fellow at the Institute of Ethnology in Academia Sinica and a joint-appointment professor of Psychology Department with National Taiwan University. He received his BA, MA and PhD from National Taiwan University. Yeh has been exploring indigenous conceptualizations, theories, and paradigms for understanding Chinese family interactions and their impact on individual development and adaptation since 1985. In his recent publications, he has proposed the Dual Filial Piety model and the Dual Autonomy Model in Chinese people. He had been the chief editor or associate editor of the Formosa Journal of Mental Health; Chinese Journal of Psychology; Asian Journal of Social Psychology. He received SU Shiang-Yeu Doctorate Dissertation Award, Taiwanese Psychological Association, 1992; Misumi Award, AASP, Best Article 2003 and Best Contribution Award 2004; Significant Research Achievement of Academia Sinica, 2006, 2008; Distinguished Research Award of National Science Council, 2007. He authored books *The Filial Piety of Chinese People: A Psychological Perspective* (2008) and *Cultivation of Chinese Characters from a Perspective of Parent-children Network* (2017); Editor-in-chief of books *Family Psychology: Exploration and Application of Systemic Thinking Perspective* (1999), *Affect, Emotion, and Culture: Anthropological and Psychological Studies in Taiwanese Society* (2002), *Chinese Indigenous Psychology in Global Context: Reflections and Future Direction* (2013), *Asian Indigenous Psychologies in the Global Context* (2019), *Global Psychology from Indigenous Perspectives: Visions Inspired by K. S. Yang* (2020) and

Reflection and Transformation: Academic Paradigm, Social Issues, and Local Development (2023).

Saengduean Yotanyamaneewong is a clinical psychologist and an Assistant Professor in the Department of Psychology at Chiang Mai University, Thailand. She obtained her B.S. from Chiang Mai University in Thailand, her MEd from Srinakharinwirot University in Thailand, and her PhD in Special Education from the University of Birmingham in the UK. Her primary research areas encompass both developmental psychology and clinical psychology, with a focus on the dynamics of childhood and adolescence as well as parenting practices. As a co-Investigator for the Parenting Across Cultures project in Thailand, she is engaged in investigating how cultural influences shape parenting and child development outcomes. Currently, she is developing a screening assessment for emotional and social development for young children in Thailand.

Jiaxi Zhou is a PhD candidate at the Graduate School of Education, University of Pennsylvania. She received a BA from Beijing Normal University and an MSED from the University of Pennsylvania. Zhou's research centers on the social relationships of children and adolescents, with a particular emphasis on the influence of social context, cultural factors, and social dynamics on developmental outcomes. She has contributed to several academic articles in these areas and is deeply engaged in research that explores the role of culture in shaping social interactions among children and adolescents.

Qing Zhou is a Professor of Psychology and the Director of Culture and Family Study Lab at University of California Berkeley. She received a M.A. in developmental psychology and a Ph.D. in clinical psychology from Arizona State University. Her research focuses on cultural, family, and temperament influences on children's executive function, socio-emotional, and academic development from preschool to young adulthood. Her team has conducted longitudinal studies of parenting and socioemotional development of Chinese children in Asia and Chinese American and Mexican American children in the U.S. She was a recipient of the Foundation for Child Development Young Scholars Award, and her research has been funded by the National Institutes of Health. She has published empirical and theoretical articles in developmental, cultural, clinical, and educational science journals and volumes. She is a member of the Society for Research in Child Development.

1

CULTURE AND PARENTING IN ASIAN SOCIETIES

Xinyin Chen

Research has shown that children and adolescents in Asian societies may display culturally distinct patterns of social, cognitive, and psychological functioning. Relative to their Western counterparts, for example, children in many Asian societies tend to engage in less active interactions and be less expressive of their emotions in challenging social settings (Camras et al., 1998; Chen et al., 2006). Chinese and Korean children display more shy and vigilant behaviors, particularly in unfamiliar situations, than Western children (Huntsinger & Jose, 2006; Kong et al., 2024; Rubin et al., 2006). Asian children also appear to be more compliant-cooperative than North American children in task-oriented or limited-resource situations (e.g., Chen et al., 2003; Oh & Lewis, 2008; Schirmbeck et al., 2020). At the same time, considerable similarities as well as differences have been revealed among children across Asian societies on behaviors, emotions, and academic performance. According to parental reports, for example, children in some South and Southeast Asian countries, particularly Malaysia, Pakistan, the Philippines, showed higher levels of negative affectivity (e.g., fear, anger, sadness) than children in East Asian countries, such as Japan and South Korea (Putnam et al., 2024). Moreover, as a result of social and cultural changes that have been occurring in many Asian countries, children and adolescents may differ on the exhibition of specific behaviors across different historical times and different regions within the society (e.g., Cai et al., 2020; Chen, 2024).

Given this background, developmental theorists and researchers have been interested in how socialization factors, particularly parenting, play a role in shaping Asian children's socioemotional and cognitive functioning

DOI: 10.4324/9781003383949-1

(Chao, 1995; Ng & Wang, 2019). As a major socialization agent, parents have the responsibility to provide care to children and exert influence on their development according to socialization goals. Research has indicated that parental socialization goals and parenting practices are determined, to large extent, by social, economic, and cultural circumstances in the society (e.g., Bornstein, 2012; Super & Harkness, 2002). In the study of Asian parenting, cultural beliefs and values, such as Confucian group-oriented principles, have received much attention (Ng & Wang, 2019 Shek et al., in this volume). It is believed that these cultural beliefs and values serve as guidance for childrearing and parent–child interaction in Asian societies (Chen et al., 2019). The cultural contexts not only shape the display of specific parental attitudes and practices, but also provide frames of reference for social judgments and evaluations of specific parenting behaviors and thus shape their significance for child development.

Authoritarian and Authoritative Parenting Styles of Asian Parents

Parenting styles and practices in some East Asian societies have been discussed over the last several decades. Ho (1986) identified salient features of parenting beliefs and behaviors of Chinese parents that are related to traditional socialization goals in China. Several studies (e.g., Chiu, 1987; Lin & Fu, 1990) with Chinese or Chinese American samples in or from Taiwan found that Chinese parents reported higher levels of parental control and restrictiveness and greater emphasis on achievement than European American parents. Based on their findings about parenting styles in samples of adolescents with different ethnic background in the United States (Dornbusch et al., 1987), Steinberg et al. (1992) indicated that Asian American adolescents rated their parents as more authoritarian and less authoritative than their European American counterparts, although Asian students had higher academic achievement than students in other ethnic groups. To address the "paradox", Chao (1994) argued that the high-power parenting of Asian parents should not be viewed as authoritarian because it is associated with care and concern, rather than coldness, rejection, or hostility. Chao (1994) adopted the concept of *guan* from Tobin et al.'s book (1989, p. 93) describing the strategy that Chinese teachers and parents used to monitor and correct the under-controlled behaviors of "only" children in China. According to Chao, *guan* or *chiao shun* (training) represents a mixture of governing, training, care, and love.

In the discussion of Asian parenting from an indigenous perspective, Chao (1994) argued that the concepts in the Western literature, such as "authoritarian" or "controlling" parenting, are embedded in Western cultures that Asian parents may not share. Thus, Baumrind's model about authoritarian and authoritative parenting styles may not be applicable to Asian contexts because these parenting styles may have different implications for the development of Asian and Western children. This argument is consistent with Steinberg et al.'s assertion (1992) that parents may be less influential on youngsters in Asian families than in Western families. To examine this view, Chen et al. (1997) conducted a study of parenting styles in a sample of school-age children in Beijing, China. Authoritative and authoritarian parenting styles were assessed using parents' reports on Block's Child Rearing Practices Report (CRPR; Block, 1981), and data on children's social and school adjustment were obtained from multiple sources including peer assessments, teacher ratings, and school records. The results showed that parental authoritarian parenting was negatively associated with peer acceptance, social competence, distinguished studentship, and academic achievement and positively associated with aggression. In contrast, parental authoritative style was associated positively with indexes of social and school competence and negatively with problems. These results indicated that, inconsistent with Chao (1994)'s and Steinberg et al. (1992)'s arguments, authoritarian and authoritative styles in Baumrind's model were relevant to children's performance in social and school domains in Chinese children. Similar results were reported in later studies with Chinese and other Asian samples (e.g., Kho et al., 2019; Lee et al., 2014; Nguyen, 2008; Shen et al., 2018; Zhou et al., 2004; also see Pinquart & Kauser, 2018 for a review).

Whereas the studies of the broad categories of authoritarian and authoritative parenting styles results help us understand their implications for child development in Asian societies, they have not resolved the so-called "paradox" in the literature. It remains unclear why Asian and Western parents consistently differ on these parenting styles and why the differences are not reflected in children's developmental outcomes at the group level. It is possible that the various components of authoritarian and authoritative parenting styles are related to child outcomes in a complicated manner in Asian and Western societies. For example, authoritarian parenting in Baumrind's theory is represented by parental high control as well as negative affect, rejection, and hostility. Indeed, the measures of authoritarian parenting typically include items that indicate, to a varying extent, negative parental attitudes and emotions (e.g., "I explode in anger towards my child," "I yell or shout when my child misbehaves," "I use threats as punishment with little or no justification"; Lee et al., 2014) in addition to items assessing high control. Given the literature on the culturally similar function of parental acceptance and rejection (e.g., Chen et al., 2000; Rohner & Lansford, 2017), it is conceivable that authoritarian parenting that is assessed using measures containing items of negative parental attitudes and emotions is similarly associated with adjustment problems and low competence in Asian and non-Asian children. However, the relatively high scores of Asian parents on authoritarian measures may be due largely to their strong endorsement of high control but not negative attitudes and emotions. In other words, whereas high control or power assertion is often accompanied with negative emotions to form an authoritarian parenting style in Western parents, the two aspects are not typically connected with each other in Asian parents (Chao, 1994; Chen et al., 2019).

Features of Asian Parenting

A number of studies have been conducted to explore specific parenting dimensions or behaviors in Asian societies in recent years (e.g., Ju et al, 2021; Yu et al., 2019). These studies appear to be effective in revealing the cultural features of Asian parenting. Several interesting patterns have emerged from the findings.

The first pattern is that relative to Western parents, Asian parents tend to be more closely involved in monitoring and directing children's social and school activities and use a higher level of control or power assertion. Asian parents' high control may be behavioral, psychological, or both. Parental behavioral control, such as supervision and requirement of rule-abiding (e.g., "I make sure I know where my child is and what he/she is doing," "I have strict, well-established rules for my child"; Block, 1981), may help children learn appropriate behaviors according to social standards and expectations, complete tasks, and regulate their deviant behaviors in most cultures. As such, a higher level of behavioral control that Asian parents exert may provide more benefits to children in social-behavioral and school performance than their Western counterparts. A more interesting question is how parental psychological control, which typically includes shaming, guilt induction, and love-withdrawal (Yu et al., 2019), affects child development in Asian societies. For example, Chinese parents are particularly inclined to use shaming (e.g., tell children that they should be ashamed when they misbehave) and guilt induction (e.g., tell children, "If you really care for me, you would not do things that cause me to worry"; Chao & Aque, 2009; Cheah et al., 2019; Louie et al., 2013; Wu et al., 2002). Social comparison (e.g., "Others are doing well on the exam, why can't you?") and telling parental sacrifice (e.g., "All dad and mom are doing is for you!") are often used to provoke shame and guilt in children. As indicated by Fung (1999, 2006), Chinese parents believe that the experiences of shaming and guilt induction can teach children right from wrong and help them learn social responsibility and develop sensitivity to the feelings of others.

More importantly, Asian children and adolescents seem to interpret and react to parental psychological control in a relatively favorable manner.

In a study with Chinese, Pilipino, Korean, and European American adolescents in the United States, Chao and Aque (2009) measured emotional reactions to parental psychological control (e.g., "If my parent brings up past mistakes when s/he criticizes me then I would feel...") and found that Asian adolescents reported lower levels of feeling angry with parental psychological control than European American adolescents did. Psychological control was positively associated with externalizing behavioral problems among European American adolescents, but not among Asian adolescents. Cheah et al. (2019) found that Chinese children and adolescents tended to interpret parental use of shaming and guilt induction positively (e.g., "For my own good"). Moreover, children's and adolescents' positive interpretations of parental psychological control buffered against the negative impact of parental psychological control on their depressive symptoms. Similarly, Yu et al. (2019) reported that parental psychological control was associated with fewer problems or more positive outcomes in social and school performance in Chinese children than in European American children. Apparently, the positive interpretations of and attitudes toward parental psychological control reduce its potentially harmful effects, allowing children to cooperate with parents to achieve socialization goals.

The second pattern from the research findings is that parental warmth may be manifested in a culturally specific form in Asian societies. Compared with Western parents, parents in at least some Asian societies exhibit less explicit positive affect, such as smiling, hugging, kissing, and telling the child "I love you", in their interaction with children. Accordingly, Aian children and adolescents tend to report fewer experiences of positive emotions with their parents than their European American counterparts (e.g., "On the phone my dad's like, 'I love you.', 'Yeah, love you too, Dad.'"; Saw & Okazaki, 2010). Relatively low levels of parental affect have been found in in multiple countries in Asia, such as China, Indonesia, India, Japan, and South Korea (e.g., Chen et al., 1998; Daga et al., 2015; Louie et al., 2013; Trommsdorff & Friedlmeier, 2010).

The difference in parental affect between Asian and Western samples is likely to be related to cultural beliefs and values. Specifically, whereas parent–child affective communication is regarded as important for children to develop a sense of security, self-confidence, and autonomy in Western societies (Maccoby & Martin, 1983), parents' expression of affection toward children is believed to undermine parental authority to exert effective training or disciplining of children in East Asian societies (Chao, 1995; Cheah & Li, 2010). Since socialization goals in Asian families focus on helping children develop group-oriented characteristics, such as compliance, responsibility, and self-control, displaying emotions may be regarded as unnecessary or undesirable in parenting. Thus, Asian parents, particularly fathers, are encouraged to constrain their emotions in their interaction with children (Li et al., in this volume). According to this argument, the utilitarian nature of group-oriented socialization goals and cultural values of emotional constraint may impede affective involvement in parenting of Asian parents.

Nevertheless, a relatively low level of affect, as indexed by outward and direct demonstrations and communications of positive emotions in the Western literature (Maccoby & Martin, 1983; Rohner, 1986), in Asian parents in their interaction with children may not necessarily indicate low parental warmth. It is possible that parental warmth in Asian societies is manifested in manners that are different from those in Western societies. Cheah et al. (2015), for example, found that Asian parents often reported that they expressed their warmth through instrumental support, such as providing guidance and educational opportunities (e.g., "I try to let her go to good schools," "I help and guide the child to develop good habits and be polite.") and satisfying daily routine needs (e.g., "I help him organize clothes and quilts," "I make him his favorite dumplings."). Thus, it seems important to define parental warmth broadly by including instrumental support and guidance that are not directly related to the expression of positive emotions.

Alternatively, as Chen (2023) argues, to avoid potential conceptual confusion, the supportive aspect of Asian parenting can be viewed as parental care. Parental care refers to attentiveness and concern arising from the responsibility to socialize children to succeed in the society, often reflected by high levels of involvement, sacrifice, and anxiety about the child's performance. From this perspective, whereas parental warmth serves to enhance children's feelings of security and confidence to explore the environment and positive self-regard in Western societies (e.g., Maccoby & Martin, 1983), parental care is integrated with power assertion to form care-based power-assertive parenting that Asian parents use to help children develop socially desirable behaviors and attain achievement (Chen, in this volume).

Heterogeneity of Parenting across Asian Societies and Communities and the Impact of Social Change

Substantial differences exist on parenting across Asian societies. As noted by Kim et al. (in this volume), the majority of the studies of Asian parenting have been conducted with families in China, Korea, and some other East Asian countries. However, researchers have been increasingly interested in parental goals, beliefs, and behaviors in other countries and regions in

Asia, particularly India, Pakistan, Indonesia, Malaysia, and the Philippines. Whereas many of the Asian societies share certain cultural values such as group orientation, respect for authority in the hierarchical system, gender norms, and emphasis on social responsibility, they differ in historical, political, economic, and ecological circumstances, religious backgrounds (e.g., Hinduism, Islam, and Confucianism), and languages. The unique features of each society are likely to affect family organization, such as the roles of fathers, mothers, and other family members in childrearing, parent–child relationships, and specific parenting practices (Li et al., in this volume).

Research has also revealed considerable variations in parenting beliefs and behaviors within an Asian society. Cole et al. (2006), for example, found that parental reactions to child emotions, such as anger, were associated with specific cultural contexts in two villages, Tamangs and Brahmans, in Nepal. Brahmans are high-caste Hindus who value dominance, power, and hierarchy. In contrast, Tamangs, with a background of Tibetan Buddhism, value compassion, social equality, and non-violence. Consistent with the cultural orientations, in response to situations in which a child displayed negative emotions, such as anger, Brahman caregivers tended to support and coax the child to make him or her to feel better. However, Tamang caregivers were more likely to criticize, rebuke, or ignore the child. The results indicated that children's expression of negative emotions was associated with disapproval and rejection among Tamang parents but was more tolerated among Brahman parents (Cole & Kim, in this volume).

Rural-urban differences within a country have been reported on parenting attitudes and behaviors. In China, for example, traditional values are more maintained in rural regions than in urban regions. Accordingly, Chen et al. (2010) found that whereas urban adolescents reported greater parental encouragement of independence/autonomy (e.g., "Lets me make many decisions for myself," "Encourage me to be independent of her/him"), rural adolescents reported a high level of parental control and power assertion ("Does not allow me to question her/his decisions," "Believes physical punishment is the best way of disciplining."). As indicated by Chen et al. (2010), rural Chinese parents may continue to endorse traditional parenting including high control to reinforce adult authority and to achieve family goals. However, parents in urban China may realize that it is important for their children to learn autonomous and initiative-taking skills in order to achieve success in the competitive environment. As such, urban Chinese parents tend to encourage their children to express their opinions and display independence in social settings.

Relatedly, rapid social changes have been occurring in many Asian societies, which have considerable implications for parenting (Okazaki et al., in this volume). In a study of the parental goals of Turkish families over three decades, for example, Kağıtçıbaşı and Ataca (2005) found that along with urbanization and socioeconomic development, parents were more likely to appreciate the "psychological value of the child" (e.g., fun to have young children around, pleasure watching children grow). At the same time, as the need for material dependence within the family declined, parents were more likely to view child autonomy positively. Chen and Chen (2010) found that parents became less controlling and more sensitive to children's feelings in China as a function of urbanization. Similar changes in parental warmth and control have been reported in other studies in east Asian countries (e.g., Park et al., 2015; Ren & Edwards, 2016; Way et al., 2013). In a study of parental beliefs in different generations in India, Lamm et al. (2008) found, relative to grandmothers, mothers placed greater emphasis on autonomy and were less concerned with maintaining their authority in parenting.

The research findings seem to be largely consistent with Greenfield (2009)'s theory of social change and human development, which suggests that the movement between *Gemeinschaft* (rural residence, substance-based economy, the use of simple technology, informal education) and *Gesellschaft* (urban residence, commercial or industrialized economy, the use of complex technology, formal education) in most countries typically results in a shift from collectivistic to individualistic values and corresponding change in socialization goals and practices. However, Chen (2015, 2024) argued from a pluralist-constructivist perspective that ongoing social changes in many countries have led to a coexistence and integration of diverse values and lifestyles, which constitutes a new context for socialization and human development. According to this perspective, values from different cultures are likely to coexist with and eventually be integrated with the traditional cultural systems, rather than being adopted completely in their original forms in the society. In the new context, parents need to help children and youth develop competencies and qualities that allow them to function effectively in adaptation to the requirements of different cultures. Ju et al. (2021), for example, examined maternal encouragement of autonomy and power assertion and children's adjustment in South Korea. Extensive social changes occurred in the last century in Korea, owing to a series of major events including war, rapid industrialization, and large-scale population migration to cities. With the changes, Western values and traditional Confucian values coexisted in Korean society and affected parents' and children's behaviors. The results of the study showed that maternal support for autonomy was positively associated with peer acceptance and school and psychological adjustment. Maternal power assertion was also positively associated with social competence and academic achievement. These results indicate that encouragement of autonomy and power assertion are not contradictory for Korean parents and that both have positive effects on children's adaptive development.

Future Directions

Interest in Asian parenting and its significance for child development has been growing rapidly in the past three decades, particularly since the publication of Amy Chua's memoir *Battle Hymn of the Tiger Mother* (2011). A number of research projects have been conducted in this area. This edited volume responds to the absence of a comprehensive and scholarly discussion of parenting in traditional and contemporary Asian societies. Leading scholars contribute to the discussion of conceptual and methodological issues in the study of Asian parenting, the role of social, economic, cultural, and ecological circumstances in shaping Asian parenting, culturally prescribed socialization processes, the influence of Asian parenting on children's and adolescents' socioemotional functioning, academic achievement, and psychological wellbeing, and the impact of social changes in Asian societies on parenting beliefs, attitudes, and behaviors. The chapters cover a variety of issues, including parental socialization goals, beliefs and values, emotion socialization practices, fathering, and gender socialization. Several chapters are concerned with the relations between Asian parenting and developmental outcomes including learning and behaviour problems. The chapters in the final section focus on parenting issues in specific contexts, such as childrearing beliefs and behaviors in Brahman and Tamang families in the rural middle hills of Nepal, filial piety and parenting in Taiwan, and parenting in majority world Asian countries. These chapters provide valuable insights into the cultural meanings, characteristics, and implications of parenting in Asian societies at different levels from different perspectives.

Several future directions for research on Asian parenting may be offered. First, most studies of Asian parenting have been conducted in East Asian countries, particularly China and South Korea. As a result, our understanding of the issues in this area remains largely limited to the contexts primarily with a traditional background of group-oriented Confucian values. Given the remarkable variations of Asian societies on social, economic, and cultural conditions, it is necessary to investigate similarities as well as differences on parenting and its developmental outcomes across regions and countries in Asia.

Second, despite the arguments about the distinct nature of socialization goals, beliefs, and practices in Asian societies (e.g., Chao & Aque, 2009; Ho, 1986), research on Asian parenting has relied mainly on Western theories, models, and concepts, such as Baumrind's model of authoritative and authoritarian parenting styles (1971), Rohner's acceptance-rejection theory (1986); Ryan and Deci's self-determination theory (2000; see Kim et al., in this volume). It will be important for researchers to identify culturally relevant issues and develop appropriate conceptual frameworks in the study of parenting in Asian societies.

Third, the existing research on Asian parenting has been mostly concerned with its descriptive features (e.g., the display of particular parenting behaviors, often in comparison of those in a Western sample) and their relations with child outcomes. The arguments about the features of Asian parenting are mostly speculative. Little is known about the developmental processes of parenting attitudes and practices and their links with child behaviors in Asian contexts. It will be important to explore how contextual factors in Asian societies are involved in shaping parenting and its implications for child development.

Finally, studies of parenting of Asian parents have often used parent or child self-report questionnaires. Self-report data, particularly from a single source, have obvious limitations, such as being subject to information biases, owing to subjective judgments and social desirability effects, which may confound the results. Relative to self-reports, observations of parent–child interactions, particularly in naturalistic home settings, can provide more objective information that allows for an in-depth understanding of parenting processes in Asian families. It may be difficult to conduct observational studies, owing to practical challenges. Nevertheless, researchers should attempt to use a multimethod approach to achieve a more accurate and comprehensive understanding of the contextual nature of parenting.

References

Baumrind, D. (1971). Current patterns of parental authority. *Developmental Psychology Monograph, 4*, 1–103.

Block, J. H. (1981). The Child-Rearing Practices Report (CRPR): *A set of Q items for the description of parental socialization attitudes and values*. Berkeley, CA: University of California, Institute of Human Development.

Bornstein, M. H. (2012). Cultural approaches to parenting. *Parenting: Science and Practice, 12*(2–3), 212–221. doi:10.1080/15295192.2012.683359.

Cai, H., Huang, Z., Lin, L., Zhang, M., Wang, X., Zhu, H.,... Jing, Y. (2020). The psychological change of the Chinese people over the past half century: A literature review. *Advances in Psychological Science, 28*(10), 1599–1618.

Camras, L. A., Oster, H., Campos, J., Campos, R., Ujiie, T., Miyake, K., Wang, L., & Meng, Z. (1998). Production of emotional facial expressions in European American, Japanese, and Chinese infants. *Developmental Psychology, 34*(4), 616–628. doi:10.1037/0012–1649.34.4.616.

Chao, R. K. (1994). Beyond parental control and authoritarian parenting style: Understanding Chinese parenting through the cultural notion of training. *Child Development, 65*(4), 1111–1119. doi:10.2307/1131308.

Chao, R. K. (1995). Chinese and European American cultural models of the self-reflected in mothers' childrearing beliefs. *Ethos, 23*(3), 328–354. doi:10.1525/eth.1995.23.3.02a00030.

Chao, R. K. & Aque, C. (2009). Interpretations of parental control by Asian immigrant and European American youth. *Journal of family psychology, 23*(3), 342–354. doi:10.1037/a0015828.

Cheah, C. S. L. & Li, J. (2010). Parenting of young immigrant Chinese children: Challenges facing their social emotional and intellectual development. In E. L. Grigorenko and R. Takanishi (Eds), *Immigration, Diversity, and Education* (pp. 225–241). New York: Routledge.

Cheah, C. S. L., Yu, J., Liu, J., & Coplan, R. J. (2019). Children's cognitive appraisal moderates associations between psychologically controlling parenting and children's depressive symptoms. *Journal of adolescence, 76*, 109–119. doi:10.1016/j.adolescence.2019.08.005.

Chen, X. (2015). Exploring the implications of social change for human development: Perspectives, issues, and future directions. *International Journal of Psychology, 50*(1), 56–59. doi:10.1002/ijop.12128.

Chen, X. (2023). *Socialization and socioemotional development in Chinese children*. Cambridge University Press. doi:10.1017/9781009072380.

Chen, X. (2024). Social change and human development in Chinese context: A pluralist-constructivist perspective. *Acta Psychologica Sinica, 56*(7), 977–993. doi:10.3724/SP.J.1041.2024.00977.

Chen, X., & Chen, H. (2010). Children's socioemotional functioning and adjustment in the changing Chinese society. In R. K. Silbereisen & X. Chen (Eds), *Social change and human development: Concepts and results* (pp. 209–226). Sage Publications.

Chen, X., Bian, Y., Xin, T., Wang, L., & Silbereisen, R. K. (2010). Perceived social change and childrearing attitudes in China. *European Psychologist, 15*(4), 260–270. doi:10.1027/1016–9040/a000060.

Chen, X., DeSouza, A. T., Chen, H., & Wang, L. (2006). Reticent behavior and experiences in peer interactions in Chinese and Canadian children. *Developmental Psychology, 42*(4), 656–665. doi:10.1037/0012–1649.42.4.656.

Chen, X., Dong, Q., & Zhou, H. (1997). Authoritative and authoritarian parenting practices and social and school performance in Chinese children. *International Journal of Behavioral Development, 21*(4), 855–873. doi:10.1080/016502597384703.

Chen, X., Fu, R., & Yiu, W. Y. V. (2019). Culture and parenting. In M. H. Bornstein (Ed.), *Handbook of parenting: Biology and ecology of parenting* (pp. 448–473). Routledge/Taylor & Francis Group. doi:10.4324/9780429401459-14.

Chen, X., Hastings, P. D., Rubin, K. H. et al. (1998). Child-rearing attitudes and behavioral inhibition in Chinese and Canadian toddlers: A cross-cultural study. *Developmental Psychology, 34*(4), 677–686. doi:10.1037/0012–1649.34.4.677.

Chen, X., Liu, M., & Li, D. (2000). Parental warmth, control, and indulgence and their relations to adjustment in Chinese children: A longitudinal study. *Journal of Family Psychology, 14*(3), 401–419. doi:10.1037/0893–3200.14.3.401.

Chen, X., Rubin, K. H., Liu, M., Chen, H., Wang, L., Li, D., Xiangping, G., Cen, G., Gu, H., & Li, B. (2003). Compliance in Chinese and Canadian toddlers: A cross-cultural study. *International Journal of Behavioral Development, 27*(5), 428–436. doi:10.1080/01650250344000046.

Chiu, L.-H. (1987). Child-rearing attitudes of Chinese, Chinese-American, and Anglo-American mothers. *International Journal of Psychology, 22*(4), 409–419. doi:10.1080/00207598708246782.

Chua, A. (2011). *Battle hymn of the tiger mother*. New York: Penguin Books.

Cole, P. M., Tamang, B. L., & Shrestha, S. (2006). Cultural variations in the socialization of young children's anger and shame. *Child development, 77*(5), 1237–1251. doi:10.1111/j.1467–8624.2006.00931.x.

Daga, S. S., Raval, V. V., & Raj, S. P. (2015). Maternal meta-emotion and child socioemotional functioning in immigrant Indian and White American families. *Asian American Journal of Psychology, 6*(3), 233–241. doi:10.1037/aap0000014.

Dornbusch, S. M., Ritter, P. L., Leiderman, P. H., Roberts, D. F., & Fraleigh, M. J. (1987). The relation of parenting style to adolescent school performance. *Child Development, 58*(5), 1244–1257. doi:10.2307/1130618.

Fung, H. (1999). Becoming a moral child: The socialization of shame among young Chinese children. *Ethos, 27*(2), 180–209. doi:10.1525/eth.1999.27.2.180.

Greenfield P. M. (2009). Linking social change and developmental change: shifting pathways of human development. *Developmental psychology, 45*(2), 401–418. doi:10.1037/a0014726.

Ho, D. Y. F. (1986). Chinese pattern of socialization: A critical review. In M. H. Bond (Ed.), *The psychology of the Chinese people* (pp. 1–37). New York: Oxford University Press.

Huntsinger, C. S. & Jose, P. E. (2006). A longitudinal investigation of personality and social adjustment among Chinese American and European American adolescents. *Child development, 77*(5), 1309–1324. doi:10.1111/j.1467–8624.2006.00936.x.

Ju, S. G., Chen, X., Chen, L., Zhao, S., & Fegley, S. G. (2021). Relations of maternal power assertion and autonomy support with children's adjustment in Korea. *Journal of Family Psychology, 35*(3), 335–344. doi:10.1037/fam0000720.

Kağıtçıbaşı, C. & Ataca, B. (2005). Value of children and family change: A three-decade portrait from Turkey. *Applied Psychology: An International Review, 54*(3), 317–337. doi:10.1111/j.1464–0597.2005.00213.x.

Kho, C., Main, A., Chung, S., & Zhou, Q. (2019). Intrusive parenting in Chinese American immigrant families: Relations with cultural orientations and children's adjustment. *Asian American Journal of Psychology, 10*(4), 341–350. doi:10.1037/aap0000165.

Kong, X., MacGowan, T. L., Wang, S., Li, Y., & Schmidt, L. A. (2024). Observed shyness-related behavioral responses to a self-presentation speech task: A study comparing Chinese and Canadian children. *Behavioral Sciences, 14*(12), 1147. https://doi.org/10.3390/bs14121147

Lamm, B., Keller, H., Yovsi, R. D., & Chaudhary, N. (2008). Grandmaternal and maternal ethnotheories about early child care. *Journal of Family Psychology, 22*(1), 80–88. doi:10.1037/0893–3200.22.1.80.

Lee, E. H., Zhou, Q., Ly, J., Main, A., Tao, A., & Chen, S. H. (2014). Neighborhood characteristics, parenting styles, and children's behavioral problems in Chinese American immigrant families. *Cultural Diversity and Ethnic Minority Psychology, 20*(2), 202–212. doi:10.1037/a0034390.

Lin, C. Y. C. & Fu, V. R. (1990). A comparison of child-rearing practices among Chinese, immigrant Chinese, and Caucasian-American parents. *Child Development, 61*, 429–433.

Louie, J. Y., Oh, B. J., & Lau, A. S. (2013). Cultural differences in the links between parental control and children's emotional expressivity. *Cultural Diversity & Ethnic Minority Psychology, 19*(4), 424–434. doi:10.1037/a0032820.

Maccoby, E. E. & Martin, J. A. (1983). Socialization in the context of the family: Parent–child interaction. In P. H. Mussen (Series Ed.) & E. M. Hetherington (Vol. Ed.), *Handbook of child psychology: Socialization, personality, and social development* (4th ed., Vol. 4., pp. 1–101). Wiley.

Ng, F. F. Y. & Wang, Q. (2019). Asian and Asian American parenting. In M. H. Bornstein (Ed.), *Handbook of parenting: Social conditions and applied parenting* (pp. 108–169). Routledge/Taylor & Francis Group.

Nguyen, P. V. (2008). Perceptions of Vietnamese fathers' acculturation levels, parenting styles, and mental health outcomes in Vietnamese American adolescent immigrants. *Social Work, 53*(4),337–346.

Oh, S. & Lewis, C. (2008). Korean preschoolers' advanced inhibitory control and its relation to other executive skills and mental state understanding. *Child development, 79*(1), 80–99. doi:10.1111/j.1467–8624.2007.01112.x.

Park, H., Joo, J., Quiroz, B., & Greenfield, P. M. (2015). Sociodemographic factors influence cultural values: Comparing European American with Korean mothers and children in three settings—rural Korea, Urban Korea, and Los Angeles. *Journal of Cross-Cultural Psychology, 46*(9), 1131–1149. doi:10.1177/0022022115600258.

Pinquart, M. & Kauser, R. (2018). Do the associations of parenting styles with behavior problems and academic achievement vary by culture? Results from a meta-analysis. *Cultural diversity & ethnic minority psychology, 24*(1), 75–100. doi:10.1037/cdp0000149.

Putnam, S. P., Sehic, E., French, B. F., Gartstein, M. A., Lira Luttges, B., & 486 Additional Partners in the Global Temperament Project. (2024). The Global Temperament Project: Parent-reported temperament in infants, toddlers, and children from 59 nations. *Developmental Psychology, 60*(5), 916–941. doi:10.1037/dev0001732.

Ren, L. & Edwards, C. (2016). Contemporary Chinese parents' socialization priorities for preschoolers: A mixed methods study. *Early Child Development and Care, 186*, 1779–1791.

Rohner, R. P. (1986). *The warmth dimension: Foundation of parental acceptance-rejection theory.* Newbury Park, CA: Sage Publications.

Rohner, R. P. & Lansford, J. E. (2017). Deep structure of the human affectional system: Introduction to interpersonal acceptance–rejection theory. *Journal of Family Theory & Review, 9*(4), 426–440. doi:10.1111/jftr.12219.

Rubin, K. H., Hemphill, S. A., Chen, X., Hastings, P., Sanson, A., Coco, A. L., Zappulla, C., Chung, O.-B., Park, S.-Y., Doh, H. S., Chen, H., Sun, L., Yoon, C.-H., & Cui, L. (2006). A cross-cultural study of behavioral inhibition in toddlers: East-West-North-South. *International Journal of Behavioral Development, 30*(3), 219–226. doi:10.1177/0165025406066723.

Ryan, R. M. & Deci, E. L. (2000). Self-determination theory and the facilitation of intrinsic motivation, social development, and well-being. *American Psychologist, 55,* 68–78. http://dx.doi.org/10.1037/0003-066X.55.1.68.
Saw, A. & Okazaki, S. (2010). Family emotion socialization and affective distress in Asian American and White American college students. *Asian American Journal of Psychology, 1*(2), 81–92. doi:10.1037/a0019638.
Schirmbeck, K., Rao, N., & Maehler, C. (2020). Similarities and differences across countries in the development of executive functions in children: A systematic review. *Infant and Child Development, 29*(1), e2164. doi:10.1002/icd.2164.
Shen, J. J., Cheah, C. S. L., & Yu, J. (2018). Asian American and European American emerging adults' perceived parenting styles and self-regulation ability. *Asian American Journal of Psychology, 9*(2), 140–148. doi:10.1037/aap0000099.
Steinberg, L., Dornbusch, S. M., & Brown, B. B. (1992). Ethnic differences in adolescent achievement: An ecological perspective. *American Psychologist, 47*(6), 723–729. doi:10.1037/0003–066X.47.6.723.
Super, C. M. & Harkness, S. (2002). Culture structures the environment for development. *Human Development, 45*(4), 270–274. doi:10.1159/000064988.
Tobin, J. J., Wu, D. Y. H., & Davidson, D. H. (1989). *Preschool in three cultures.* New Haven, CT: Yale University Press.
Trommsdorff, G. & Friedlmeier, W. (2010). Preschool girls' distress and mothers' sensitivity in Japan and Germany. *European Journal of Developmental Psychology, 7,* 350–370.
Way, N., Okazaki, S., Zhao, J., Kim, J. J., Chen, X., Yoshikawa, H., Jia, Y., & Deng, H. (2013). Social and emotional parenting: Mothering in a changing Chinese society. *Asian American Journal of Psychology, 4*(1), 61–70. doi:10.1037/a0031204.
Wu, P., Robinson, C. C., Yang, C., Hart, C. H., Olsen, S. F., Porter, C. L., Jin, S., Wo, J., & Wu, X. (2002). Similarities and differences in mothers' parenting of preschoolers in China and the United States. *International Journal of Behavioral Development, 26*(6), 481–491. doi:10.1080/01650250143000436.
Yu, J., Cheah, C. S., Hart, C. H., Yang, C., & Olsen, J. A. (2019). Longitudinal effects of maternal love withdrawal and guilt induction on Chinese American preschoolers' bullying aggressive behavior. *Development and Psychopathology, 31*(4), 1467–1475. doi:10.1017/S0954579418001049.
Zhou, Q., Eisenberg, N., Wang, Y., & Reiser, M. (2004). Chinese children's effortful control and dispositional anger/frustration: Relations to parenting styles and children's social functioning. *Developmental Psychology, 40*(3), 352–366. doi:10.1037/0012–1649.40.3.352.

2

ASIAN PARENTING

Concepts and Measurement

Su Yeong Kim, María Paula Yávar Calderón, Albert Y. H. Lo, Wen Wen, and Jinjin Yan

Parents' cultural values can shape their own behaviors and roles as caretakers (Chao, 2000; Darling & Steinberg, 1993). According to parental ethnotheories (i.e., parents' ideas about themselves, their families, and their children that are shared by a cultural community). parents tend to follow cultural patterns of their environment to make decisions as caretakers (Harkness & Super, 2020). The dominant cultural patterns found in the extant parenting literature come from a Western perspective. Although Asians represent 60 percent of the global population (United Nations, 2022; Wikipedia, 2023), studies tend to focus on Western parenting measures and constructs. A common Western perception of Asian parents is that they are predominantly authoritarian (i.e., high in demandingness that can be expressed through discipline, and low in responsiveness of the child's needs, Maccoby & Martin, 1983). Contrary to this perception, empirical research reveals that only about 10 percent of Chinese mothers fit an authoritarian classification (Zhang et al., 2017). Moreover, research on parenting ideals shows that Asian parents tend to highly value interactions with their children and responsibilities toward their families; in addition, their beliefs focus on their family and children, specifically on teaching, guiding, caring, and loving their children and family (Lin et al., 2023). The mismatch between stereotypes about Asian parents and research findings about them demonstrates a need for studies to consider cultural variations more carefully by examining Asian parenting practices and styles. This mismatch also highlights the need to adapt existing parenting measures or create new ones that have more validity in the Asian context. To provide

DOI: 10.4324/9781003383949-2

a more comprehensive and accurate overview of parenting among Asians, this chapter seeks to further examine the main concepts and measures of parenting as applied within the Asian context.

Based on the extant literature on parenting, we present a conceptual framework (Figure 2.1) comprising four categories: family characteristics, parenting cognitions, family climate, and parenting behaviors. Family characteristics include parent characteristics such as emotional state (e.g., depression, stress, and burnout), status (e.g., divorce and immigration), demographic characteristics (e.g., age, sex, ethnicity), and culture. It also includes demographic characteristics (e.g., age, sex, and ethnicity) for children and grandparents or other parental figures. Parenting cognitions refer to parents' mental processes about childrearing such as goals, beliefs, and values (Bornstein & Cote, 2006). Family climate examines the quality of the interactions between family members in terms of cohesion and conflict. Parenting behaviors encompass parenting styles (e.g., authoritative), parenting practices (e.g., parenting control), parent–child relationship (e.g., attachment), and parenting specific to a situation (e.g., academic involvement).

Our conceptual framework also examines how the characteristics of the parent, child, grandparents, or other parental figures may influence parenting behaviors (*Path 1*), as well as influence parents' cognitions and vice versa (*Path 2*). Despite the conceptual importance of children and grandparents or other parental figures' characteristics, few papers consider them empirically. Therefore, we focus exclusively on parent characteristics in this chapter. The lower part of the figure shows how parents' cognitions can impact parenting behaviors (*Path 3*). Furthermore, family climate may influence parenting behaviors (*Path 4*). After reviewing the

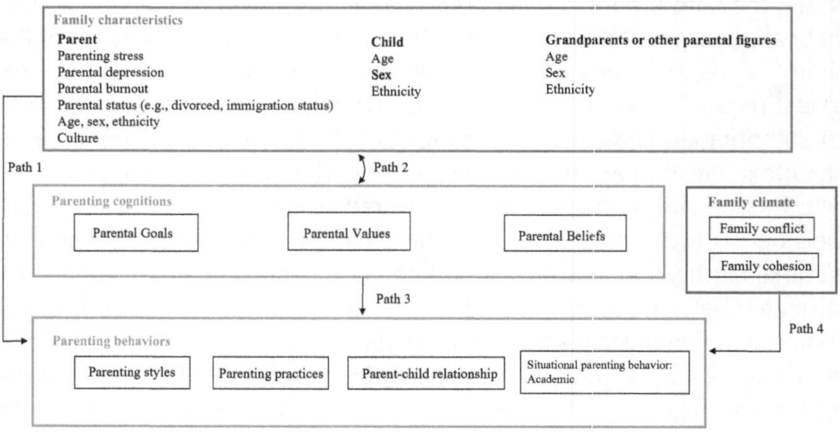

FIGURE 2.1 Conceptual Framework of Parenting Constructs.

parenting constructs in our conceptual framework, we then present the top measures of parenting and their application in Asian parents across the studies reviewed.

This review focuses on English-language journal articles from the past decade (2013–23) on the topic of Asian parenting with samples from South, Southeast, and East Asia, as well as samples including individuals who identify as having an Asian ethnic background and living in countries outside of Asia. We also reviewed studies that included different parenting figures (e.g., grandparents, only mother, and only father) and observers as reporters of the child and parent experience to better comprehend parenting experiences that go beyond the parent–child dyad. We present studies that consider the status of the parents (e.g., marital or immigration status, etc.), as well as studies that focus on specific parenting constructs, and how they represent parents' characteristics, parenting cognitions, behaviors, and family climate. We also take a lifespan perspective, including studies that focus on developmental phases from infancy to late adulthood, to examine how parenting is conceptualized and measured. Based on the articles that met inclusion criteria, we provide information such as the frequencies of the countries in which these parenting measures are studied, age groups, and reporters of the parenting concepts and measures. We close with a discussion of implications and suggest future research directions presented in the studies.

Inclusion Criteria and Characteristics of the Studies' Samples

For this review, we included countries in East Asia, Southeast Asia, South Asia, and samples including people who identified as belonging to a specific ethnic group from these regions but who live in countries outside of Asia (e.g., Chinese Americans living in the United States) (Table 2.1). We excluded countries in Central Asia, West Asia, and North Asia, as their residents are sometimes classified as White and/or Middle Eastern according to the United States Census.

To conduct our search we used EBSCO PsycINFO between May 9 and May 14, 2023, by using the word "parent" (for those living in an Asian region such as "Chinese AND parent"), and the term "Asian AND parent" in the "Title" search field to capture studies that did not specify a country of origin for their Asian sample or to capture samples such as Asian parents living in the U.S. We then refined this initial search by coding the identified articles according to our three inclusion criteria. An initial coder determined whether an article (1) was an empirical, quantitative study; (2) measured at least one aspect of Asian parenting; and (3) included participants who were Asian or of Asian origin. Then, two additional coders reviewed this first round of coding; the first author resolved discrepancies. A total of 881 articles met inclusion criteria. Each of the included articles were coded for parenting measures and constructs. Once the coding process was completed, articles with the most common parenting constructs and measures were further coded to quantify their frequency across the articles.

Among the 881 articles that were coded, Chinese was the most studied racial/ethnic group (47.8 percent) followed by South Korean (14.2 percent, Table 2.1). Most studies involved children/youth as participants (84.3 percent, Table 2.2), who were typically between 13 and 18 years old (Table 2.3). Other common participants were mothers (33.8 percent) and parents (non-specific) (28.7 percent). The most common age for mothers and parents was between 30 and 39 years old (Table 2.3). The most

TABLE 2.1 Race-ethnicity of Sample in Study

Race-ethnicity of Sample in Study	*Number*
China	421
Japan	61
South Korea	125
Hong Kong	99
Taiwan	57
Macao	2
Mongolia	4
India	72
Pakistan	35
Bangladesh	19
Bhutan	4
Maldives	1
Nepal	9
Sri Lanka	10
Brunei	1
Cambodia	13
Indonesia	26
Laos	4
Philippines	39
Singapore	20
Vietnam	37
Thailand	16
Myanmar/Burma	7
Malaysia	29
East Timor	1
Asians in the United States	110
Asians in Canada	4
Asians in Europe	13
Other (e.g., Rohingya, Asians in Australia, Hmong)	39

TABLE 2.2 Type of Participant in the Study

Type of Participant	*Number*
Children	743
Parent(s)	253
Mother	298
Father	206
Grandparents	26
Other (e.g., teacher)	17

TABLE 2.3 Age of Participants

Age of Participants	*Child/Youth Participant*	*Parent Participant*	*Mother*	*Father*	*Grandparents*
Ages 0–4	157	0	0	0	0
Ages 5–9	258	0	0	0	0
Ages 10–12	321	0	0	0	0
Ages 13–18	374	0	1	0	0
Ages 18–29	147	54	84	34	1
Ages 30–39	30	107	180	82	2
Ages 40–49	19	102	151	102	4
Ages 50–59	11	57	48	57	5
Ages 60–69	7	37	7	9	6
Ages 70–79	0	18	1	2	3
Ages 80–89	0	14	0	0	2
Ages 90–99	0	6	0	0	0
Ages 100–109	0	0	0	0	0
Ages 110–119	0	0	0	0	0
Age not specified	47	121	101	91	18

common types of research were studies in which parenting was examined as a predictor variable (59.3 percent), followed distantly by studies that assessed parenting as an outcome variable (22.4 percent).

Parenting Constructs

Various parenting constructs (Table 2.4a and Table 2.4b) play an important role in understanding Asian parenting experiences. This section focuses on defining key parenting constructs, which have been grouped into categories to reflect our conceptual framework (Figure 2.1): family characteristics, parenting cognitions, parenting behaviors, and family climate. We provide examples of specific studies to illustrate how these constructs were used in the study of Asian parenting experiences.

TABLE 2.4A Parenting Constructs

	Experience reported by:						
	Parent(s)	*Mother*	*Father*	*Child*	*Grandparents*	*Observer*	*Other*
Family Characteristics							
Parent Characteristics							
Parenting Stress	46	49	21	2	0	0	0
Parental Depression	14	16	5	1	0	0	0
Parental Burnout	3	3	1	1	0	0	0
Parental Status	15	5	2	12	0	2	4
Parenting Cognitions							
Parental Goals							
Parental Expectation	7	5	4	13	0	0	0
Parental Values							
Filial Piety	9	1	1	12	1	1	1
Parental Sacrifice	0	3	3	3	0	1	0
Parental Beliefs							
Parental Efficacy	22	25	5	2	0	0	0
Parental Beliefs	25	16	10	2	1	0	1
Family Climate							
Family Conflict							
Conflict	17	9	8	34	0	0	0
Family Cohesion							
Co-parenting	6	10	9	0	0	1	0
Cohesion	3	1	1	8	0	0	0
Family functioning	11	5	4	5	1	0	0

TABLE 2.4B Parenting Constructs

	Experience reported by:						
	Parent(s)	*Mother*	*Father*	*Child*	*Grandparents*	*Observer*	*Other*
Parenting Behaviors							
Parenting Styles							
Parenting style	17	16	6	25	0	1	1
Authoritarian Parenting	25	21	10	34	1	0	0
Authoritative Parenting	27	20	10	28	1	0	0
Permissive/Indulgent Parenting	14	7	3	18	0	0	0
Neglectful/Uninvolved Parenting	6	2	2	18	0	0	0
Parenting Practices							
Parenting practices	22	12	6	8	0	1	0
Parental Warmth	16	26	17	52	0	1	0
Parental Support	15	11	5	42	1	2	2
Positive Parenting	13	5	4	10	0	0	0
Parental Involvement	21	13	9	21	0	5	3
Parental Control	14	10	7	30	0	1	0
Behavior Control	2	2	2	15	0	0	0
Psychological Control	5	9	4	41	0	0	0
Guilt Induction	1	3	0	8	0	0	0
Love Withdrawal	1	5	2	8	0	0	0
Shaming	0	7	3	5	0	0	0
Parental Rejection	7	2	1	24	0	0	0
Parental Acceptance	6	2	1	17	0	0	0
Parental Monitoring	12	1	1	32	0	0	0
Parental Knowledge	2	5	1	12	0	0	0

(Continued)

TABLE 2.4B (Continued)

	Experience reported by:						
	Parent(s)	*Mother*	*Father*	*Child*	*Grandparents*	*Observer*	*Other*
Solicitation	0	0	0	4	0	0	0
Overprotection	4	5	3	27	0	0	0
Care	1	3	4	18	0	0	1
Autonomy Support	6	8	3	26	0	1	0
Punitiveness	4	7	5	12	0	0	0
Harsh or Hostile Parenting	10	14	12	24	0	0	0
Alienation	0	2	2	11	0	0	0
Responsiveness	2	4	1	5	0	1	0
Helicopter Parenting	0	0	0	6	0	0	0
Inconsistent Parenting	8	3	2	0	0	0	0
Inductive Reasoning/Parenting	4	5	3	2	0	0	0
Mindful Parenting	8	3	3	0	0	1	0
Coercion	4	2	2	2	0	0	0
Parent–child Relationship							
Parent–child Relationship	25	6	5	46	1	0	1
Parent–child Attachment	4	2	1	43	0	1	0
Parent–child Communication	9	7	3	23	0	3	0
Parent–child Interaction	8	8	5	6	0	10	0
Situational Parenting Behaviors							
Academic Involvement	9	2	1	8	0	2	1

Parent Characteristics

The most common parent characteristics across studies were parenting stress, parental depression, parental burnout, and parental status. As shown in Figure 2.1, these parent characteristics can influence parents' behaviors and mutually influence parents' cognitions (*Path 1* and *Path 2*). Oftentimes, Asian parents have a strong sense of responsibility in their parental role and highly value childrearing to foster family harmony (Kouros et al., 2014; Lam et al., 2012). Research on parenting stress, parental depression, and burnout indicates that Asian parents experience high parenting demands that can be rooted in parenting beliefs and traditional perceptions of parenting roles (Cheng et al., 2020; Ding et al., 2022). Specifically, Asian parents may be more likely to develop depressive symptoms when they experience high parenting demands, owing to not being able to share frustrations with their spouse (Ding et al., 2022). Furthermore, Asian mothers may present higher levels of parental burnout when they hold traditional expectations in terms of the mother (versus the father) assuming more responsibilities and having higher expectations for themselves as a parent (*Path 2*) (Cheng et al., 2020). Cultural expectations and beliefs that Asian parents hold for themselves in their role as parents may thus lead to parents experiencing higher parenting demands, which could increase their levels of parenting stress, parental depression, and burnout (*Path 2*).

Parents' characteristics (e.g., parental marital status) can also influence the parent–child relationship (*Path 1*), which plays a prominent role in children's development. For instance, research on Hong Kong Chinese families suggests that although children from divorced families may experience negative outcomes (e.g., lower life satisfaction), they can also experience positive development in certain areas such as self-esteem and purpose in life (Chui & Wong, 2017). Nevertheless, it is not clear whether those positive outcomes may be related to cultural factors, such as family support, that characterize Asian cultures and may help adolescents cope with the outcomes of a divorce (*Path 1*) (Chui & Wong, 2017).

Family Climate

The studies included in this review also examined the impact of family cohesion (i.e., emotional bond between family members, Zhang & Fuligni, 2006) and family conflict (i.e., verbal or physical opposition between family members, Marta & Alfieri, 2014) on parent–child relationships and youth outcomes (*Path 4*). Research on family conflict showed that sometimes conflicts arise within a family, owing to discrepancies around autonomy and authority, with families experiencing higher levels of conflict when the parents endorsed more authority than their adolescents (*Path 4*) (Jensen & Dost-Gözkan, 2015). In contrast, parent–child cohesion may help prevent risk-taking behaviors, given that adolescents' closeness with their parents may meet their emotional needs and thus reduce their adoption of these behaviors (*Path 4*) (Wang et al., 2020). These results may suggest that authority and autonomy are important concepts in understanding the dynamics of Asian families as it appears that discrepancies around how much authority parents should exert and how much autonomy adolescents should have may lead to higher levels of conflict among Asian families. Moreover, closeness seems to be another important factor in understanding how Asian parents meet their children's needs and promote family cohesion.

Parenting Cognitions

Parenting cognitions, that is, goals, values, and beliefs can be influenced by the parents' culture during the child rearing process (*Path 2*). Parenting cognitions can also influence parenting behaviors (e.g., parenting practices, parent–child relationship) as parents may have certain motivations (e.g., socialization goals) and desires for their children (e.g., qualities the child should possess) (*Path 3*) (Chen-Bouck et al., 2019; Darling & Steinberg, 1993; Dornbusch et al., 1987; Symonds, 1939).

Parenting goals can be highly influenced by cultural values, owing to parents raising their children in ways that meet the expectations of their cultural backgrounds (*Path 2*). For example, Chinese culture traditionally values collectivism; thus, parents who adhere to collectivistic socialization goals and "training" goals (i.e., educating children to adopt appropriate and expected behaviors, Chao, 1994) may adopt parenting strategies that ensure that their children will become self-sufficient in an evolving social environment while also remaining obedient and respectful (*Path 3*) (Chen-Bouck et al., 2019).

Further, a common parenting value in Asian culture is filial piety. Research on filial piety (i.e., refers to the respect, obedience, and love a child shows towards their parents, Nelson & Chen, 2007) has shown that this family value can lead to both positive and negative outcomes for children. According to Yeh's (2003) Dual Filial Piety model, filial piety embodies two focal attributes. The first, authoritarian filial piety (i.e., child suppressing their own wishes to please parents because of their seniority and to maintain the family's reputation), is associated with negative outcomes. The second, reciprocal filial piety (i.e., child attending to parents financially and emotionally out of gratitude for raising them), is associated with positive outcomes. For instance, when Chinese emerging adults endorse high levels of authoritarian filial piety, they may experience lower self-esteem because they perceive a sense of duty to their parents, but resent their parents' intrusion, leading to a lack of autonomy, and hindering the development of positive self-esteem (*Path 3*) (Jorgensen et al., 2017). However, when Chinese adolescents endorse reciprocal filial piety beliefs, they tend to use compromise and compatibility strategies to improve their mutual understanding about their parents' expectations (*Path 3*) (Wu & Yeh, 2021). These contradictory results highlight the duality of filial piety and highlight a need for researchers to deeply examine Asian parenting constructs given that the two attributes of filial piety affect the parent–child relationship in different ways. While authoritarian filial piety seems to harm the parent–child relationship by generating a sense of resentment from the child towards the parent, reciprocal filial piety has the opposite effect as it increases communication and understanding between parent and child. Despite these clear differences, studies continue to define filial piety as a unidimensional construct (e.g., Nelson & Chen, 2007) and fail to address the contrasting effects of authoritarian and reciprocal filial piety.

Parenting beliefs such as parental efficacy (i.e., parents' beliefs about their competence to raise their children, Chung et al., 2015) are also related to cultural expectations regarding parenting roles and the child's education (*Path 2*). For example, South Korean mothers are expected to be highly involved in their children's education, which is an important source of parental efficacy (Byun, 2009). In fact, higher involvement in the child's education was associated with a higher sense of parental efficacy in South Korean mothers when their children are in elementary school (*Path 2*) (Chung et al., 2015).

Parenting Behaviors

Based on the studies included in this review, we grouped parenting behaviors into four categories: parenting styles, parenting practices, parent–child relationship, and situational parenting behaviors. These parenting behaviors can be influenced by parents' characteristics (*Path 1*), parenting cognitions (*Path 3*), and family climate (*Path 4*).

According to Baumrind's (1971) conceptualization based on Western populations, parenting styles encompass three types: authoritarian (e.g., punitive technique with a strict set of standards), permissive/indulgent (e.g., fewer boundaries and rules for the child), and authoritative (e.g., appropriate levels of discipline and affection). Later, a fourth style, neglectful or uninvolved (e.g., neglecting the child's needs) was introduced by Maccoby and Martin (1983).

However, culture and ethnicity can influence these styles and create variations that are culturally meaningful for Asian families. One example would be a form of authoritarian parenting that goes beyond the Western style by including a mixture of control, care, and concern found in Asian parenting (chiao shun or "training"), leading to different outcomes in Asian children compared to Western children (Ang, 2006; Chao, 1994). Specifically, that mixture may be responsible for the little to no impact of authoritarian parenting on Chinese children's depressive symptoms, whereas research on Western children has often shown that authoritarian parenting fosters helplessness and heightens children's negative emotions (*Path 1*) (Chan & Oi Poon, 2016).

On the other hand, authoritative parenting seems to have a similarly positive effect in both Asian and Western cultures. For American adolescents in the U.S., authoritative parenting predicted better emotional functioning because parents provided autonomy and support (*Path 1*) (Wang et al., 2007). Similar results were found in Singaporean adolescents of authoritative parents, who presented higher levels of emotional intelligence and emotional regulation, owing to their parents promoting warmth and supportiveness through communication as part of their authoritative parenting (*Path 1*) (Chong & Chan, 2015).

Studies also examined components of parenting styles by examining the two major dimensions of parenting practices, that is, parental control and parental warmth (Deater-Deckard et al., 2011). Parental control can be exercised in different forms, including behavioral control (i.e., limitation of child's behavior) and/or psychological control (i.e., intrusion and dominance in ways that minimize child autonomy) over their children (Barber, 1996; Steinberg et al., 1992), and it is often found to be higher in Asian samples than in Western samples. For instance, Japanese college students reported that parental control was more relevant in their assessment of future romantic partners, in comparison to White Canadian and Dutch college students, who were not as influenced by parental control when choosing their romantic partners (Dubbs et al., 2013). Moreover, parents may exercise behavioral and psychological control by intruding in their child's personal choices and dictating what they should eat or wear, which may lead to higher scores in internalizing disorders (depression) in Chinese adolescents and more intense parent–child daily conflicts (*Path 4*). (Chen-Gaddini et al., 2020). These negative outcomes stem from strict control over the child, whereas other components of control such as monitoring (i.e., parent knows about child's whereabouts and affiliations, Pettit et al., 2001) are associated with positive outcomes in Asian adolescents, for example, reducing aggressive behavior as this practice promotes closeness and awareness of the youth's whereabouts, which limits adolescents' chances of engaging in antisocial behavior (Han & Grogan-Kaylor, 2013). Given that different forms of control may lead to either negative or positive outcomes for Asian youth, researchers must distinguish strict control from other components of control that lead to positive developmental outcomes and increase closeness within the family.

Further, studies on parental warmth (i.e., parental affection, understanding, and responsiveness to the child, Baumrind, 1971; Maccoby & Martin, 1983) show that warmth can provide the child with the confidence and security to explore academic domains (e.g., math) as the parents approach the child with love, acceptance, and support (B.-B. Chen et al., 2019). Academic exploration and success are expectations that some Asian parents (e.g., Chinese) hold when it comes to their children, which emphasizes the influence that parenting goals have on parenting practices (*Path 3*). Specifically, Chinese children who reported higher levels of parental warmth and lower levels of parental hostility had higher levels of math engagement because they were more likely to develop effortful control (i.e., ability to persist in a task and retain attention,Rothbart & Bates, 2006) (Tian & Chen, 2020).

Moreover, parent–child relationship quality plays a prominent role in family cohesion and the child's development as secure relationships can function as a protective factor against risk behaviors in adolescents (e.g., delinquent behavior) and can promote family resilience in the face of stress (*Path 4*) (Bao et al., 2015; Chen et al., 2018). Parent–child relationships can comprise different aspects, for example, parent–child attachment (i.e., bond between parent and child, Bowlby, 2008), parent–child communication (i.e., listening and exchanging verbal and non-verbal information, Epstein et al., 2003), and parent–child interaction (i.e., a process of reciprocity and synchrony between parent and child, Feldman, 2007; Harrist & Waugh, 2002). Research on parent–child attachment in Chinese adolescents found that those with a secure attachment style were less likely to engage in delinquent behaviors, as their positive experiences with their parents shaped their moral development by making them more likely to adopt the parents' values, thus reducing morally disengaged attitudes (i.e., justifying immoral behaviors and freeing oneself from guilt and self-sanctions, Bandura et al., 1996) (*Path 3*) (Bao et al., 2015).

Lastly, studies also examined parenting behaviors that are specific to a situation, namely parents becoming involved in their children's academics. For instance, Chan et al.'s (2021) study identified that Chinese parents highly value their children's education and are willing to work with schools and teachers to improve their programs, particularly when they are dissatisfied with the education quality at school (*Path 3*).

Measures of Parenting

In this section, we describe the types of parenting measures applied in the studies that were reviewed. We follow that with a discussion on the validity of using these parenting measures with Asian populations.

The studies included in this review used a variety of parenting measures to assess different components of the parenting experience such as parenting styles, practices, control, and the relationship between parent and child, as well as family and stress (Table 2.5). Many studies utilized measures that assessed different parenting styles. For example, the Parenting Practices Questionnaire and Parenting Styles and Dimensions Questionnaire (PSDQ) (Robinson et al., 2001; Robinson et al., 1995), and the Parental Authority Questionnaire (Buri, 1991) were commonly used to examine authoritarian, permissive, and authoritative parenting styles based on Baumrind's (1971) conceptualization. Buri's (1991) scale relies on children's perceptions of their parents, while Robinson's questionnaires rely on a parent report to indicate how frequently they engage in those behaviors.

Studies also measured parenting practices. For instance, the Alabama Parenting Questionnaire (Elgar et al., 2007; Frick, 1991; Shelton et al., 1996) assesses five parenting qualities: positive involvement with children, supervision and monitoring, use of positive discipline techniques, consistency in the use of positive discipline, and use of corporal punishment. The Parenting Scale (Arnold et al., 1993) measures three domains of dysfunctional parenting: laxness, over-reactivity, and hostility. The Parental Bonding Instrument (Parker et al., 1979) is used to examine parental bonding by either combining scores of two dimensions (care and overprotection) or by using them separately. The Parental Acceptance Rejection Questionnaire (Rohner et al., 1980; Rohner, 2004) measures the child's perceptions of the degree to which they experienced parental acceptance or rejection during childhood. The Child Rearing Practices Report (Block, 1965; Chen et al., 2000) examines parents' attitudes about childrearing and parenting practices (e.g., parental warmth).

Some studies assessed specific parenting practices such as mindfulness and parental self-efficacy. Mindfulness (i.e., being aware of your parenting and staying in the present with your child) was measured with the Interpersonal Mindfulness in Parenting Scale (Duncan, 2007). The Child Adjustment and Parent Efficacy Scale (Morawska et al., 2014) is a measure with two subscales: one assesses children's behavior problems and emotional

TABLE 2.5 Measures

Parenting Styles	*Number*
Parenting Styles and Dimensions Questionnaire (PSDQ)/Parenting Practices Questionnaire (PPQ) (Robinson et al., 2001; Robinson et al., 1995)	65
Parental Authority Questionnaire (Buri, 1991)	19
Parenting Practices	
Alabama Parenting Questionnaire (Elgar et al., 2006; Frick, 1991; Shelton et al., 1996)	17
Parenting Scale (Arnold et al., 1993)	11
Parental Bonding Instrument (Parker et al., 1979)	27
Parental Acceptance Rejection Questionnaire (Rohner, 2004; Rohner et al., 1980)	28
Child Rearing Practices Report (Block, 1965; Chen et al., 2000)	12
Specific Parenting Practices	
Interpersonal Mindfulness in Parenting Scale (Duncan, 2007)	8
Child Adjustment and Parent Efficacy Scale (Morawska et al., 2014)	10
Parental Control	
Psychological Control Scale (Barber, 1996)	18
Parental Control Questionnaire (Wang et al., 2007)*	24
Family	
Parenting and Family Adjustment Scale (Sanders et al., 2014)	8
Chinese Family Assessment Instrument (Shek, 2002; Shek, 2003; Shek & Ma, 2010; Siu & Shek, 2005)*	6
Coparenting Relationship Scale (Feinberg, 2003; Feinberg et al., 2012)	7
Conflict Tactics Scale (Straus, 1979; Straus et al., 1998)	19
Asian American Family Conflict Scale (Lee et al., 2000)*	18
Parent–Child Relationship	
Inventory of Parent and Peer Attachment (Armsden & Greenberg, 1987)	33
Parenting Stress	
Parenting Stress Index/Inventory (Abidin, 1995)	57
Other	
Coping with Children's Negative Emotions Scale (Fabes et al., 2002)	7
Egna Minnen Bertäffande Uppfostran (My Memories of Upbringing) (Perris et al., 1980)	20

Note. **Measures originally created for Asian sample.*

maladjustment, and the other assesses the parent's self-efficacy to manage the child's behavioral problems.

Parental control is a prominent parenting construct with several measures dedicated for its assessment. Studies used the Psychological Control

Scale (Barber, 1996), which assesses adolescents' perceptions of parental control. Other studies employed the Parental Control Questionnaire (Wang et al., 2007), which measures Chinese and American adolescents' perceptions of the parent's behavioral and psychological control.

Studies also attended to the importance of family to capture different parenting experiences. For instance, the Parenting and Family Adjustment Scale (Sanders et al., 2014) assesses changes in parental adjustment and parenting practices. In addition, the Chinese Family Assessment Instrument (Shek, 2002, 2003; Shek & Ma, 2010; Siu & Shek, 2005) measures family interaction and parenting divided into five dimensions: communication, mutuality, conflict and harmony, parental concern, and parental control. Another common measure of the family was the Coparenting Relationship Scale (Feinberg, 2003; Feinberg et al., 2012), which examines seven coparenting domains in dual-parent relationships (e.g., coparenting agreement, coparenting closeness, exposure of child to conflict, coparenting support, undermining coparenting, endorsement of partner's parenting, and division of labor). The Conflict Tactics Scale (Straus, 1979; Straus et al., 1998) has two different versions, one that examines conflict (verbal aggression, violence, and reasoning) within the family and another that assesses parent to child conflict by measuring four types of abuse: neglect, physical abuse, sexual abuse, and emotional abuse. Another common scale is the Asian American Family Conflict Scale (Lee et al., 2000), which assesses conflicts and disagreements on aspects of acculturative values and practices between Asian immigrant parents and their U.S.-raised children.

The Inventory of Parent and Peer Attachment (Armsden & Greenberg, 1987) is a self-report measure for adolescents that assesses two subscales of attachment: parental attachment and peer attachment. Another common measure was the Parenting Stress Index/Inventory (Abidin, 1995), which examines parental stress with three subscales: parental distress, parent–child dysfunctional interactions, and the difficult child subscale. Other studies incorporated measures of the parent–child relationship. Some studies also assessed other parenting dimensions. For example, the Egna Minnen Bertäffande Uppfostran (My Memories of Upbringing) (Perris et al., 1980) evaluates parents' memories of their own parents' rearing behaviors, which are divided into three dimensions: rejection, emotional warmth, and overprotection. Lastly, parents' different responses to their children's negative emotions were measured with the Coping with Children's Negative Emotions Scale (Fabes et al., 2002).

Application of Parenting Measures in Asian Parents

Parenting measures were used in multiple ways among the studies included in this review, including testing their validity or modifying them for use with Asian samples. First, some studies tested the validity and psychometric properties of Western measures for use with samples of Asian parents. For instance, Guo et al. (2017) and Sumargi et al. (2018) tested the Parenting and Family Adjustment Scale's validity in Indonesian and Chinese families, respectively. Both studies showed acceptable or good internal consistencies. The only exception was the parental consistency subscale, which showed low internal reliability, owing to cultural factors, such that parents perceived items in this subscale as ineffective parenting practices. However, the results still indicate that this scale could be used with Indonesian and Chinese samples. Two other studies focused on testing the psychometric properties and validity of the Interpersonal Mindfulness in Parenting (IM-P) to be used with Hong Kong Chinese and Korean samples (Kim et al., 2019; Lo et al., 2018). These tests had acceptable internal consistency but presented some differences from the original scale. Specifically, Lo et al.'s (2018) study found that coping strategies related to the subscales of emotional awareness of self and emotional awareness of child were not endorsed by Chinese parents. Moreover, Kim et al. (2019) divided the "emotional awareness of self" subscale into two (noticing child's feelings and insight into the effect of mood) to better assess how much attention parents pay to their own emotions and the child's mood. After considering these differences, the results showed that the Chinese and Korean versions of the IM-P can be used to assess mindfulness as a parenting practice in these populations.

Second, other studies focused on the development of new measures for Asian parents and used Western measures for comparison. For example, Choi et al.'s (2013) study developed the new Korean *ga-jung-kyo-yuk* measure of parenting and tested its association with the Parent Acceptance Rejection Questionnaire. The results showed that the new measures for Korean parenting constructs may not be similar to the original Western measures because Korean parents tend to combine different parenting styles such as authoritative and authoritarian styles.

Third, studies modified Western measures to be valid for use with Asian parents. Shi et al. (2021) excluded one of the subscales (minimization reactions) from the Coping with Children's Negative Emotions Scale as it showed different results when used in Asian samples in comparison to European-American samples. In Asian samples, that subscale was positively correlated with non-supportive and supportive reactions. However, in European-American samples, it correlated positively only with subscales that showed non-supportive reactions. Similarly, Chen et al. (2017) excluded the permissive parenting dimension from the PSDQ (Robinson et al., 1995) because previous research shows that such categories are not reliable in Chinese samples (McBride-Chang & Chang, 1998).

Fourth, studies employed Western measures and Asian versions of original scales that showed good validity in Asian samples. For example, Chen et al. (2019) used the Inventory of Parent and Peer Attachment as it showed good reliability and validity in a previous study with Chinese adolescents (e.g., Chen et al., 2016). In addition, Guo et al. (2017) and Chen et al. (2020) used the Chinese version of s-EMBU (the short-form Egna Minnen Beträffande Uppfostran, Arrindell et al., 2005; Jiang et al., 2010; Li et al., 2012), which has shown adequate construct validity and reliability in Western and Asian populations. Guo et al. (2019) used the Chinese version of the Inventory of Parent and Peer Attachment, which also shows good validity in Chinese samples (e.g., Song et al., 2009). Other examples include Kim and Kim (2019) using the Korean version of the Parental Acceptance and Rejection Questionnaire to assess family and peer rejection in Korean adolescents, and Hu et al. (2019) using a Chinese version of the Parental Bonding Instrument to measure the behaviors of parents with autism spectrum disorder.

Lastly, other studies used measures designed for Asian samples. However, these measures are scarce. Our review showed that most measures focus on Western samples and parenting constructs, despite culture being an essential component of parenting (Chao, 2000; Darling & Steinberg, 1993). Out of the 20 most common measures used by the studies included in this review, only three scales were designed specifically for Asian samples. These measures are particularly important for the understanding of Asian parenting experiences as they were specifically designed to be used in Asian populations and they consider the role of culture in parenting experiences. For instance, Kiang et al. (2017) and Choi et al. (2020) used the Asian American Family Conflict Scale to assess the role of immigration on family conflict, for instance, acculturation gaps, owing to U.S.-born children endorsing U.S. values and practices to a stronger degree than their immigrant parents. The Parental Control Questionnaire used by Li et al. (2013) and Li et al. (2016) considers cultural aspects such as Asian parents' focus on control over academic work (e.g., "How often do your parents require you to let them know how you are doing in school?"). The Chinese Family Assessment Instrument was used by Leung and Shek (2013) and it examines harmony as a domain of Asian family interactions and parenting.

Implications from Studies on Asian Parenting

Studies included in this review focused on the importance of parent characteristics (e.g., stress and depression) and parenting practices (e.g., involvement) in the well-being of Asian parents and their families. Thus, some studies recommend implementing intervention programs and policies that can improve how Asian parents cope with parental stress, lack of resources, and lower levels of education. For instance, summing up their studies of parents raising a child with emotional and behavioral problems, Sumargi et al. (2015) and Hou et al. (2018) suggested implementing intervention programs that focus on child management strategies and reducing externalizing behaviors that aim to prevent dysfunctional parenting practices, parental stress, and parental depression. Moreover, given that parental involvement in education is an important component of Asian parenting practices, some studies discussed implementing education policies to help close achievement gaps. For example, Matsuoka et al. (2015) found an "effort inequality" between lesser and higher educated Japanese parents, with less educated parents having fewer resources to provide supplemental instruction for their children. Therefore, these authors recommended adopting policies in Japan that are similar to policies in other countries, such as the Supplemental Educational Services provided by the U.S. No Child Left Behind Act. These policies would provide children with additional instruction (e.g., supplemental lessons) and close the effort gap between families.

Conclusion

Research on Asian parenting over the past decade has examined multiple aspects of parents' experiences, including the influence of the parents' own characteristics, the overall family climate, parents' cognitive processes, and parents' behaviors. Such work has been valuable in clarifying a model linking Asian parents' cultural and social experiences to both their interactions with their children and their children's outcomes. In pursuit of generating findings that can be responsibly applied to practice and policy, future research requires the continued validation and cultural adaptation of existing parenting measures by recognizing the cultural context of parenting constructs, as well as the creation of measures that reflect constructs not represented in the Western parenting literature. As described in this chapter, multiple Western measures have been found to demonstrate insufficient reliability within Asian samples, to measure constructs that may not be applicable to Asian parents' experiences, or to measure constructs that are not comparable to those derived using Western samples. There may also be publication bias surrounding Asian parenting measures, as measures with low validity and reliability among Asians were unlikely to be published and not included in this review. Moreover, the studies reviewed in this chapter were written in English, which could also limit our comprehension of Asian parenting measures and concepts. Centering Asian families in studies using both established and emerging parenting theories would be beneficial for the well-being of Asian parents and their children.

References

Abidin R., R. (1995). *Parenting Stress Index* (3rd ed.). Psychological Assessment Resources.

Ang, R. P. (2006). Effects of parenting style on personal and social variables for Asian adolescents. *American Journal of Orthopsychiatry, 76*(4), 503–511. https://doi.org/10.1037/0002-9432.76.4.503.

Armsden, G. C. & Greenberg, M. T. (1987). The inventory of parent and peer attachment: Individual differences and their relationship to psychological well-being in adolescence. *Journal of Youth and Adolescence, 16*(5), 427–454. https://doi.org/10.1007/bf02202939.

Arnold, D. S., O'Leary, S. G., Wolff, L. S., & Acker, M. M. (1993). The Parenting Scale: A measure of dysfunctional parenting in discipline situations. *Psychological Assessment, 5*(2), 137–144. https://doi.org/10.1037/1040-3590.5.2.137.

Arrindell, W., Akkerman, A., Bages, N., Feldman, L., Caballo, V., Oei, T. P., Torres, B., Canalda, G., Castro, J., Montgomery, I., Davis, M., Calvo, M., Kenardy, J., Palenzuela, D., Richards, J., Leong, C. C., Simón, M., & Zaldívar, F. (2005). The Short-EMBU in Australia, Spain, and Venezuela: Factorial invariance, and associations with sex roles, self-esteem, and Eysenckian personality dimensions. *European Journal of Psychological Assessment, 21*, 56–66. https://doi.org/10.1027/1015-5759.21.1.56.

Bandura, A., Barbaranelli, C., Caprara, G. V., & Pastorelli, C. (1996). Mechanisms of moral disengagement in the exercise of moral agency. *Journal of Personality and Social Psychology, 71*(2), 364–374. https://doi.org/10.1037/0022-3514.71.2.364.

Bao, Z., Zhang, W., Lai, X., Sun, W., & Wang, Y. (2015). Parental attachment and Chinese adolescents' delinquency: The mediating role of moral disengagement. *Journal of Adolescence, 44*(1), 37–47. https://doi.org/10.1016/j.adolescence.2015.06.002.

Barber, B. K. (1996). Parental psychological control: Revisiting a neglected construct. *Child Development, 67*(6), 3296–3319. https://doi.org/10.2307/1131780.

Baumrind, D. (1971). Current patterns of parental authority. *Developmental Psychology, 4*(1), 1–103. https://doi.org/10.1037/h0030372.

Block, J. H. (1965). *The Child-Rearing Practices Report (CRPR): A set of Q items for the description of parental socialization attitudes and values*. University of California, Berkeley.

Bornstein, M. H. & Cote, L. R. (2006). Parenting cognitions and practices in the acculturative process. In M. H. Bornstein & L. R. Cote (Eds), *Acculturation and parent–child relationships: Measurement and development* (pp. 173–196). Erlbaum. https://doi.org/10.4324/9780415963589-9.

Bowlby, J. (2008). *A secure base: Parent–child attachment and healthy human development*. Basic Books.

Buri, J. R. (1991). Parental Authority Questionnaire. *Journal of Personality Assessment, 57*(1), 110–119. https://doi.org/10.1207/s15327752jpa5701_13.

Byun, Y. (2009). A study of practical meaning in the Korean moms' education for their children. *Journal of Adolescent Welfare, 11*(4), 51–72.

Chan, S. M., & Oi Poon, S. F. (2016). Depressive symptoms in Chinese elementary school children: Child social-cognitive factors and parenting factors. *Early Child Development and Care, 186*(3), 353–368. https://doi.org/10.1080/03004430.2015.1030635.

Chan, T. C., Shu, Z., & Xiao, H. Y. (2021). Perception of Chinese parents toward school and family collaboration. *School Community Journal, 31*(1), 233–258.

Chao, R. K. (1994). Beyond parental control and authoritarian parenting style: Understanding Chinese parenting through the cultural notion of training. *Child Development, 65*(4), 1111–1119. https://doi.org/10.2307/1131308.

Chao, R. K. (2000). The parenting of immigrant Chinese and European American mothers: Relations between parenting styles, socialization goals, and parental practices. *Journal of Applied Developmental Psychology, 21*(2), 233–248. https://doi.org/10.1016/S0193-3973(99)00037-4.

Chen-Bouck, L., Patterson, M. M., & Chen, J. (2019). Relations of collectivism socialization goals and training beliefs to Chinese parenting. *Journal of Cross-Cultural Psychology, 50*(3), 396–418. https://doi.org/10.1177/0022022118822046.

Chen-Gaddini, M., Liu, J., & Nucci, L. (2020). "It's my own business!": Parental control over personal issues in the context of everyday adolescent–parent conflicts and internalizing disorders among urban Chinese adolescents. *Developmental Psychology, 56*(9), 1775–1786. https://doi.org/10.1037/dev0001053.

Chen, B.-B., Wiium, N., Dimitrova, R., & Chen, N. (2019). The relationships between family, school and community support and boundaries and student engagement among Chinese adolescents. *Current Psychology, 38*, 705–714. https://doi.org/10.1007/s12144-017-9646-0.

Chen, C. M., Du, B. F., Ho, C. L., Ou, W. J., Chang, Y. C., & Chen, W. C. (2018). Perceived stress, parent-adolescent/young adult communication, and family resilience among adolescents/young adults who have a parent with cancer in Taiwan: A longitudinal study. *Cancer Nursing, 41*(2), 100–108. https://doi.org/10.1097/ncc.0000000000000488.

Chen, G., He, J., Cai, Z., & Fan, X. (2020). Perceived parenting styles and body appreciation among Chinese adolescents: Exploring the mediating roles of dispositional mindfulness and self-compassion. *Children and Youth Services Review, 119*, 105698. https://doi.org/10.1016/j.childyouth.2020.105698.

Chen, J. J., Sun, P., & Yu, Z. (2017). A comparative study on parenting of preschool children between the Chinese in China and Chinese immigrants in the United States. *Journal of Family Issues, 38*(9), 1262–1287. https://doi.org/10.1177/0192513x15619460.

Chen, W., Zhang, D., Liu, J., Pan, Y., & Sang, B. (2019). Parental attachment and depressive symptoms in Chinese adolescents: The mediation effect of emotion regulation. *Australian Journal of Psychology, 71*(3), 241–248. https://doi.org/10.1111/ajpy.12239.

Chen, W., Zhang, D., Pan, Y., Cheng, G., & Liu, G. (2016). Research on parental attachment and depression of adolescents: Mediating role of psychological Suzhi. *Journal of Psychological Science, 39*(6), 1282–1289. https://doi.org/10.16719/j.cnki.1671-6981.20160601.

Chen, X., Liu, M., Li, B., Cen, G., Chen, H., & Wang, L. (2000). Maternal authoritative and authoritarian attitudes and mother–child interactions and relationships in urban China. *International Journal of Behavioral Development, 24*(1), 119–126. https://doi.org/10.1080/016502500383557.

Cheng, H., Wang, W., Wang, S., Li, Y., Liu, X., & Li, Y. (2020). Validation of a Chinese version of the Parental Burnout Assessment. *Frontiers in Psychology, 11*. https://doi.org/10.3389/fpsyg.2020.00321.

Choi, Y., Kim, Y. S., Kim, S. Y., & Park, I. J. K. (2013). Is Asian American parenting controlling and harsh? Empirical testing of relationships between Korean American and Western parenting measures. *Asian American Journal of Psychology, 4*(1), 19–29. https://doi.org/10.1037/a0031220.

Choi, Y., Lee, M., Lee, J. P., Park, M., Lee, S. Y., & Hahm, H. C. (2020). Disempowering parenting and mental health among Asian American youth: Immigration and ethnicity. *Journal of Applied Developmental Psychology, 66*, 101077. https://doi.org/10.1016/j.appdev.2019.101077.

Chong, W. H. & Chan, C. S. Y. (2015). The mediating role of self-talk between parenting styles and emotional intelligence: An Asian perspective with Singaporean adolescents. *International Perspectives in Psychology, 4*(3), 195–208. https://doi.org/10.1037/ipp0000034.

Chui, W. H. & Wong, M. Y. H. (2017). Association between parents' marital status and the development of purpose, hope, and self-esteem in adolescents in Hong Kong. *Journal of Family Issues, 38*(6), 820–838. https://doi.org/10.1177/0192513x15606490.

Chung, G. H., Lee, H., Lee, J., & Lee, K. (2015). A mediational model of school involvement, knowledge about a child's school life, and parental efficacy among South Korean mothers. *Journal of Child and Family Studies, 24*(4), 899–908. https://doi.org/10.1007/s10826-014-9900-0.

Darling, N. & Steinberg, L. (1993). Parenting style as context: An integrative model. *Psychological Bulletin, 113*(3), 487–496. https://doi.org/10.1037/0033-2909.113.3.487.

Deater-Deckard, K., Lansford, J. E., Malone, P. S., Alampay, L. P., Sorbring, E., Bacchini, D., Bombi, A. S., Bornstein, M. H., Chang, L., Di Giunta, L., Dodge, K. A., Oburu, P., Pastorelli, C., Skinner, A. T., Tapanya, S., Tirado, L. M. U., Zelli, A., & Al-Hassan, S. M. (2011). The association between parental warmth and control in thirteen cultural groups. *Journal of Family Psychology, 25*(5), 790–794. https://doi.org/10.1037/a0025120.

Ding, W., Lin, X., Hinshaw, S. P., Liu, X., Tan, Y., & Meza, J. I. (2022). Reciprocal influences between marital quality, parenting stress, and parental depression in Chinese families of children with oppositional defiant disorder symptoms. *Children and Youth Services Review, 136*, 106389. https://doi.org/10.1016/j.childyouth.2022.106389.

Dornbusch, S. M., Ritter, P. L., Leiderman, P. H., Roberts, D. F., & Fraleigh, M. J. (1987). The relation of parenting style to adolescent school performance. *Child Development, 58*(5), 1244–1257. https://doi.org/10.2307/1130618.

Dubbs, S. L., Buunk, A. P., & Taniguchi, H. (2013). Parent-offspring conflict in Japan and parental influence across six cultures. *Japanese Psychological Research, 55*(3), 241–253. https://doi.org/10.1111/jpr.12003.

Duncan, L. G. (2007). *Assessment of mindful parenting among parents of early adolescents: Development and validation of the Interpersonal Mindfulness in Parenting scale*. The Pennsylvania State University.

Elgar, F. J., Waschbusch, D. A., Dadds, M. R., & Sigvaldason, N. (2007). Development and validation of a short form of the Alabama Parenting Questionnaire. *Journal of Child and Family Studies, 16*(2), 243–259. https://doi.org/10.1007/s10826-006-9082-5.

Epstein, N. B., Ryan, C. E., Bishop, D. S., Miller, I. W., & Keitner, G. I. (2003). *The McMaster model: A view of healthy family functioning*. Guilford.

Fabes, R. A., Poulin, R. E., Eisenberg, N., & Madden-Derdich, D. A. (2002). The coping with Children's Negative Emotions Scale (CCNES): Psychometric properties and relations with children's emotional competence. *Marriage & Family Review, 34*(3–4), 285–310. https://doi.org/10.1300/J002v34n03_05.

Feinberg, M. E. (2003). The internal structure and ecological context of coparenting: A framework for research and intervention. *Parenting: Science and Practice, 3*(2), 95–131. https://doi.org/10.1207/S15327922PAR0302_01.

Feinberg, M. E., Brown, L. D., & Kan, M. L. (2012). A multi-domain self-report measure of coparenting. *Parenting, 12*(1), 1–21. https://doi.org/10.1080/15295192.2012.638870.

Feldman, R. (2007). Parent-infant synchrony: Biological foundations and developmental outcomes. *Current Directions in Psychological Science, 16*(6), 340–345. https://doi.org/10.1111/j.1467-8721.2007.00532.x.

Frick, P. J. (1991). *The Alabama parenting questionnaire*. University of Alabama.

Guo, M., Morawska, A., & Filus, A. (2017). Validation of the parenting and family adjustment scales to measure parenting skills and family adjustment in Chinese parents. *Measurement and Evaluation in Counseling and Development, 50*(3), 139–154. https://doi.org/10.1080/07481756.2017.1327290.

Guo, Q. & Feng, L. (2017). The associations between perceived parenting styles, empathy, and altruistic choices in economic games: A study of Chinese children. *Frontiers in Psychology, 8*. https://doi.org/10.3389/fpsyg.2017.01843.

Guo, X. (2019). Coping as a mediator between parental attachment and resilience: An examination of differential effects between Chinese adolescents from single parent families versus those from intact families. *Psychological Reports, 122*(2), 506–524. https://doi.org/10.1177/0033294118765418.

Han, Y. & Grogan-Kaylor, A. (2013). Parenting and youth psychosocial well-being in South Korea using fixed-effects models. *Journal of Family Issues, 34*(5), 689–715. https://doi.org/10.1177/0192513x12440091.

Harkness, S. & Super, C. M. (2020). Why understanding culture is essential for supporting children and families. *Applied Developmental Science, 25*(1), 14–25. https://doi.org/10.1080/10888691.2020.1789354.

Harrist, A. W. & Waugh, R. M. (2002). Dyadic synchrony: Its structure and function in children's development. *Developmental Review, 22*(4), 555–592. https://doi.org/10.1016/S0273-2297(02)00500-2.

Hou, Y. M., Stewart, L., Iao, L. S., & Wu, C. C. (2018). Parenting stress and depressive symptoms in Taiwanese mothers of young children with autism spectrum disorder: Association with children's behavioural problems. *Journal of Applied Research in Intellectual Disabilities, 31*(6), 1113–1121. https://doi.org/10.1111/jar.12471.

Hu, X., Han, Z. R., Bai, L., & Gao, M. M. (2019). The mediating role of parenting stress in the relations between parental emotion regulation and parenting behaviors in Chinese families of children with autism spectrum disorders: A dyadic analysis. *Journal of Autism and Developmental Disorders, 49*(10), 3983–3998. https://doi.org/10.1007/s10803-019-04103-z.

Jensen, L. A. & Dost-Gözkan, A. (2015). Adolescent-parent relations in Asian Indian and Salvadoran immigrant families: A cultural-developmental analysis of autonomy, authority, conflict, and cohesion. *Journal of Research on Adolescence, 25*(2), 340–351. https://doi.org/10.1111/jora.12116.

Jiang, J., Lu, Z., Jiang, B., & Xu, Y. (2010). Revision of the Short-form Egna Minnenav Barndoms Uppfostran for Chinese. *Psychological Development and Education, 26*(1), 94–99.

Jorgensen, N. A., Nelson, L. J., & Duan, X. (2017). Perceived parenting practices and adjustment: Moderation by cultural values in Chinese emerging adults. *Emerging Adulthood, 5*(5), 371–376. https://doi.org/10.1177/2167696817694800.

Kiang, L., Glatz, T., & Buchanan, C. M. (2017). Acculturation conflict, cultural parenting self-efficacy, and perceived parenting competence in Asian American and Latino/a Families. *Family Process, 56*(4), 943–961. https://doi.org/10.1111/famp.12266.

Kim, E., Krägeloh, C. U., Medvedev, O. N., Duncan, L. G., & Singh, N. N. (2019). Interpersonal Mindfulness in Parenting Scale: Testing the psychometric properties of a Korean version. *Mindfulness, 10*(3), 516–528. https://doi.org/10.1007/s12671-018-0993-1.

Kim, J. & Kim, E. (2019). Bullied by siblings and peers: The role of rejecting/neglecting parenting and friendship quality among Korean Children. *Journal of Interpersonal Violence, 34*(11), 2203–2226. https://doi.org/10.1177/0886260516659659.

Kouros, C. D., Papp, L. M., Goeke-Morey, M. C., & Cummings, E. M. (2014). Spillover between marital quality and parent–child relationship quality: Parental depressive symptoms as moderators. *Journal of Family Psychology, 28*(3), 315. https://doi.org/10.1037/a0036804.

Lam, W., Fielding, R., McDowell, I., Johnston, J., Chan, S., Leung, G., & Lam, T. (2012). Perspectives on family health, happiness and harmony (3H) among Hong Kong Chinese people: A qualitative study. *Health Education Research, 27*(5), 767–779. https://doi.org/10.1093/her/cys087.

Lee, R. M., Choe, J., Kim, G., & Ngo, V. (2000). Construction of the Asian American Family Conflicts Scale. *Journal of Counseling Psychology, 47*(2), 211–222. https://doi.org/10.1037/0022-0167.47.2.211.

Leung, J. T. Y. & Shek, D. T. L. (2013). Parental beliefs and family functioning in Chinese families experiencing economic disadvantage in Hong Kong. *International Journal on Disability and Human Development, 12*(2), 151–161. https://doi.org/doi:10.1515/ijdhd-2013-0006.

Li, D., Li, X., Wang, Y., & Bao, Z. (2016). Parenting and Chinese adolescent suicidal ideation and suicide attempts: The mediating role of hopelessness. *Journal of Child and Family Studies, 25*(5), 1397–1407. https://doi.org/10.1007/s10826-015-0334-0.

Li, X., Li, D., & Newman, J. (2013). Parental behavioral and psychological control and problematic internet use among Chinese adolescents: the mediating role of self-control. *Cyberpsychology, Behavior, and Social Networking, 16*(6), 442–447. https://doi.org/10.1089/cyber.2012.0293.

Li, Z., Wang, L., & Zhang, L. (2012). Exploratory and confirmatory factor analysis of a short-form of the EMBU among Chinese adolescents. *Psychological Reports, 110*(1), 263–275. https://doi.org/10.2466/02.08.09.21.Pr0.110.1.263-275.

Lin, G.-X., Mikolajczak, M., Keller, H., Akgun, E., Arikan, G., Aunola, K., Barham, E., Besson, E., Blanchard, M. A., Boujut, E., Brianda, M. E., Brytek-Matera, A., César, F., Chen, B.-B., Dorard, G., dos Santos Elias, L. C., Dunsmuir, S., Egorova, N., Escobar, M. J., . . . Roskam, I. (2023). Parenting culture(s): Ideal-parent beliefs across 37 countries. *Journal of Cross-Cultural Psychology, 54*(1), 4–24. https://doi.org/10.1177/00220221221123043.

Lo, H. H. M., Yeung, J. W. K., Duncan, L. G., Ma, Y., Siu, A. F. Y., Chan, S. K. C., Choi, C. W., Szeto, M. P., Chow, K. K. W., & Ng, S. M. (2018). Validating of the Interpersonal Mindfulness in Parenting Scale in Hong Kong Chinese. *Mindfulness, 9*(5), 1390–1401. https://doi.org/10.1007/s12671-017-0879-7.

Maccoby, E. & Martin, J. A. (1983). Socialization in the context of the family: Parent–child interaction. In E. M. Hetherington & P. H. Mussen (Eds), *Handbook of child psychology* (Vol. 4, pp. 1–101). Wiley.

Marta, E. & Alfieri, S. (2014). Family conflicts. In A. C. Michalos (Ed.), *Encyclopedia of quality of life and well-being research* (pp. 2164–2167). Springer Netherlands. https://doi.org/10.1007/978-94-007-0753-5_997.

Matsuoka, R., Nakamuro, M., & Inui, T. (2015). Emerging inequality in effort: A longitudinal investigation of parental involvement and early elementary school-aged children's learning time in Japan. *Social Science Research, 54*, 159–176. https://doi.org/10.1016/j.ssresearch.2015.06.009.

McBride-Chang, C. & Chang, L. (1998). Adolescent-parent relations in Hong Kong: Parenting styles, emotional autonomy, and school achievement. *The Journal of Genetic Psychology, 159*(4), 421–436. https://doi.org/10.1080/00221329809596162.

Morawska, A., Sanders, M. R., Haslam, D., Filus, A., & Fletcher, R. (2014). Child adjustment and parent efficacy scale: Development and initial validation of a parent report measure. *Australian Psychologist, 49*(4), 241–252. https://doi.org/10.1111/ap.12057.

Nelson, L. J. & Chen, X. (2007). Emerging adulthood in China: The role of social and cultural factors. *Child Development Perspectives, 1*(2), 86–91. https://doi.org/10.1111/j.1750-8606.2007.00020.x.

Parker, G., Tupling, H., & Brown, L. B. (1979). A Parental Bonding Instrument. *British Journal of Medical Psychology, 52*(1), 1–10. https://doi.org/10.1111/j.2044-8341.1979.tb02487.x

Perris, C., Jacobsson, L., Linndström, H., von Knorring, L., & Perris, H. (1980). Development of a new inventory for assessing memories of parental rearing behaviour. *Acta Psychiatrica Scandinavica, 61*(4), 265–274. https://doi.org/10.1111/j.1600-0447.1980.tb00581.x.

Pettit, G. S., Laird, R. D., Dodge, K. A., Bates, J. E., & Criss, M. M. (2001). Antecedents and behavior-problem outcomes of parental monitoring and psychological control in early adolescence. *Child Development, 72*(2), 583–598. https://doi.org/10.1111/1467-8624.00298.

Robinson, C., Mandleco, B., Olsen, F., & Hart, C. (2001). The parenting styles and dimensions questionnaire (PSDQ). In B. F. Perlmutter, J. Touliatos, & M. A. Straus (Eds), *Handbook of family measures techniques* (pp. 319–321). Sage Publications.

Robinson, C. C., Mandleco, B., Olsen, S. F., & Hart, C. H. (1995). Authoritative, authoritarian, and permissive parenting practices: Development of a new measure. *Psychological Reports, 77*(3), 819–830. https://doi.org/10.2466/pr0.1995.77.3.819.

Rohner, E. C., Chaille, C., & Rohner, R. P. (1980). Perceived parental acceptance-rejection and the development of children's locus of control. *The Journal of Psychology: Interdisciplinary and Applied, 104*(1), 83–86. https://doi.org/10.1080/00223980.1980.12062952.

Rohner, R. P. (2004). The parental "acceptance-rejection syndrome": Universal correlates of perceived rejection. *American Psychologist, 59*(8), 830–840. https://doi.org/10.1037/0003-066X.59.8.830.

Rothbart, M. K. & Bates, J. E. (2006). Temperament. In N. Eisenberg (Ed.), *Handbook of child psychology: Social, emotional, and personality development* (6th ed., Vol. 3, pp. 99–166). Wiley.

Sanders, M. R., Morawska, A., Haslam, D. M., Filus, A., & Fletcher, R. (2014). Parenting and Family Adjustment Scales (PAFAS): Validation of a brief parent-report measure for use in assessment of parenting skills and family relationships. *Child Psychiatry & Human Development, 45*(3), 255–272. https://doi.org/10.1007/s10578-013-0397-3.

Shek, D. T. L. (2002). Assessment of family functioning in chinese adolescents: The Chinese family assessment instrument. In N. N. Singh, T. H. Ollendick, & A. N. Singh (Eds), *International perspectives on child and adolescent mental health* (Vol. 2, pp. 297–316). Elsevier. https://doi.org/10.1016/S1874-5911(02)80013-6.

Shek, D. T. L. (2003). Family functioning and psychological well-being, school adjustment, and substance abuse in Chinese adolescents: Are findings based on multiple studies consistent? In S. P. Shohov (Ed.), *Advances in psychology research* (Vol. 20, pp. 163–184). Nova Science Publishers.

Shek, D. T. L. & Ma, C. M. S. (2010). The Chinese Family Assessment Instrument (C-FAI): Hierarchical confirmatory factor analyses and factorial invariance. *Research on Social Work Practice, 20*(1), 112–123. https://doi.org/10.1177/1049731509355145.

Shelton, K. K., Frick, P. J., & Wootton, J. (1996). Assessment of parenting practices in families of elementary school-age children. *Journal of Clinical Child Psychology, 25*(3), 317–329. https://doi.org/10.1207/s15374424jccp2503_8.

Shi, Z. & Wang, Q. (2021). Chinese adolescents' coping with COVID-19: Relationships with emotional maladjustment and parental reactions to negative emotions. *Journal of Research on Adolescence, 31*(3), 645–656. https://doi.org/10.1111/jora.12649.

Siu, A. M. & Shek, D. T. (2005). Psychometric properties of the Chinese Family Assessment Instrument in Chinese adolescents in Hong Kong. *Adolescence, 40*(160), 817–830.

Song, H., Thompson, R. A., & Ferrer, E. (2009). Attachment and self-evaluation in Chinese adolescents: Age and gender differences. *Journal of Adolescence, 32*(5), 1267–1286. https://doi.org/10.1016/j.adolescence.2009.01.001.

Steinberg, L., Lamborn, S. D., Dornbusch, S. M., & Darling, N. (1992). Impact of parenting practices on adolescent achievement: authoritative parenting, school involvement, and encouragement to succeed. *Child Development, 63*(5), 1266–1281. https://doi.org/10.1111/j.1467-8624.1992.tb01694.x.

Straus, M. A. (1979). Measuring intrafamily conflict and violence: The Conflict Tactics (CT) Scales. *Journal of Marriage and the Family, 41*(1), 75–88. https://doi.org/10.2307/351733.

Straus, M. A., Hamby, S. L., Finkelhor, D., Moore, D. W., & Runyan, D. (1998). Identification of child maltreatment with the Parent–child Conflict Tactics Scales: Development and psychometric data for a national sample of American parents. *Child Abuse & Neglect, 22*(4), 249–270. https://doi.org/10.1016/S0145-2134(97)00174-9.

Sumargi, A., Filus, A., Morawska, A., & Sofronoff, K. (2018). The parenting and family adjustment scales (PAFAS): An Indonesian validation study. *Journal of Child and Family Studies, 27*(3), 756–770. https://doi.org/10.1007/s10826-017-0926-y.

Sumargi, A., Sofronoff, K., & Morawska, A. (2015). Understanding parenting practices and parents' views of parenting programs: A survey among Indonesian parents residing in Indonesia and Australia. *Journal of Child and Family Studies, 24*, 141–160. https://doi.org/10.1007/s10826-013-9821-3.

Symonds, P. W. (1939). *The psychology of parent–child relationships*. Appleton-Century.

Tian, Q. & Chen, B. B. (2020). The associations among parental warmth and hostility and student engagement in math and the mediating role of effortful control among Chinese children. *PsyCh Journal, 9*(3), 339–349. https://doi.org/10.1002/pchj.337.

United Nations (2022). *Word Population Prospects 2022*. Retrieved December 5, 2023 from https://population.un.org/wpp/Graphs/Probabilistic/POP/TOT/935.

Wang, Q., Pomerantz, E. M., & Huichang, C. (2007). The role of parents' control in early adolescents' psychological functioning: A longitudinal investigation in the United States and China. *Child Development, 78*(5), 1592–1610. https://doi.org/10.1111/j.1467-8624.2007.01085.x.

Wang, Q., Wang, H., & Liu, X. (2020). Loneliness, non-suicidal self-injury, and friendship quality among Chinese left-behind adolescents: The role of parent–child cohesion. *Journal of Affective Disorders, 271*, 193–200. https://doi.org/10.1016/j.jad.2020.03.112.

Wikipedia (2023). *Demographics of Asia*. Retrieved December 5, 2023 from https://en.wikipedia.org/wiki/Demographics_of_Asia.

Wu, C.-W. & Yeh, K.-H. (2021). Self-sacrifice is not the only way to practice filial piety for Chinese adolescents in conflict with their parents. *Frontiers in Psychology, 12*. https://doi.org/10.3389/fpsyg.2021.661335.

Yeh, K.-H. (2003). The beneficial and harmful effects of filial piety: An integrative analysis. In K.-S. Yang, K.-K. Hwang, P. B. Pedersen, & I. Daibo (Eds), *Progress in Asian social psychology: Conceptual and empirical contributions* (pp. 67–82). Greenwood.

Zhang, W. & Fuligni, A. J. (2006). Authority, autonomy, and family relationships among adolescents in urban and rural China. *Journal of Research on Adolescence, 16*(4), 527–537. https://doi.org/10.1111/j.1532-7795.2006.00506.x.

Zhang, W., Wei, X., Ji, L., Chen, L., & Deater-Deckard, K. (2017). Reconsidering parenting in Chinese culture: Subtypes, stability, and change of maternal parenting style during early adolescence. *Journal of Youth and Adolescence, 46*(5), 1117–1136. https://doi.org/10.1007/s10964-017-0664-x.

3

PARENTING GOALS AND VALUES IN ASIAN CULTURES

Florrie Fei-Yin Ng and Yan Li

Introduction

Children do not come with a manual, but parents are not unguided when it comes to rearing their children. In every culture, there are shared ideas regarding child development, parenting and parenthood, as well as the family, which constitute parents' ethnotheories (Harkness & Super, 2006; Olson et al., 2019). Although parents' ethnotheories may never be articulated by parents themselves and may even be contradictory when scrutinized, they serve as powerful guides as parents develop goals for children and make decisions—big and small, well-planned and spontaneous—about every aspect of children's lives from the moment children enter the world. These ethnotheories are miniatures of the culture (Harkness & Super, 2006). On the one hand, they reflect deep-seated cultural values that are eventually passed on to the next generation via parental socialization; on the other hand, they continuously evolve in adaptation to changes in the social ecologies (Bornstein, 2012; Greenfield, 2016).

As research on parenting was spearheaded in Western countries—mostly by White researchers from North America and Western Europe, it is unsurprising that most studies have focused on families from these countries, yielding Western models of parental socialization. These models reflect and perpetuate assumptions about the fundamentals of parentings that are widely shared among the general public and perhaps the research community in Western countries. For instance, it is often assumed that all parents consider their children's happiness a primary socialization goal, but this is not necessarily true in Asia, where personal happiness

DOI: 10.4324/9781003383949-3

may not be a salient concept and interpersonal harmony as well as fulfilment of family obligations are more important in the Asian ethnotheory of child development. Through a Western cultural lens, one may prejudge Asian parents who do not prioritize children's happiness as negligent and unloving at best and harsh and selfish at worst. Decolonizing parenting science requires us to consider the sociocultural contexts and the associated parental ethnotheories that give meaning to Asian parents' goals and behaviors (Raval, 2023).

This chapter aims to highlight major parental socialization goals that are characteristic of Asian cultures, including parents' goals for children as a member of the family, a member of the community, and a future contributing member of the society. We consider Asian parents' goals as a mirror of their values and beliefs, which need to be understood in relation to the dominant values and norms of their cultures. A caveat to note is that we will only be able to present Asian parents' goals and values in broad strokes; it is impossible for a chapter to do justice to the rich diversity and nuances in parents' goals and values across the thousands of ethnic groups in Asia. Also of note is that the literature to date on Asian parenting is highly unevenly distributed and studies on parenting in Central Asian countries are scant. The scope of this chapter will be restricted to East Asia, Southeast Asia, and South Asia, drawing evidence disproportionately from countries in which there has been more research on parents' goals and values.

To understand Asian parents' socialization goals, it is important to recognize the influence of two related systems that permeate all aspects of life in Asia. Religious systems are prominent in Asia, where Buddhism and Hinduism originated, and which is home to the largest Muslim population (Indonesia) and the third largest Catholic population (the Philippines) in the world. Doctrines concerning the family in sacred texts serve as the ultimate authority on parenting and imbue this life task with spiritual significance. Confucianism, which tends to be considered as a philosophy more than a religion, is also influential in Asia, with China, Japan, Korea, Singapore, and Vietnam known collectively as Confucian heritage cultures. Another system that is important for understanding parenting goals is the gender system, which is intertwined with religion due to religious doctrines that delineate gender roles. The gender system includes gendered power relations, gender roles, gender norms, and gender stereotypes that are deep-rooted in the society (Ridgeway & Correll, 2004). Gender roles and beliefs shape parents' goals for children and are socialized to children—both implicitly and explicitly—from a young age, often constituting the ground for justifying gender imparity both at home and in the larger society (Leaper, 2015).

The Child as a Member of the Family

Asian children are typically born into a large family. Multi-generational households remain common in Asia in spite of urbanization, albeit with regional variations. In South Asia, more than half of all households are multi-generational, often with six members or more; such households are slightly less common in Southeast Asia, but still make up nearly half of all households in Cambodia, Myanmar, and the Philippines (United Nations, 2019). In contrast, the nuclear household is the norm in East Asia, where the average household comprises only two or three members (United Nations, 2019). However, East Asian children have frequent contact with the extended family, and grandparents are often one of their primary caregivers, especially in the early years (Xu & Chi, 2015; Zhang et al., 2024). Across Asian cultures, inherent in the strong family ties is the hierarchy in the extended family network: The old is placed above the young and in most Asian cultures, the male is placed above the female, reflecting their centuries- and millennia-long patriarchal culture. This clear hierarchy and the corresponding norms and expectations weave the tapestry of interpersonal dynamics in Asian families, serving the critical function of maintaining harmony in the family and ensuring its smooth functioning. It is in this intricate tapestry that Asian children develop their sense of self as defined by their relationships with others and learn to place the family and community above themselves, as are characteristic of the collectivistic Asian cultures in which the interdependent self is dominant (Markus & Kitayama, 1991).

The role of parents

All parents are expected to provide for and nourish their children. This expectation is codified in laws against child neglect and abuse worldwide. However, Asian parents are traditionally held to a much higher standard that requires them to fully dedicate themselves to the proper upbringing of their children. A study that examined cultural norms in 33 economies found that Asian cultures are tight cultures with strong norms and low tolerance for deviant behavior compared to Western and Latin American cultures, which are loose cultures with weak norms and high tolerance for norm deviation (Gelfand et al., 2011). Among the 11 Asian economies included in the study, those in South Asia (e.g., Pakistan) and Southeast Asia (e.g., Malaysia) were particularly high in cultural tightness compared to those in East Asia (e.g., China). Tight cultures are characterized by clear, rigid rules governing one's behavior in innumerable daily situations; one is expected to adhere to norms or else face sanction for norm violation (Gelfand et al.,

2011). In the collectivistic Asian cultures, where the family rather than the individual is the basic unit of the community, cultural tightness means not only monitoring one's own behavior but also the behavior of one's family members, especially those under one's authority such as children.

The tight and collectivistic nature of Asian cultures translates into well-defined roles for every family member. Just as children are expected to be "good" children and behave with propriety, Asian parents are expected to be "good" parents and held responsible for ensuring that their children meet societal expectations. A recent study of parents from 37 countries found that, when asked what it meant to be an ideal parent, Asian (China, Japan, Thailand, and Vietnam) parents held similar beliefs and tended to mention concepts such as "family" and "responsibility," which shared some similarities with parents from Africa but differed from the emphasis on being "loving" among parents from Russia as well as Hispanic and other Western countries (Lin et al., 2023). The strong sense of responsibility among contemporary Asian parents can be traced back to their religious teachings and traditional systems of thought. Confucian heritage cultures emphasize parents' training of children, which is captured by the indigenous notion of *chiao shun* (Chao, 1994). In the ancient Chinese classic text *Three Character Classic*, which has been used to educate children in China for centuries, the famous verse that states that a father is at fault for not teaching a child is still widely known by heart among Chinese today. In Islamic teaching, the training of children is considered a holy duty of parents, with *tarbiat* as the Urdu equivalent of *chiao shun* (Stewart et al., 1999). Similarly, the teaching of Hinduism requires parents to train their children, with punishment in the next world for parents who fail to discharge this duty (Sriram & Navalkar, 2012). In the Philippines, of which Christianity is the official religion, the Biblical teaching "Train up a child in the way he should go; even when he is old he will not depart from it" (Crossway Bibles, 2001, Proverbs 22:6) is well known when it comes to parenting. These enduring religious teachings and ideologies make it clear to Asian parents and those around them that they are accountable for training children to be well-behaved.

Respect and obedience

The traditional, often divine, mandate for parents in Asian cultures to train children means that they place utmost importance on ensuring that their children's behavior lives up to societal standards. This requires that parents establish authority over children and instill a sense of respect in them. One of the earliest goals of Asian parents is to teach their young children to show proper respect to elders as well as other members of the family according to their seniority (e.g., Graf et al., 2014; Jocson, 2020; Riany et al., 2017; see Ng & Wang, 2019, for a review). Many Asian cultures have a large, complex system of kinship appellation. From a young age, Asian children learn to greet each family member using kinship terms that are highly specific—terms that reflect not only the person's generation and gender but, in some cultures, their birth order and lineage to the child as well (Fung & Thu, 2019). The overt display of respect for parents and the elders is exemplified by ritualized gestures that are common across Asian cultures (Tan et al., 2021). For example, in India, where the head is considered sacred and the foot is considered to be at heightened risk of contamination, children and adolescents are taught to touch the foot of parents and other senior members of the family with the head to ask for their blessings (*charan sparsh*). Similarly, Filipino children are expected to honor their parents and senior family members by bowing to and touching the hand of the senior members with their forehead (*mano*). In China, there are still occasional reports of families requesting children to prostrate before (kowtow) more senior family members during special occasions such as the Chinese New Year.

Whereas kinship terms and rituals serve as constant reminders to Asian children of the family hierarchy, it is the unquestioned obedience of children that Asian parents traditionally emphasize (Riany et al., 2017). Training for obedience begins early on, although Asian parents may indulge children until they reach the age of understanding at about six years of age (Riany et al., 2017; see also Barth & Wikan, 2011), after which they are expected to submit to and obey their parents. Directives and controlling practices are regularly used by parents to regulate children's behavior in Asia (e.g., Louie et al., 2013; Ng et al., 2014; Rudy et al., 2014; see Ng & Wang, 2019, for a review). Children also learn of traditional sayings—such as "Walk behind a grown-up and dogs will not bite you" in Thai culture and "If you do not listen to an elder, you will surely suffer" in Chinese culture—that warn them of the repercussions of disobedience (Tapanya, 2011). Asian children are traditionally prohibited from negotiating with their parents; talking back and other signs of disobedience are to be punished severely (Alampay & Rothenberg, 2021). It is not uncommon for Asian children, especially boys, to receive corporal punishment at home (End Corporal Punishment, 2014; Graf et al., 2014; Jasmine & Nduna, 2022; Lin, 2020; Raj & Raval, 2013), although this varies by culture and parental education. Such punishment has been found to be more common in India and the Philippines than in China and Thailand (Lansford et al., 2005; see also Raj & Raval, 2013) and among less educated parents (Jocson et al., 2012).

Asian parents' use of power-assertive and controlling practices to enforce obedience may appear to the average person in the West as insensitive and harsh. However, it is crucial to understand these practices through an Asian cultural lens. Compared to their peers in many Western cultures, how Asian parents bring up their children is much less of a personal choice because they live in tight, collectivistic cultures, in which individuals are interconnected and their fates are intertwined in the case of norm adherence or violation (Gelfand et al., 2011; Markus & Kitayama, 1991). A child who grows up disobedient and unruly may not only bring disgrace to the parents and the extended family, but also to the entire community and even to generations of ancestors; the parents themselves would be considered non-filial to their own parents and ancestors for failing to bring up "good" children. Mindful of the limitations of Western ideas of parenting, Chao (1994) argued three decades ago that the concept of authoritarian parenting cannot accurately represent Chinese parenting. She introduced the indigenous Chinese notion of *guan* and pointed out the centrality of love and care in Chinese parents' seemingly harsh parenting (Chao, 1994). Echoing Chao's views but noting conceptual and measurement limitations with *guan*, Chen (2023) put forth the term "care-based power-assertive parenting" and suggested that power assertion and care are the two core, inseparable, and complementary components at the heart of Chinese parenting. This dual emphasis of power assertion and loving care actually characterizes parenting across Asian cultures (Ang & Sin, 2021; Gan et al., 2022; Joscon, 2020). Importantly, Asian parents' care for children goes beyond meeting children's various needs; it calls for devotion to and sacrifice for children on the part of parents. Just as Asian children are expected to put aside their personal desires and obey their parents, Asian parents are expected to sacrifice their self-interest for the sake of the family.

Filial piety

The indebtedness that children feel toward their parents for making sacrifices to nurture them forms the underpinning of filial piety—one of the most important socialization goals of parents in Asia. Indeed, Asian children's filial piety, along with Asian parents' devotion to their children, exemplify the mutual role obligations that function as the bedrock of the collectivistic Asian cultures. Filial piety, which Confucius considered as the foundation of morality, requires children's lifetime commitment to honor and care for their parents; it also extends to include grandparents, other elders in the family, and ancestors (Bedford & Yeh, 2019; Luo et al., 2013). Whether in China or other Asian cultures, paramount importance is placed on filial piety and related concepts (e.g., *seva* in Hindi, *hyo* in Korean, and *bekti* in Indonesian; Kim, 2006; Nguyen et al., 2014; Riany et al., 2017; Stewart et al., 1999; Tan et al., 2021). Across Asia, children are expected to show filial piety to their parents for as long as they live, but the forms of their filial obligations change as they progress through different life stages. During childhood, filial piety is primarily manifested in children's obedience to their parents so that they do not cause grief to the latter. As children grow up, they are expected to assist their parents to ease the latter's burden. After children come of age, they are still obliged to obey their parents but increasingly shoulder the responsibility to provide for and attend to the needs of their parents as the latter become frail and dependent. After parents pass away, children are expected to honor them with a proper funeral and visit the graves regularly (Riany et al., 2017). In ancient China, Confucian teaching even specified a three-year mourning period following the death of a parent as a parallel to the first three years of life when a child is completely dependent on the parent (Foust, 2009).

Of note is the regional diversity in Asia regarding whether parents expect sons or daughters to provide old-age support, which shows a pattern that mirrors the dominance of patrilocal residence in East and South Asia and the mix of both patrilocal and matrilocal residence in Southeast Asia (Global Data Lab, 2024). In East and South Asian countries such as China and India, traditionally, sons and their wives shoulder the primary responsibility to provide old-age support; daughters are no longer considered a core member of their natal family and not expected to care for their parents after they get married and move out, although they are still expected to perform their filial duty by behaving with propriety and not bringing shame to their parents (Ng & Wang, 2019). These traditional ideas continue to be influential in East and South Asia in the modern times, but daughters have become more involved in caring for their parents due to socioeconomic development (e.g., increased female workforce participation means married daughters are more ready to provide financial support to their parents) and demographic changes (e.g., under the One Child Policy, sons and daughters became equally important for old-age care in China; Dhar, 2012; Sun & Wang, 2019). For example, 58 percent of adults in India indicated that both sons and daughters have the primary responsibility to care for their aging parents, whereas 39 percent and 2 percent indicated that only sons and daughters are responsible, respectively (Pew Research Center, 2022). In contrast, there is historically considerable heterogeneity in the arrangement of old-age support in Southeast Asia. In some Southeast Asian countries such as the Lao PDR and Thailand, the dutiful daughter tends to be the primary caregiver of the elderly parents (Angeles & Sunanta, 2009; see Ng & Wang, 2019, for a review). Yet in other Southeast Asian communities, this responsibility may be shared among sons and daughters, members of the extended family (e.g., nephews, nieces, and younger siblings of the elderly parents), and other members of the community (e.g., friends, neighbors), with the geographical proximity and availability of the adult children being an important factor (e.g., Guilmoto, 2015; see Wongboonsin & Tan, 2018).

According to the Dual Filial Piety model by Yeh and Bedford (2003), two types of filial piety coexist. Authoritarian filial piety is embedded in the household hierarchy and obliges children to provide support and obey their parents according to social norms, whereas reciprocal filial piety builds on the intimacy in the parent–child relationship and entails children's heartfelt concerns for their parents' well-being out of love and gratitude. Although there appears to be a decline in authoritarian filial piety, possibly because the absolute authority of parents has been undermined by the remarkable socioeconomic development in Asia and the associated changes such as increased educational attainment and exposure to Western ideas, reciprocal filial piety continues to be emphasized in Asia, with no sign of decline (Bedford & Yeh, 2019). Religion may have contributed to the continued emphasis of filial piety in Asian families. There are clear religious doctrines that state that children should revere their parents or else face divine retribution (Riany et al., 2017; see Tan et al., 2021, for a review). Teachings in Buddhism stress children's debt to their parents and the Buddha is said to have specified ways in which children should repay their parents, including supporting them in this life and honoring them in the afterlife (Guang, 2016). In Burma and Thailand, for example, it remains customary for young men to take temporary ordination to acquire merit for their parents and ancestors (Wilson, 2014). As in Buddhism, Hinduism elevates parents to the level of gods and requires children to show them utmost respect (Guang, 2016; Tan et al., 2021), with Shravan Kumar—a filial son devoted to his parents—celebrated in Hindi mythology as the epitome of filial piety. In Islam, parents are considered second only to God (Stewart et al., 1999) and children are taught that paradise lies at the feet of the mother (Zaman, 2014). Together these religious teachings make children's deference to their parents an unquestionable mandate in Asian families, providing a strong moral and spiritual foundation for parents' emphasis on filial piety across Asia.

The Child as a Junior Member of the Community

The collectivistic nature of Asian cultures means that just as Asian children are considered as a part of the family more than as individuals, their families are also embedded in the community in an interwoven social network. Compared to many Western communities, boundaries between families tend to be less defined in Asia. For instance, in regions of Asia where multi-generational households are still prevalent, it is not unusual to find a family friend residing in the household or neighbors being part of the daily family life (Fung & Thu, 2019). Moreover, given tight social norms that delineate how children should behave, Asian children's conduct is never a private matter of the family. The extent to which each child lives up to societal standards is constantly scrutinized by members of the community in Asian cultures, who may feel "entitled as moral socializers" (Fung & Thu, 2019, p. 285) and openly convey their approval or disapproval of children and their parents in public.

In East Asia, one of the biggest fears of parents is to have their children criticized by others as lacking in "family education". Most East Asian societies have face cultures, in which one's sense of worth is based on one's face—that is, one's respectability as conferred by others based on one's fulfillment of role expectations in the social hierarchy (Kim et al., 2010; Severance et al., 2013). This means that when parents are criticized or implied as having failed their responsibility to train children well, it results in the humiliating loss of face for the parents and the entire family. A parallel to the concept of face in East Asia is the concept of honor (*izzat* in Hindi and Urdu) in many South Asian and Islamic societies (UNICEF, 2018), where there is an honor culture (Severance et al., 2013; Stewart et al., 1999). In these societies, honor can be earned or lost depending on the social evaluation of the behavior of oneself or one's close others (Severance et al., 2013). Children who fail to behave with propriety would lead to the loss of honor for the family, which would require immediate corrective action for the restoration of honor.

Manners and etiquette

Given that Asian children's misbehavior may incur a social reputation cost for the family, Asian parents consider it important for children to be well-mannered. This requires Asian parents to train children to be attuned to the social hierarchy in the community, which reflects some of the same determining factors of social hierarchy in the household such as age and gender. Interestingly, and attesting to the hazy boundary between families in Asia, Asian children can transfer their knowledge about interactions with their family members to their interactions with community members. In Asian cultures, the etiquette for greeting someone outside the family involves some of the same kinship terms and gestures used within the family. For instance, a Filipino girl who meets a younger boy and an old woman for the first time would be asked by her parents to address them using the same kinship terms for her own younger brother and grandmother and perform the *mano* to the old woman as she would to senior members of the family.

The importance that Asian parents place on their children's manners towards others is nicely illustrated in an ethnographic study by Fung and Thu (2019), which documented the meticulous care with which Vietnamese parents train their young children to utter respectful greetings at arrival and departure as well as perform the postural display of respect by folding their arms across their chest (*vòng tay/ khoanh tay*). These researchers found that such training begins as early as the first year of life even before infants speak their first word or take their first step, peaking in early childhood. In daily occasions of greeting, leave-taking, thanking, and apology, young children frequently practice conveying respect to each community member they encounter according to the member's seniority under the guidance of their parents (Fung & Thu, 2019). These researchers noted that Asian children's good manners serve to foster affective relationships between children and others in the community, thereby promoting group harmony (Fung & Thu, 2019).

Interpersonal harmony

Interpersonal harmony has long been of import in the collectivistic Asian cultures and parents place a premium on ensuring that children maintain harmonious relationships with others (e.g., Luo et al., 2013; Markus & Kitayama, 1991; Mestechkina et al., 2014; Riany et al., 2017; Stewart et al., 1999). Across Asia, children are socialized to be oriented toward the group and to be sensitive to how their behavior may disrupt group harmony. For instance, Filipino children are trained to view themselves as interdependent with others and admonished for acting without regard for others (Alampay, 2014). In the same vein, researchers have reported that Japanese parents consider being uncooperative and socially insensitive as the most undesirable attributes of young children (Olson et al., 2019). To preserve interpersonal harmony, Asian parents emphasize self-control in children (Hossain & Eisberg, 2020; Luo et al., 2013; Olson et al., 2019). In particular, Asian parents stress children's emotion regulation, given that the expression of strong emotions can cause tension and strife. In fact, Asians have been found to be less expressive of their emotions than their Western peers are, with neurological evidence that Asians exhibit a readiness to down-regulate their emotional arousal (Matsumoto et al., 2008; Murata et al., 2013). Moreover, Asians are found to prefer low-arousal emotions to high-arousal emotions and this preference is linked to their interpersonal goals of suppressing the self and conforming to the group as opposed to asserting themselves and influencing others (Tsai et al., 2007).

Cultural norms of emotions are reflected in Asian parents' emotional socialization, with the preservation of social harmony as the overarching goal. Research shows that East and South Asian parents often respond to children's negative emotions by explaining to children why they need to adjust to the situation, punishing them, or ignoring the emotions (see Raval, 2023, for a review). Importantly, although considered nonsupportive from a Western perspective, these responses are not necessarily maladaptive in Asia (Raval, 2023). Moreover, although the expression of negative emotions is generally discouraged across Asian cultures, emotional socialization in specific Asian cultures also reflect the influence of other factors such as religion and majority or minority group status. In rural Nepal, Hindu Brahman caregivers attend to children more in response to their anger than do Buddhist Tamang caregivers, who tend to downplay and ignore it; this is presumably because anger is linked to social dominance and thus less undesirable for the Brahmans—the majority group of the country— than for the Tamang, who as Buddhists value inner peace and view intense emotions as harmful (Cole et al., 2006).

Although much research on Asian parents' emotional socialization has focused on negative emotions, these parents are also wary of children's positive emotions. One positive emotion that is particularly discouraged by Asian parents is pride. Pride, which is often associated with accomplishment, connotes risk for arousing jealousy and disrupting social harmony in Asia. This may explain why Asian parents are apprehensive about praising children for fear of making them too proud and primarily use it to reinforce children's positive behavior (Chen, 2023; Raj & Raval, 2013). East Asian parents, in particular, tend to socialize children to self-efface and focus on their shortcomings rather than celebrating their strengths and accomplishments (Heine et al., 1999; Heyman et al., 2011; Luo et al., 2013; Ng et al., 2007). This may partly reflect their face culture, which expects individuals to show modesty and maintain harmony by not claiming higher status in the social hierarchy than warranted (Kim et al., 2010).

Religiosity and morality

Religion is prominent in the lives of Asians and bringing up children in their religion is a major, if not most important, goal of most Asian parents (Abidin et al., 2017; Tapanya, 2011). However, this goal has been understudied in the literature on parental socialization, which has been dominated by studies on Western populations. In most Asian countries, one's religion is inseparable from one's upbringing and loyalty to the family, and conversion to other religions is typically considered unacceptable (Pew Research Center, 2023). A study by the Pew Research Center found that in Cambodia, Sri Lanka, and Thailand, where Buddhists are the majority, about 90 percent of Buddhists believe that their religion represents a family tradition that one must follow; in Indonesia and Malaysia, in which Islam is the official religion, about three quarters of Muslims hold the same view about their religion (Pew Research Center, 2023).

Across major religions in Asia, parents are held responsible for ensuring that children follow their parents' faith. For instance, in India, it is considered the fathers' duty to teach their children to be good Hindus (Sriram & Navalkar, 2012; see also Cole et al., 2006). Islam also charges parents and family members with the responsibility to teach children to read the Quran (Zaman, 2014). The aforementioned Pew study found that across the five countries studied, parents overwhelmingly choose to bring up their children in their religion and almost all individuals continue to identify with the religion in which they were brought up. Parents' religious socialization may involve educating their children about the values of their religion, sending children to religious schools, as well as engaging in religious activities (e.g., praying and reading sacred text) with their children (Park et al., 2012). By bringing up children in their religion, Asian parents will also have the assurance that their children will arrange funeral rites according to their religion upon their death, which is of central import in their cultures (Pew Research Center, 2023).

Of note is that religiosity is viewed as the foundation of morality in most Asian cultures, with sacred texts and religious teachings functioning as moral codes of conduct. The vast majority of Muslims in Asia believe that it is necessary to believe in God to be a moral person (Pew Research Center, 2013). Morality also lies at the center of Buddhism, which teaches that one's rebirth in the next life is influenced by the merits and demerits that one accrues from moral and immoral acts in this life, respectively (Guang, 2016). This implies that the cultural mandate for Asian parents to train their children to be "good" actually requires them to bring up their children in their religion *so that* their children can be moral and upright. In China, one of the least religious countries in Asia, parents similarly place importance on the development of virtues in their children, reflecting the centuries-long influence of Confucianism, which considers moral self-perfection to be the ultimate goal in life (Luo et al., 2013; Ng & Wang, 2019).

The Child as a Future Contributing Member of the Society

Being a "good" parent requires Asian parents to rear children who are not only obedient and filial at home as well as well-mannered and religious as a community member who gets along with others, but also ready to contribute to the society in the future as a self-sufficient and productive adult. While all parents may support their children to become active, contributing members of their society, coaching children for their future roles has added significance in the Asian context. For example, the prestige of young adults' achievement and the social status brought along by their occupations affect the social standing of their immediate as well as extended families. The income that they earn also represents a major source of resource for the entire family in Asia, where resource pooling is common in family networks.

Education and achievement

There is a narrow definition of success in Asia that is closely tied to academic achievement. For many Asian parents, the "script" for success for their children entails performing well academically, graduating from prestigious universities, working a respectable job, earning high income, and having a family. In fact, the high esteem attached to academic achievement distinguishes Asia from other regions in the world. Academic achievement is valued in Asia not only because it allows one to enter a reputable and high-paying profession, but also because of the honor it brings to the family and the belief—especially in Confucian heritage cultures—that an educated person is more virtuous (Jasmine & Nduna, 2022; Ng & Wei, 2020; Nguyen et al., 2014; Park et al., 2012; Raj & Raval, 2013; Sovet & Metz, 2014; Tapanya, 2011). Given the financial, social, and moral significance of academic achievement, Asian parents are obliged to support children in their academic endeavor. The sacrifice that Asian parents are expected to make for their children is exemplified in their investment of resources in children's learning. Across Asia, myriads of parents enroll their children in private tutoring or extra-curricular activities after school to increase their children's chances of entering prestigious schools, and the related expenses take up a substantial proportion of their income (Sovet & Metz, 2014; Tapanya, 2011; see Ng & Wang, 2019, for a review). Besides the investment of financial resources, Asian parents also sacrifice their time, energy, as well as personal comfort to support their children's learning (Leung, 2020). Many of them are actively involved in their children's education, from collecting information for identifying the best tutors to providing academic assistance themselves (Ng et al., 2007; Park et al., 2011; Wei et al., 2019).

Cognizant of their parents' sacrifice and financial investment in their education, many Asian children feel obliged to commit themselves to their studies. One study found that the more Chinese children perceived their parents as involved in their learning, the more they reported parent-oriented motivation in school, which predicted their greater use of self-regulated learning strategies and ultimately higher academic performance (Cheung & Pomerantz, 2012). In some Asian households, children are spared from all household chores as well as economically productive activities and told to focus exclusively on their studies. It is not uncommon for these children to spend nearly every waking moment on their studies, especially as high-stakes public exams approach. Paralleling their parents' sacrifice, many Asian children sacrifice their comfort, entertainment, and social life, in the hope that attaining high academic achievement would lead to honor and upward mobility for the family (Finnan, 2022; Minza & Herlusia, 2022).

Nevertheless, not all Asian parents have high expectations for their children's academic performance and center their family life around school. Parents' economic hardship represents one of the biggest impediments to their investment in children's education in Asia. In rural areas of less developed Asia countries, where child labor is common and education can be costly, parents may need their children, especially the first-born, to quit school and work full-time to contribute to household income (Heissler, 2012). Children's gender also affects whether their parents choose to invest in their education when financial resources are limited. Across East and Southeast Asian countries such as Mongolia and Myanmar, boys are more likely than girls to be pulled out of school, especially as they progress through school, because parents believe boys are more able to generate income for the family and do not need as much education for their future livelihood (UNICEF, 2019). Gender stereotypes matter, as well. For example, Mongolia parents may choose to keep girls rather than boys in school because they see girls as more vulnerable and needing to stay in school for protection, and Filipino parents may do so because they believe girls are more engaged in school than boys are (UNICEF, 2019).

The obedient wife and daughter-in-law

Asian cultures are largely patriarchal despite some regional variations. Traditionally, males have enjoyed higher status than females do both at home and in the society, and women have been viewed as "born to serve men" (Borovoy, 2005; Nguyen et al., 2014; Rajadhyaksha & Bhatnagar, 2000; Riany et al., 2017, p. 215). Although the rapid socioeconomic development in Asia has brought about greater gender parity across the region, there are still notable variations in this regard among the many cultures in Asia. According to the 2023 Global Gender Gap Report, the Asian countries that scored highest on gender parity were in Southeast Asia, with the Philippines ranking highest at 16th out of 146 countries around the world, followed by Singapore (49th), whereas the lowest ranking Asian countries were India (127th) and Pakistan (142nd) in South Asia (World Economic Forum, 2023). Such variations in gender parity are also reflected in the career prospects available to girls in Asia. In Japan, despite entrenched stereotypical beliefs that women should find fulfillment only in their role as a dutiful wife and mother (Borovoy, 2005), young women are increasingly prioritizing their career and postponing marriage and childbearing (Nemoto, 2008). In stark contrast, in South Asia, especially the rural areas, girls are often expected to be housewives when they grow up. Parents in rural India have been found to see little value in their daughters' education, believing that it may be a disadvantage in the marriage market (Raj & Raval, 2013). Paradoxically, there has been a notable increase in girls' years of education in India in recent years, but it has been largely driven by the perceived utility of education in the marriage market (Adams-Prassl & Andrew, 2019; see also Stewart et al., 1999).

In rural, if not urban, areas of South Asian countries such as Bangladesh and India, the primary goal that many parents have for their daughters is to prepare them for their future role as a housewife and make them attractive for the marriage market. Not surprisingly, South Asian girls tend to be actively involved in household chores (Jasmine & Nduna, 2022; Zaman, 2014), but this is also true for girls in other Asian countries and many Asian boys are asked to help with physical labor around the house as well (Alampay, 2014). Of note is that unlike their peers in other Asian cultures, as South Asian girls approach puberty, concerns about their honor and chastity loom large such that their parents often choose to keep them at home (Stewart et al., 1999; UNICEF, 2018). Such concerns also underlie the prevalence of child marriage in South Asia, where one in four young women are child brides, albeit with substantial differences between (50 percent young women in Bangladesh versus 2 percent in Maldives) and within (ranging from nearly 0 percent to over 40 percent across provinces in India) countries (UNICEF, 2023). Because girls' chastity translates into the honor of the family or even the community, girls who are perceived as having violated chastity norm are often victims of domestic violence or even murder ("honor killing"), with fathers and other male relatives or community members as perpetrators with the goal of restoring their own honor (UNICEF, 2018; Raval et al., 2010).

Aside from domesticating girls and protecting their chastity, many South Asian parents also aim to train their daughters to become obedient wives and daughters-in-law. In India, 87 percent of adults agreed that a wife must always obey her husband; the level of agreement was only slightly lower among women, younger adults, and college graduates, and it varied among the provinces with a range of 32 percent to 90 percent of adults indicating complete agreement with this view (Pew Research Center, 2022). Such a view is also shared by 88 percent of Muslims in Bangladesh and Pakistan and over 90 percent of Muslims in Malaysia and Indonesia (Pew Research Center, 2013). The patrilocal tradition dominant in South Asia means that as soon as daughters are married, many of them move to their in-law's home. As the person with the lowest position in the family hierarchy, they are expected to shoulder the responsibility for housekeeping and care of all members of their new family. Evidence shows that domestic violence against wives is common in South Asia and widely accepted by women themselves, with mothers-in-law as one of the perpetrators (UNICEF, 2018). Mindful of the harsh and oppressive environment that their daughters will face in the future, South Asian mothers not only seek to train their daughters to be submissive and obedient but also lavish their daughters with love so that they may be able to endure hardship in their in-law's house in the future (Zaman, 2014).

Future Directions

For a long time, scientific knowledge about parenting was predominantly based on studies examining parents in a few Western countries conducted by researchers from the same countries. There has been a danger of over-generalizing Western models of parenting to non-Western populations. In the last three decades, the field has made great strides in expanding research to examine parents in Asia. Nevertheless, there are notable methodological limitations in the growing literature on Asian parents' goals and values.

A major limitation concerns the populations that have been studied. Even without considering the sparse research on Central Asia, the uneven distribution of parenting research across East, Southeast, and South Asia is astonishing. In contrast to the exponential growth in empirical studies on parenting in countries such as Bangladesh and China, there are hardly any publications accessible to the international research community on countries such as North Korea and the Maldives. Within Asian countries where there has been more research, families from the ethnic majority group, especially those who are from the middle class and reside in urban areas, tend to be overrepresented; families from thousands of ethnic groups across Asia remain largely invisible in the international literature. The result is a gross misrepresentation of Asian families as a largely homogeneous group both within and across Asian cultures, neglecting the contextual factors that give rise to the rich diversity in Asian parents' goals and values, including parents' cultural heritage, religion, majority and minority group status, immigration history, exposure to Western cultures, and socioeconomic status, among others. Comparing parents who vary on these factors within Asian countries or who are similar on these factors across Asian countries would bring us closer to disentangling the effects of such factors in future studies (Bornstein, 2012). A notable example in the literature is the comparison of Tamang and Brahman communities in rural Nepal by

Cole and colleagues (2006), which shed light on how religious values and majority or minority group status may shape parents' values and goals for children within the same society. Another good example is the work of Chen and colleagues on children's shyness (see Chen, 2019, for a review). By comparing rural, urbanized, and urban parents as well as parents from different historical periods, these researchers showed that parents' views and practices regarding children's shyness reflect the sociocultural changes around them.

Another major limitation in the literature on Asian parents' goals and values concerns the methods that have been used and the constructs that have been examined by researchers. Whether conducted by researchers who are based or trained in Asia or the West, many empirical studies assessed parenting cognitions in Asia by relying on survey measures originally developed for Western parents. These measures are often unable to capture the nuances in Asian parents' beliefs—such as the beliefs by some Indian parents that education is important for their daughters due to potential returns in the marriage market, nor are they relevant for understanding concepts that are not as salient in Western families, such as the concept of family honor. In contrast, qualitative methods such as ethnography and interviews are well suited for these purposes as they can provide rich information about parents' goals, values, and beliefs, which is particularly important for exploratory research on understudied topics related to parenting or with understudied populations in Asia. The aforementioned work by Fung and Thu (2019) on the socialization of deference rituals by Vietnamese parents of young children is an excellent example of how ethnography can reveal what Asian parents value in their children and how their parenting goals are instantiated in their daily practices in a community setting. The use of in-depth interviews by Way and colleagues (2013) to examine urban Chinese mothers' socialization goals is another notable example. The study illustrated how qualitative methods can provide a window into parents' beliefs and concerns, as they formulate their ideas of what is best for their children based on deep-rooted values in the culture as well as newly emerged values in a changing world.

In spite of substantial progress in the last few decades, our understanding of Asian parenting continues to be fragmented due to the methodological issues discussed above. The field is in dire need of research that goes beyond the populations and topics that have received substantial empirical attention. More importantly, the time has come for researchers to decolonize the study of Asian parenting (Raval, 2023). It is imperative that we seek to understand Asian parents' socialization goals and practices in relation to their ethnotheories as well as their experience as parents and as members of their family, community, and society. This does not mean ignoring the large corpus of literature on parenting from Western countries, however. Rather, we need to build on this literature and identify new or overlooked research questions about parenting by examining Asian parenting from an indigenous perspective. The ultimate goal is to develop models of socialization and human development that more accurately reflect the diverse pathways in which parents bring up their children to be adaptive in their sociocultural ecologies.

References

Abidin, F. A., Siregar, J. R., Joefiani, P., & Koesma, R. E. (2017). Parenting goals among Moslem parents in Bandung, Indonesia. *Proceedings of the Advances in Social Science, Education and Humanities Research, 58*, 225–227. https://doi.org/10.2991/icece-16.2017.39.

Adams-Prassl, A. & Andrew, A. (2019). *Preferences and beliefs in the marriage market for young brides*. CEPR Discussion Paper No. DP13567. https://ssrn.com/abstract=3346358.

Alampay, L. P. (2014). Parenting in the Philippines. In H. Selin (Ed.), *Parenting across cultures: Childrearing, motherhood and fatherhood in non-Western cultures* (pp. 105–121). Springer Netherlands. https://doi.org/10.1007/978-94-007-7503-9_9.

Alampay, L. P. & Rothenberg, W. A. (2021). Four domains of parenting in the Philippines. In J. E. Lansford, W. A. Rothenberg, & M. H. Bornstein (Eds), *Parenting across cultures from childhood to adolescence* (pp. 132–151). Routledge. https://doi.org/10.4324/9781003027652-7.

Ang, C.-S. & Sin, A. B.-J. (2021). Retrospective reports of perceived 'guan' parenting: Relationships to adult attachment styles, emotion regulation, and self-esteem. *The Journal of Genetic Psychology, 182*(3), 163–173. https://doi.org/10.1080/00221325.2021.1903831.

Angeles, L. C. & Sunanta, S. (2009). Demanding daughter duty: Gender, community, village transformation, and transnational marriages in Northeast Thailand. *Critical Asian Studies, 41*(4), 549–574. https://doi.org/10.1080/14672710903328021.

Barth, F. & Wikan, U. (2011). *Situation of children in Bhutan: An anthropological perspective*. The Centre for Bhutan Studies. https://doi.org/10.11588/xarep.00002607.

Bedford, O. & Yeh, K.-H. (2019). The history and the future of the psychology of filial piety: Chinese norms to contextualized personality construct. *Frontiers in Psychology, 10*, 100. https://doi.org/10.3389/fpsyg.2019.00100.

Bornstein, M. H. (2012). Cultural approaches to parenting. *Parenting, Science and Practice, 12*(2–3), 212–221. https://doi.org/10.1080/15295192.2012.683359.

Borovoy, A. B. (2005). *The too-good wife: Alcohol, codependency, and the politics of nurturance in postwar Japan*. University of California Press.

Chao, R. K. (1994). Beyond parental control and authoritarian parenting style: Understanding Chinese parenting through the cultural notion of training. *Child Development, 65*(4), 1111–1119. https://doi.org/10.2307/1131308.

Chen. X. (2019). Culture and shyness in childhood and adolescence. *New Ideas in Psychology, 53*, 58–66. https://doi.org/10.1016/j.newideapsych.2018.04.007.
Chen, X. (2023). *Socialization and socioemotional development in Chinese children*. Cambridge University Press. https://doi.org/10.1017/9781009072380.
Cheung, C. S. S. & Pomerantz, E. M. (2012). Why does parents' involvement enhance children's achievement? The role of parent-oriented motivation. *Journal of Educational Psychology, 104*(3), 820–832. https://doi.org/10.1037/a0027183.
Cole, P. M., Tamang, B. L., & Shrestha, S. (2006). Cultural variations in the socialization of young children's anger and shame. *Child Development, 77*(5), 1237–1251. https://doi.org/10.1111/j.1467-8624.2006.00931.x.
Crossway Bibles (2001). *Proverbs 22, English standard version*. Bible Gateway. www.biblegateway.com/passage/?search=Proverbs%2022&version=ESV.
Dhar, R. L. (2012). Caregiving for elderly parents: A study from the Indian perspective. *Home Health Care Management & Practice, 24*(5), 242–254. https://doi.org/10.1177/1084822312439466.
End Corporal Punishment (2014). *Prohibiting corporal punishment of children in Central Asia, South East Asia and the Pacific: Progress report 2014*. Global Initiative to End All Corporal Punishment of Children & Save the Children. https://endcorporalpunishment.org/resources/regional-progress-publications/central-asia-south-east-asia-and-the-pacific-progress-report-2014.
Finnan, C. (2022). Affective experiences and expressions in institutional context: The case of a boarding school for Indigenous students in India. *Ethnography and Education, 17*(3), 186–205. https://doi.org/10.1080/17457823.2022.2072690.
Foust, M. A. (2009). Grief and mourning in Confucius's Analects. *Journal of Chinese Philosophy, 36*(2), 348–358. https://doi.org/10.1111/j.1540-6253.2009.01523.x.
Fung, H. & Thu, M. T. (2019). Cultivating affection-laden hierarchy: Embodied moral socialization of Vòng Tay (Khoanh Tay) with children in Southern Vietnam. *Ethos, 47*(3), 281–306. https://doi.org/10.1111/etho.12247.
Gan, S.-W., Tan, J.-P., Ang, C.-S., Cheah, C. S. L., Yaacob, S. N., & Abu Talib, M. (2022). Examining a conceptual model of maternal and paternal warmth, emotion regulation and social competence among preadolescent children in Malaysia. *The Journal of Genetic Psychology, 183*(4), 312–327. https://doi.org/10.1080/00221325.2022.2076580.
Gelfand, M. J., Raver, J. L., Nishii, L., Leslie, L. M., Lun, J., Lim, B. C., … & Yamaguchi, S. (2011). Differences between tight and loose cultures: A 33-nation study. *Science, 332*(6033), 1100–1104. https://doi.org/10.1126/science.1197754.
Global Data Lab. (2024). *Patrilocality index (positive values patrilocal, negative values matrilocal)* [Data set]. https://globaldatalab.org/areadata/table/patrilocal.
Graf, F. A., Röder, M., Hein, S., Müller, A. R., & Ganzorig, O. (2014). Cultural influences on socialization goals and parenting behaviors of Mongolian parents. *Journal of Cross-Cultural Psychology, 45*(8), 1317–1327. https://doi.org/10.1177/0022022114537702.
Greenfield, P. M. (2016). Social change, cultural evolution, and human development. *Current Opinion in Psychology, 8*, 84–92. https://doi.org/10.1016/j.copsyc.2015.10.012.

Guang, X. (2016). The teaching and practice of filial piety in Buddhism. *Journal of Law and Religion, 31*(2), 212–226. https://doi.org/10.1017/jlr.2016.20.

Guilmoto, C. Z. (2015). Mapping the diversity of gender preferences and sex imbalances in Indonesia in 2010. *Population Studies, 69*(3), 299–315. https://doi.org/10.1080/00324728.2015.1091603.

Harkness, S. & Super, C. M. (2006). Themes and variations: Parental ethnotheories in Western cultures. In K. H. Rubin, & Chung, O. B. (Eds), *Parenting beliefs, behaviors, and parent–child relations: A cross-cultural perspective* (pp. 61–79). Psychology Press. https://doi.org/10.4324/9780203942901.

Heine, S. J., Lehman, D. R., Markus, H. R., & Kitayama, S. (1999). Is there a universal need for positive self-regard? *Psychological Review, 106*(4), 766–794. https://doi.org/10.1037/0033-295X.106.4.766.

Heissler, K. (2012). Children's migration for work in Bangladesh: The policy implications of intra-household relations. *Development in Practice, 22*(4), 498–509. https://doi.org/10.1080/09614524.2012.673555.

Heyman, G. D., Itakura, S., & Lee, K. (2011). Japanese and American children's reasoning about accepting credit for prosocial behavior. *Social Development, 20*(1), 171–184. https://doi.org/10.1111/j.1467-9507.2010.00578.x.

Hossain, Z. & Eisberg, G. (2020). Parenting and academic socialization of young children: Sociocultural context for early childhood development in South Asian Families. In B. K. Ashdown, & A. N. Faherty (Eds), *Parents and caregivers across cultures: Positive development from infancy through adulthood* (pp. 89–103). Springer. https://doi.org/10.1007/978-3-030-35590-6_7.

Jasmine, U. H. & Nduna, M. (2022). Parenting in Bangladesh: A review of the literature from 2006 to 2018. *Journal of Comparative Family Studies, 53*(1), 76–103. https://doi.org/10.3138/jcfs-2021-0071.

Jocson, R. M. (2020). Filipino fathers' parenting in the context of household and neighborhood risk: Familism as a protective factor. *Cultural Diversity & Ethnic Minority Psychology, 26*(4), 472–482. https://doi.org/10.1037/cdp0000332.

Jocson, R. M., Alampay, L. P., & Lansford, J. E. (2012). Predicting Filipino mothers' and fathers' reported use of corporal punishment from education, authoritarian attitudes, and endorsement of corporal punishment. *International Journal of Behavioral Development, 36*(2), 137–145. https://doi.org/10.1177/0165025411428249.

Kim, K.-W. (2006). Hyo and parenting in Korea. In Rubin, K. H., & Chung, O. B. (Eds), *Parenting beliefs, behaviors, and parent–child relations: A cross-cultural perspective* (pp. 207–222). Psychology Press. https://doi.org/10.4324/9780203942901.

Kim, Y.-H., Cohen, D., & Au, W.-T. (2010). The jury and abjury of my peers: The self in face and dignity cultures. *Journal of Personality and Social Psychology, 98*(6), 904–916. https://doi.org/10.1037/a0017936.

Lansford, J. E., Chang, L., Dodge, K. A., Malone, P. S., Oburu, P., Palmérus, K., … & Quinn, N. (2005). Physical discipline and children's adjustment: Cultural normativeness as a moderator. *Child Development, 76*, 1234–1246. https://doi.org/10.1111/j.1467-8624.2005.00847.x.

Leaper, C. (2015). Gender and social-cognitive development. In R. M. Lerner (Series Ed.), L. S. Liben, & U. Muller (Vol. Eds), *Handbook of child psychology and developmental science* (Vol. 2, 7th ed., pp. 806–853). Wiley. https://doi.org/10.1002/9781118963418.childpsy219.

Leung, J. T. Y. (2020). Perceived parental sacrifice, filial piety and hopelessness among Chinese adolescents: A cross-lagged panel study. *Journal of Adolescence, 81*, 39–51. https://doi.org/10.1016/j.adolescence.2020.04.005.

Lin, G.-X., Mikolajczak, M., Keller, H., Akgun, E., Arikan, G., Aunola, K., ... & Roskam, I. (2023). Parenting culture(s): Ideal-parent beliefs across 37 countries. *Journal of Cross-Cultural Psychology, 54*(1), 4–24. https://doi.org/10.1177/00220221221123043.

Lin, J. (2020). The conditions that promote or discourage physical punishment as described by Taiwanese and Taiwanese American mothers. *Journal of Cross-Cultural Psychology, 51*(3–4), 222–240. https://doi.org/10.1177/0022022120913615.

Louie, J. Y., Oh, B. J., & Lau, A. S. (2013). Cultural differences in the links between parental control and children's emotional expressivity. *Cultural Diversity & Ethnic Minority Psychology, 19*(4), 424–434. https://doi.org/10.1037/a0032820.

Luo, R., Tamis-LeMonda, C. S., & Song, L. (2013). Chinese parents' goals and practices in early childhood. *Early Childhood Research Quarterly, 28*(4), 843–857. https://doi.org/10.1016/j.ecresq.2013.08.001.

Markus, H. R. & Kitayama, S. (1991). Cultural variation in the self-concept. In J. Strauss, & G. R. Goethals (Eds), *The self: Interdisciplinary approaches* (pp. 18–48). New York: Springer. https://doi.org/10.1007/978-1-4684-8264-5_2.

Matsumoto, D., Yoo, S. H., & Fontaine, J. (2008). Mapping expressive differences around the world: The relationship between emotional display rules and individualism versus collectivism. *Journal of Cross-Cultural Psychology, 39*(1), 55–74. https://doi.org/10.1177/0022022107311854.

Mestechkina, T., Son, N. D., & Shin, J. Y. (2014). Parenting in Vietnam. In H. Selin (Ed.), *Parenting across cultures: Childrearing, motherhood and fatherhood in non-Western cultures* (pp. 47–57). Springer Netherlands. https://doi.org/10.1007/978-94-007-7503-9_5.

Minza, W. M. & Herlusia, S. I. (2022). Affect and trust in educational migration of young people from provincial towns in Indonesia. *Ethnography and Education, 17*(3), 206–223. https://doi.org/10.1080/17457823.2022.2071590.

Murata, A., Moser, J. S., & Kitayama, S. (2013). Culture shapes electrocortical responses during emotion suppression. *Social Cognitive and Affective Neuroscience, 8*(5), 595–601. https://doi.org/10.1093/scan/nss036.

Nemoto, K. (2008). Postponed marriage: Exploring women's views of matrimony and work in Japan. *Gender & Society, 22*(2), 219–237. https://doi.org/10.1177/0891243208315868.

Ng, F. F.-Y., Pomerantz, E. M., & Deng, C. (2014). Why are Chinese mothers more controlling than American mothers? "My child is my report card." *Child Development, 85*(1), 355–369. https://doi.org/10.1111/cdev.12102.

Ng, F. F.-Y., Pomerantz, E. M., & Lam, S.-F. (2007). European American and Chinese parents' responses to Children's success and failure: Implications for children's responses. *Developmental Psychology, 43*(5), 1239–1255. https://doi.org/10.1037/0012-1649.43.5.1239.

Ng, F. F.-Y. & Wang, Q. (2019). Asian and Asian American parenting. In M. H. Bornstein (Ed.), *Handbook of parenting* (3rd ed., pp. 108–169). Routledge. https://doi.org/10.4324/9780429398995-4.

Ng, F. F.-Y. & Wei, J. (2020). Delving into the minds of Chinese parents: What beliefs motivate their learning-related practices? *Child Development Perspectives, 14*(1), 61–67. https://doi.org/10.1111/cdep.12358.

Nguyen, T., Chang, P. P. W., & Loh, J. M. I. (2014). The psychology of Vietnamese tiger mothers: Qualitative insights into the parenting beliefs and practices of Vietnamese-Australian mothers. *Journal of Family Studies, 20*(1), 48–65. https://doi.org/10.5172/jfs.2014.20.1.48.

Olson, S. L., Lansford, J. E., Evans, E. M., Blumstein, K. P., & Ip, K. I. (2019). Parents' ethnotheories of maladaptive behavior in young children. *Child Development Perspectives, 13*(3), 153–158. https://doi.org/10.1111/cdep.12330.

Park, H., Byun, S., & Kim, K. (2011). Parental involvement and students' cognitive outcomes in Korea: Focusing on private tutoring. *Sociology of Education, 84*(1), 3–22. https://doi.org/10.1177/0038040710392719

Park, H.-J., Yi, S.-H., Lee, K.-Y., Kim, B.-K., & Park, S.-R. (2012). Parenting values and practices among Muslim parents in Indonesia. *Child Studies in Asia-Pacific Contexts, 2*(2), 109–122. https://doi.org/10.5723/csdc.2012.2.2.109.

Pew Research Center (2013, April 30). *The world's Muslims: Religion, politics and society.* www.pewforum.org/Muslim/the-worlds-muslims-religion-politics-society.aspx.

Pew Research Center (2022, March 2). *How Indians view gender roles in families and society*. https://www.pewresearch.org/religion/2022/03/02/gender-roles-in-the-family.

Pew Research Center (2023). *Buddhism, Islam and religious pluralism in South and Southeast Asia*. http://www.pewresearch.org/religion/2023/09/12/buddhism-islam-and-religious-pluralism-in-south-and-southeast-asia.

Raj, S. P., & Raval V. V. (2013). Parenting and family socialization within a cultural context. In E. L. Anderson, & S. Thomas (Eds), *Socialization: Theories, processes and impact* (pp. 57–78). Nova Science Publishers, Inc.

Rajadhyaksha, U. & Bhatnagar, D. (2000). Life role salience: A study of dual-career couples in the Indian context. *Human Relations, 53*(4), 489–511. https://doi.org/10.1177/0018726700534002.

Raval, V. V. (2023). Toward a decolonial parenting science through centering majority world parenting: A commentary on "Parenting culture(s): Ideal-parent beliefs across 37 countries". *Journal of Cross-Cultural Psychology, 54*(1), 30–35. https://doi.org/10.1177/00220221221134915.

Raval, V. V., Raval, P. H., & Raj, S. P. (2010). Damned if they flee, doomed if they don't: Narratives of runaway adolescent females from rural India. *Journal of Family Violence, 25*(8), 755–764. https://doi.org/10.1007/s10896-010-9333-5.

Riany, Y. E., Meredith, P., & Cuskelly, M. (2017). Understanding the influence of traditional cultural values on Indonesian parenting. *Marriage & Family Review, 53*(3), 207–226. https://doi.org/10.1080/01494929.2016.1157561.

Ridgeway, C. L. & Correll, S. J. (2004). Unpacking the gender system: A theoretical perspective on gender beliefs and social relations. *Gender & Society, 18*(4), 510–531. https://doi.org/10.1177/0891243204265269.

Rudy, D., Carlo, G., Lambert, M. C., & Awong, T. (2014). Undergraduates' perceptions of parental relationship-oriented guilt induction versus harsh psychological control: Does cultural group status moderate their associations with self-esteem? *Journal of Cross-Cultural Psychology, 45*(6). 905–920. https://doi.org/10.1177/0022022114532354.

Severance, L., Bui-Wrzosinska, L., Gelfand, M. J., Lyons, S., Nowak, A., Borkowski, W., … & Yamaguchi, S. (2013). The psychological structure of aggression across cultures. *Journal of Organizational Behavior, 34*(6), 835–865. https://doi.org/10.1002/job.1873.

Sovet, L. & Metz, A. J. (2014). Parenting styles and career decision-making among French and Korean adolescents. *Journal of Vocational Behavior, 84*(3), 345–355. https://doi.org/10.1016/j.jvb.2014.02.002.

Sriram, R. & Navalkar, P. G. (2012). Who is an 'ideal' father? Father, mother and children's views. *Psychology and Developing Societies, 24*(2), 205–237. https://doi.org/10.1177/097133361202400206.

Stewart, S. M., Bond, M. H., Zaman, R. M., McBride-Chang, C., Rao, N., Ho, L. M., & Fielding, R. (1999). Functional parenting in Pakistan. *International Journal of Behavioral Development, 23*(3), 747–770. https://doi.org/10.1080/016502599383784

Sun, R. & Wang, H. (2019). Worry about eldercare in China: The role of family relations, socio-economic resources, and community services in 2000 and 2010. *International Journal of Population Studies, 5*(2), 1–13. https://doi.org/10.18063/ijps.v5i2.1046.

Tan, S.-A., Nainee, S., & Tan, C.-S. (2021). The mediating role of reciprocal filial piety in the relationship between parental autonomy support and life satisfaction among adolescents in Malaysia. *Current Psychology, 40*(2), 804–812. https://doi.org/10.1007/s12144-018-0004-7.

Tapanya, S. (2011). Attributions and attitudes of mothers and fathers in Thailand. *Parenting: Science and Practice, 11*(2–3), 190–198. https://doi.org/10.1080/15295192.2011.585566.

Tsai, J. L., Miao, F. F., Seppala, E., Fung, H. H., & Yeung, D. Y. (2007). Influence and adjustment goals: Sources of cultural differences in ideal affect. *Journal of Personality and Social Psychology, 92*(6), 1102–1117. https://doi.org/10.1037/0022-3514.92.6.1102

United Nations Children's Fund (UNICEF). (2018). *Structural violence against children in South Asia.* UNICEF, Kathmandu. www.unicef.org/rosa/sites/unicef.org.rosa/files/2018-08/SVACS%20report%28web%29August%202.pdf.

United Nations Children's Fund (UNICEF) (2019). *Gender Counts: A quantitative assessment of gender inequality and its impact on girls and boys in East and Southeast Asia.* UNICEF East Asia and the Pacific, Bangkok. https://www.unicef.org/eap/media/3601/file/EAP%20gender%20count.pdf

United Nations Children's Fund (UNICEF) (2023). *A profile of child marriage in South Asia.* UNICEF, New York, 2023. www.unicef.org/rosa/reports/profile-child-marriage-south-asia#:~:text=Around%20one%20in%20four%20young,while%20they%20are%20still%20adolescents.

United Nations, Department of Economic and Social Affairs, Population Division (2019). *Patterns and trends in household size and composition: Evidence from a United Nations dataset.* (ST/ESA/SER.A/433). www.un.org/en/development/

desa/population/publications/pdf/ageing/household_size_and_composition_technical_report.pdf.

Way, N., Okazaki, S., Zhao, J., Kim, J. J., Chen, X., Yoshikawa, H., ... & Deng, H (2013). Social and emotional parenting: Mothering in a changing Chinese society. *Asian American Journal of Psychology, 4*(1), 61–70. https://doi.org/10.1037/a0031204.

Wei, J., Pomerantz, E. M., Ng, F. F.-Y., Yu, Y., Wang, M., & Wang, Q. (2019). Why does parents' involvement in youth's learning vary across elementary, middle, and high school? *Contemporary Educational Psychology, 56*, 262–274. https://doi.org/10.1016/j.cedpsych.2018.12.007.

Wilson, L. (2014). Buddhism and family. *Religion Compass, 8*(6), 188–198. https://doi.org/10.1111/rec3.12107.

Wongboonsin, P. & Tan, J.-P. (Eds) (2018). *Care relations in Southeast Asia: The family and beyond*. Brill. https://doi.org/10.1163/9789004384330.

World Economic Forum (2023). *Global gender gap report 2023.* www.weforum.org/publications/global-gender-gap-report-2023.

Xu, L. & Chi, I. (2015). Ageing and grandparenting in Asia. In S. R. Quah (Ed.), Routledge *handbook of families in Asia* (pp. 246–258). Routledge. https://doi.org/10.4324/9781315881706.

Yeh, K.-H. & Bedford, O. (2003). A test of the dual filial piety model. *Asian Journal of Social Psychology, 6*(3), 215–228. https://doi.org/10.1046/j.1467-839X.2003.00122.x.

Zaman, R. M. (2014). Parenting in Pakistan: An overview. In H. Selin (Ed.), *Parenting across cultures: Childrearing, motherhood and fatherhood in non-Western cultures* (pp. 91–104). Springer Netherlands. https://doi.org/10.1007/978-94-007-7503-9_8.

Zhang, M.-R., Ng, F. F.-Y., Yu, D., & Von Suchodoletz, A. (2024). Granny and mama: Grandmothers' and mothers' interactions with toddlers during block play in urban China. *Early Childhood Research Quarterly, 67*, 148–158. https://doi.org/10.1016/j.ecresq.2023.12.004.

4

PARENTAL SOCIALIZATION BELIEFS AND PRACTICES IN THE CHINESE CONTEXT

Daniel T. L. Shek, Janet T. Y. Leung, Moon Y. M. Law, and Ginger C. C. Chau

Introduction

In every society, parents hold certain parental socialization beliefs, such as "children should honour their father and mother" and "children should have good academic achievement." To achieve such socialization goals, parents adopt corresponding parenting practices such as "harsh punishment is the key to parenting success" or "democratic parenting can promote creativity in children" (Shek et al., 2022). In this chapter, we focus on Chinese parental socialization beliefs and practices with particular reference to Hong Kong. There are several reasons why we focus on Chinese parental socialization beliefs and practices. First, the size of the Chinese population is huge (roughly 1.4 billion in 2023). As such, researchers cannot ignore Chinese people if they want to formulate theories on parenting beliefs and practices that are generalizable across cultures. Second, it is noteworthy that existing studies on parental socialization beliefs and practices are "WEIRD" research, which mainly selected the research targets from Western, educated, industrialized, rich, and democratic societies. Third, the political system of China, "Socialism with Chinese characteristics," with a delicate blending of the State-driven and market-driven economies, is obviously unique. Fourth, with a history of more than 5,000 years, Chinese cultural beliefs based on Confucian, Buddhist, and Taoist thoughts have much to offer to enrich our understanding of parenting beliefs and practices. In fact, these cultural beliefs are rooted in collectivistic values, which are in sharp contrast to Western concepts of parenting, focusing on the importance of individual autonomy, competition, and achievement in

DOI: 10.4324/9781003383949-4

defining parental socialization goals (Shek, 2003). Besides, research findings show that Chinese parenting attributes are different from Western parenting attributes. For example, Chinese parents focus strongly on academic excellence in their conception of an "ideal child" (Shek & Chan, 1999), and they embrace the belief of "do not lose at the starting line," hence pushing their children to achieve good examination results morbidly (Shek & Siu, 2019). Besides, compared with Western people who desire open communication and non-avoidance of interpersonal conflict, communication patterns in Chinese families are more subtle and non-expressive, particularly when children are expected to act in a filial manner (Shek & Law, 2019; Shek et al., 2022).

Specifically, there are several reasons to focus on Chinese socialization beliefs and practices in Hong Kong. First, as a city where the "East meets West," Hong Kong, as an international city, is still strongly influenced by traditional Chinese culture, such as the emphases on filial piety and academic excellence. Second, Hong Kong adopts a Capitalist system with intense competition, which translates into parental expectations such as morbid emphases on academic excellence and outstanding achievement. Finally, as there is no family policy in Hong Kong, and its parent education is loosely organized (Shek et al., 2022), it is time to review parenting socialization expectations and practices in Hong Kong to generate family policy and practice implications.

This chapter first examines the salient parental socialization beliefs and practices in traditional Chinese culture, with particular reference to two classic family instruction books (*Di Zi Gui* and *Master Chu's Homilies for Families*). Based on the review, we will tease out the basic themes intrinsic to parental socialization beliefs and practices in traditional Chinese thoughts. Second, we review empirical work on parental socialization beliefs in Hong Kong and their impact on adolescent developmental outcomes and family processes. Third, we briefly review how parenting practices (e.g., parental psychological control, Shek, 2003) influence the developmental outcomes of young people. Fourth, based on the review, we propose several future directions for research. Finally, we make some practice and policy recommendations based on the review.

Parental socialization beliefs and practices in the traditional Chinese culture

Pepitone (1994) conceived beliefs as "concepts about the nature, the causes, and the consequences of things, persons, events and processes" and are "social constructions that are part of a culture and have guided the socialization of those who share that culture" (p. 140). With specific reference to parenting, Ridao et al. (2021) defined parental beliefs as "a set of naive theories about developmental achievements: what is important for childrearing and those aspects that influence child development" (p. 3). From the above perspectives, Chinese parenting beliefs involve cognitive knowledge (i.e., concepts) about the nature of Chinese parenting and its causes and results. In particular, beliefs about the attributes of the child and the parent and the practice that helps to achieve the developmental goals are important aspects to be considered. For parenting practice, it is common to include rules and regulations on children's behaviour.

There are many parental beliefs in the traditional Chinese culture (Shek et al., 2022). Some examples are shown in Table 4.1, which can be grouped into several categories. First, in terms of socialization goals, children are expected to be filial (*"bai hang xiao wei xian"*: put filial piety in all actions) and to take care of their parents when they get old (*"fan bu zhi en"*: the gift of returning the favour). Second, children are expected to make their family illustrious (*"guang zong yao zu"*: bring glory to one's ancestors) and not to do things that make the family shameful (*"you ru jia men"*: disgraceful to the family). Third, training is indispensable to achieve such socialization goals, as shown by the saying, *"yu bu zhuo, bu cheng qi, ren bu xue, bu zhi li"* (a jade without polishing will be worthless; a person without learning will know nothing). Fourth, emphases on diligence (*"shao zhuang bu nu li, lao da tu shang bei"*: young idlers, an older beggar; *"qing you gong, xi wu yi"*: diligence has its reward while the play has no benefit); harsh punishment (*"bang xia chu xiao zi"*: spare the rod and spoil the child); academic excellence (*"shu zhong zi you huang jin wu"*: a book does hold a house of gold); and cultivation of patience and endurance (*"chi de ku zhong ku, fang wei ren shang ren"*: only those who endure the most challenging hardships will be the best of the best) are highlighted. However, there are gender differences involved in socialization goals where boys are expected to be successful (*"wang zi cheng long"*: hope one's son becomes a dragon), whereas girls are not expected to possess good talents (*"nv zi wu cai bian shi de"*: it is a virtue for a woman to have no talent). Besides, parents are expected to play different roles in the socialization process, as exemplified by the sayings, *"yang bu jiao, fu zhi guo"* (it is wrong for a father only to feed but not teach his child) and *"ci mu duo bai er"* (where there is a kind mother, there is a useless son).

In addition to the above Chinese socialization expectations and goals, related parental expectations in the socialization process also exist in "family instruction books" in Chinese culture. The first example is *Di Zi Gui* (Standards for Being a Good Student and Child), which outlines the expectations and socialization goals for raising children (Shek et al., 2021), such as expectations about filial piety, respect and love for siblings, adoption

TABLE 4.1 Examples of Chinese cultural beliefs on parenting and child development

Traditional Chinese beliefs (Traditional Chinese characters)	*English translation*
兒孫自有兒孫福 (er sun zi you er sun fu)	Younger generations will do all right on their own
家家有本難念的經 (jia jia you ben nan nian de jing)	Each family has its problems /We all have a cross to bear
清官難斷家務事 (qing guan nan duan jia wu shi)	Even an upright official finds it hard to settle a family quarrel
家醜不可外傳 (jia chou bu ke wai chuan)	Every family has a skeleton in the closet
光宗耀祖 (guang zong yao zu)	Bring honour to one's ancestors
有辱家門 (you ru jia men)	Be a scandal to the family /Humiliate the family
玉不琢，不成器，人不學，不知理 (yu bu zhuo, bu cheng qi, ren bu xue, bu zhi li)	A jade without polishing will not become a functional object; a man without learning will not know the way
少壯不努力，老大徒傷悲 (shao zhuang bu nu li, lao da tu shang bei)	A young idler, an old beggar
勤有功，戲無益 (qing you gong, xi wu yi)	Diligence has its reward, while play has no benefit
百行孝為先 ((bai hang xiao wei xian)	Piety is the foundation of all virtues
反哺之恩 (fan bu zhi en)	The grace of giving back
學海無涯，唯勤是岸 (xue hai wu ya, wei qin shi an)	Knowledge is infinite, like a boundless ocean
棒下出孝子 (bang xia chu xiao zi)	Spare the rod and spoil the child
書中自有黃金屋 (shu zhong zi you huang jin wu)	A book holds a house of gold
吃得苦中苦，方為人上人 (chi de ku zhong ku, fang wei ren shang ren)	No pain, no gain
望子成龍 (wang zi cheng long)	Putting great effort and hope into the child's future
女子無才便是德 (nv zi wu cai bian shi de)	The good woman is an illiterate one
養不教，父之過 (yang bu jiao, fu zhi guo)	To feed without teaching is the father's fault
慈母多敗兒 (ci mu duo bai er)	A loving mother causes a spoiled child
故天將降大任於斯人也，必先苦其心志，勞其筋骨，餓其體膚，空乏其身，行拂亂其所為，所以動心忍性，曾益其所不能。 (gu tian jiang jiang da ren yu si ren ye, bi xian ku qi xin zhi, lao qi jin gu, e qi ti fu, kong fa qi shen, xing fu luan qi suo wei, suo yi dong xin ren xing, zeng yi qi suo bu neng)	When Heaven is about to confer a great office on any man, it first exercises his mind and will with suffering, exhausts his muscles and bones, exposes him to starvation and poverty, harasses him with troubles and setbacks so as to stimulate his spirit, toughen his nature, and enhance his abilities

of serious attitudes to people and things, trustworthiness, learning from the saints, speaking the truth, keeping one's promise, self-reflection, and non-comparison with others as socialization ideals. The second example is the family instruction book written by Master Zhu (Jordan, 1998; Shek & Law, 2019; Zhang, 1993), which also outlines different expectations for socialization.

Integration of the materials in the two family instruction books mentioned above reveals several categories of parental socialization beliefs and parenting expectations. The first category is expectations about general intrapersonal qualities, such as keeping good hygiene, having a healthy lifestyle and safety mentality, preparation for crises and emergencies, patience, reflection, avoidance of extreme behaviour (doctrine of the mean), staying away from egocentrism, not giving up oneself, fulfilling one's duties, and fulfilling one's civic responsibility. The second category of expectations surrounds spirituality and character. Some examples include being thrift, keeping a simple life, not focusing on material beauty and female beauty, controlling one's lust, not killing animals to satisfy oral satisfaction, respecting one's fate, following the course of life, learning the teaching of the Sages, valuing the classic teaching, and not transgressing human ethics.

The third category contains family-related beliefs and expectations. These include respecting the elderly and older members of the family, teaching children to be "righteous," respecting order in family relationships, valuing family bondage, avoiding family and interpersonal conflicts, and upholding the importance of family harmony. The final category of parenting beliefs and expectations is interpersonal. These include not "over-admiring" the rich, not despising the poor, protecting the powerless and helping those with needs, not oppressing the poor and widowed, not having the mindset of envy and gloat, not hurting others with tricks, and not being too mean. Besides, children are expected not to hang around with peers with problems but mix with those with morals and experience, help others without expectation of repayment, remember those who have offered help, and be grateful.

Theoretically, the socialization goals in the expectations mentioned above resemble the desired socialization goals highlighted in contemporary models of adolescent development (Shek et al., 2022). For example, the focus on hygiene and health is in line with the socialization goals in physical development. Besides, the emphases on simple life, character, and spiritual development are in line with the emphases of positive psychology (e.g., character strengths) and existential psychology. Empirically, the expected qualities of children and adolescents in the family instruction books are generally consistent with the research findings. For example, based on the study of Chinese families, an ideal child should achieve academic excellence, be obedient, and exhibit proper behaviour from the parents' perspectives (Shek & Chan, 1999). The analyses are also consistent with Wu's view (2022) that several parental expectations are common, including *"guan,"* *"jiao,"* *"achievement,"* and *"chi."*

Parental socialization beliefs in Hong Kong

Parental expectations across five cohorts of parents

In the survey adopting a non-random quota sampling to collect data from five cohorts across different generations (N=5,707), research findings revealed parents' expectations and beliefs in several domains (Lam et al., 2020). In the first domain, the Hong Kong Chinese Parental Expectation Scale was applied to assess 24 parental expectations for their children's attributes with reference to parental socialization goals in the traditional Chinese culture (e.g., being a well-bred person, respecting the elderly, and being an honest person) and contemporary Western cultural values (e.g., pursue equality, pursue justice, and respect human rights). Results showed two interesting observations. First, parents showed endorsement of "traditional" expectations such as respect for old people, respect for justice, and possession of a sense of responsibility. Second, parents also held "modern" expectations, such as engagement in politics and endorsement of the importance of justice, human rights, and equality, although the responses were diverse. For example, around 35 percent of parents agreed that children should not be involved in politics. For socio-demographic correlates of traditional expectations about the future of children, several correlates were identified. These include being mothers, being older, having lower educational attainment, being retired, and having a lower family income, such as receiving social security (Shek, Lam, & Zhu, 2019).

The second domain is expectations for boys and girls (i.e., gendered expectations) based on the Chinese Parental Gendered Expectations for Sons and Daughters Scale. Some expectations include "sons are more responsible than daughters," "daughters are decent and virtuous," and "a marriage is more important than a successful career for daughters." There are three observations based on the findings. First, some parents expect their children to follow some traditional rules and social customs, such as the expectation that daughters should be able to get married, although such beliefs are not overwhelming. Second, fathers and mothers are expected to differentiate their roles in raising sons and daughters, such as "mothers take a more important role to take care of the daughters." Third, traditional expectations about sons and daughters are transforming. For example, only around 30 percent of the respondents agreed that "if possible, I wish to have a son" and "if daughters are too capable, it will be difficult for them to find a partner." Regarding socioeconomic correlates of gendered expectations, fathers did not differ from mothers in gendered expectations. However, higher educational levels, higher occupational status, and higher household income were related to parents' lower gender expectations of the traditional roles of their children. In other words, lower socioeconomic status was related to higher gender expectations of traditional roles of their children (Shek, Kwong, et al., 2019).

Closely related to the concept of gender expectations for sons and daughters is the expected division of labour between fathers and mothers within the family, which constitutes the third domain under study. In this study, Shek, Lam, and Yang (2019) used the five-item Parental Division of Labor Scale. The items include "In the domestic division of labour, I take charge of childcare," "In the domestic division of labour, I assist in childcare," "I am an implementer in childcare," "I am a decision-maker in childcare," and "I agree with the perspective that men are breadwinners and women are homemakers." There are several findings based on the study. First, compared with mothers, fathers showed a lower endorsement of taking up the "main role" of childrearing. Second, relative to mothers, fathers played a stronger "assisting" role. Third, regarding the traditional Chinese belief that men serve as breadwinners and women serve as homemakers, fathers showed a stronger endorsement of this belief than mothers. There were also several socio-demographic correlates of perceived parental division of labour. Generally speaking, parental educational attainment, parental occupation, and family income were related to participation in childcare duties. For example, parents with higher educational attainment were less likely to play the "assisting role," and they had a weaker endorsement of the traditional form of parental division.

The fourth domain is parental beliefs about parental roles and responsibilities (Shek, To, et al., 2019). The researchers used the 23-item Chinese Parental Beliefs Scale on Parental Roles and Responsibilities with five dimensions, including "parental love and nurturing" (seven items), "parenthood as a normative life stage" (four items), "readiness to relax and restrict parental control" (four items), "parental guidance of the young" (four items), and "fulfilment of children's needs" (four items). With reference to "parental love and nurturing," parents generally agreed that parents should be loving and nurturing, such as paying close attention to the emotions of the children and spending enough effort on parent–child time. Nevertheless, about 20 percent of the parents were neutral about teaching their children knowledge about sex. Regarding the perception of "parenthood as a normative life stage," there are some interesting patterns. Surprisingly, roughly one-fourth of the respondents viewed parenthood as occurring naturally and that there was no need to learn. Besides, only one-fifth of the participants believed that bringing up offspring would enable parents to be looked after in old age. Obviously, the old belief that "save for the rainy days" no longer works. Concerning "readiness to relax and restrict parental control," parents generally acknowledged that they should recognize their children's choices and desires and should not force their expectations upon the children. Nevertheless, only around 44 percent of the parents supported the idea that parents should recognize their children's sexual orientation.

Regarding "parental guidance to the young," results showed that parents generally agreed that "parents' responsibility is to educate (to teach and to nurture) their children," "to teach is to discipline," and "to nurture is to provide them with needs such as food and clothing." Besides, parents agreed that "parents are responsible for preventing their children from getting into bad company," "when children do not meet the requirements, parents ought to provide appropriate guidance," and "if circumstances allow, parents have to provide resources and opportunities so as to lay a good foundation for their children." The above views are consistent with the traditional Chinese belief that parents have to shoulder responsibility for taking care of their children.

Finally, regarding the "fulfilment of children's needs," parents agreed that parents should "assist their children in preventing them from running into obstacles on important matters" and that they are "responsible for providing financial support for their children to complete university education." Only roughly one-third of the parents agreed that "parents should meet the needs of their children as far as possible." Regarding socio-demographic correlates, mothers showed stronger parental beliefs on parental roles and responsibilities than fathers did. However, compared with mothers, fathers had a stronger endorsement of "parents should meet the needs of their children as far as possible." Compared with parents with higher educational levels, parents with lower educational levels showed a higher endorsement of beliefs about the roles and responsibilities of parents. Employment status is also related to prenatal beliefs about parental roles and responsibilities. Compared with the fathers and mothers who have retired and those receiving social security, working parents (full-time and part-time) showed lower levels of traditional parental beliefs. Similarly, parents with lower household incomes were inclined to show higher endorsement of parental beliefs on parental roles and responsibilities.

Parental expectations on children's future

Chinese parents strongly emphasize their children's future (particularly their achievements), and there are several reasons for this. First, probably because of political and social instability in the past two centuries, having a "secure" future is vital for children, and academic excellence is usually the ladder to fulfil this expectation. Second, when children have a "good" future, they can have adequate resources to take care of their parents, and there is no need for parents to take care of the children. Third, pursuing children's "bright" future is also an essential strategy to establish family honour.

Leung and Shek (2011b) developed the Parental Expectation on Child's Future Scale. Using data collected through a focus group, the researchers proposed five domains surrounding parental expectations on children's future, including "educational achievement," "self-reliance," "occupation," "family obligation," and "conduct," which formed the 23-item Chinese Expectation on Child's Future Scale. To validate the scale, Leung and Shek (2011c) collected data from 125 Hong Kong parents, with findings supporting the psychometric properties of the scale. Studies showed that Chinese parents' expectation about their children's future was linked to children's developmental outcomes. Leung (2016) examined maternal beliefs (including "Chinese cultural beliefs of familism," "expectations of children's prospects," and "attrition of children's accomplishment"), perceived maternal control, and psychological competence of young people in 337 divorced mothers experiencing economic disadvantage. They reported that adolescents' perceived maternal beliefs predicted adolescent developmental outcomes, with perceived maternal control as a mediator. Leung and Shek (2019b) further examined the role of parental expectations of children's future and parental control on adolescent cognitive competence and self-identity in 275 Chinese families with financial difficulties. While parental expectations of children's future and adolescents' perceived parental control had direct effects on adolescent cognitive competence and self-identity, perceived maternal control moderated the relationship between paternal expectations and adolescent cognitive competence and self-identity.

Parental expectations about children's future are also associated with other family processes. Leung and Shek (2013) collected data from 550 poor Chinese parents in Hong Kong who responded to measures of parental beliefs (including expectations about children's future) and parenting characteristics. The finding showed that more substantial parental expectations about children's future were related to higher levels of positive parenting styles and parental control in fathers and mothers. In a study based on

275 poor Chinese parents, Leung and Shek (2015b) reported that positive parental child-specific beliefs (i.e., positive family beliefs), particularly parents' expectations of the future of children, were positively associated with parents' sacrifice for children's education. In another research, Leung and Shek (2016) studied the predictive relationships between parental beliefs ("Chinese beliefs about hardships," "attribution of children's achievement," and "expectations of the future of children") and parental control on adolescent development in 275 families with financial difficulties. Expectations of fathers on children's future also predicted perceived maternal control and positive youth development. Besides, maternal control mediated the effect of parental beliefs on youth positive development. The findings highlighted the triadic interaction of fathers, mothers, and children.

Parental attributions of children's success and failure

In the study involving 275 Chinese couples with adolescent children, Leung and Shek (2015a) examined the linkages between parental attributions of children's success and failure and family processes of low-income households. The parents were assessed in terms of parental attributions, parenting style, parental control, parental sacrifice for the child's education, and family functioning. Paternal attribution of children's success and failure to effort predicted paternal control, paternal sacrifice for children's education, and fathers' perceived family functioning. Similarly, maternal attribution of children's success and failure to effort predicted maternal control and maternal sacrifice for children's education. While paternal and maternal attribution of children's success and failure to ability predicted parental and maternal control, there was no effect of attribution of children's success and failure to luck.

Parental socialization practices in Hong Kong

Parental control: behaviour control, psychological control, and indigenous parental control

Previous studies have reviewed parental socialization practices in parents in Hong Kong (Shek, 2004; Shek & Law, 2019; Shek et al., 2022). Generally speaking, parents in Hong Kong mainly control their children's conduct when it is closely related to academic performance, but the parents put less emphasis on children's behaviours in the non-academic domain, such as knowledge of their children's peers. Besides, Chinese parents also used psychological control and behavioural control according to indigenous concepts of parenting in Chinese culture. For example, parents expected their children to be filial and have good virtues. Besides, some findings suggested that the classical parenting style of "strict father, kind mother" has been changed to "strict mother, kind father" (i.e., tiger mom and panda dad).

Previous studies generally showed that parental behavioural control generated positive developmental outcomes, and psychological control was related to negative developmental effects (Shek, 2004; Shek & Law, 2019; Shek et al., 2022). Recent studies have also shown that while parental behavioural control protected adolescents from developmental problems, parental psychological control was related to adolescent problem behaviour, such as Internet addiction (Shek, Zhu, et al., 2019; Shek et al., 2018), substance abuse (Shek, Zhu, et al., 2019) and delinquency (Shek & Zhu, 2019). Shek et al. (2021) also reported that parental attributes are antecedents of adolescent spirituality.

Besides, studies have shown that parental control interacts with other family processes and/or across parents in influencing child developmental outcomes. Leung (2016) examined maternal beliefs (including cultural beliefs of familism, expectations of children's future, attrition of children's achievement), perceived maternal control, and adolescent psychological competence in 337 divorced mothers experiencing economic disadvantage. They reported that adolescents' perceived maternal beliefs predicted adolescent developmental outcomes, with perceived maternal control as a mediator. In another study, Leung and Shek (2020a) examined the interaction effect of parental behavioural control and psychological control on adolescent developmental outcomes (N=2,369). There was a stronger relationship between paternal behavioural control and adolescent life satisfaction under high paternal psychological control. Besides, the life satisfaction of boys was more strongly influenced by parental behavioural control than that of girls. However, girls were negatively influenced by maternal psychological control in terms of life satisfaction, but the negative effects were not evident in boys. Paternal and maternal psychological control also showed interaction effects on adolescent hopelessness.

Leung et al. (2017) showed that mother- and adolescent-reported maternal control interacted to predict filial piety (N=432). While high adolescent-perceived parental control was related to higher filial piety when mother-related maternal control was high, filial piety gradually dropped when adolescents reported higher levels of maternal control but lower mother-reported maternal control. Based on multiple group analyses, these associations were stable across gender and age groups.

Leung (2020a) studied the linkage between concerted cultivation (i.e., intensive nurturing of children with enrichment) and adolescent depression and anxiety, with parent–child conflict proposed as a mediator (N=1,570 young adolescents). She reported that paternal concerted cultivation predicted adolescent psychopathology with father-child conflict as a mediator. In contrast, although maternal concerted cultivation positively predicted adolescent mental health issues through increased mother–child conflict, there was a reduction in father-child conflict.

Regarding the antecedents of parental control, Leung, Shek, Kwok, and Cheung (2022) examined the relationships between parenting perfectionism and parental control (monitoring and psychological control) in 386 intact Chinese families. They found an actor-only effect pattern in the relationship between socially prescribed parenting perfectionism and paternal monitoring. A couple effect in the relationship between socially prescribed parenting perfectionism and maternal monitoring was also observed. They concluded that prescribed social expectations about parenting in fathers influence parental control practice in Chinese contexts. Using the same data set, Leung, Shek, Kwok, and Yung (2022) examined the inter-relationships between marital dissatisfaction, psychological control and parent–child conflict. While father-perceived marital dissatisfaction positively predicted parental psychological control, mother-perceived marital dissatisfaction did not. This finding also suggested that the spillover effect from marital dissatisfaction triggers psychological control in their spouse. Moreover, when the parents are not satisfied with their marriage, parents and children will have more disputes in their daily lives.

Parental sacrifice for child's education

The concept of parental sacrifice is deep-rooted in the Chinese culture. It is a culturally reinforced concept that parents would sacrifice their own interests to facilitate the academic development of children. Using focus group interviews as a methodology, Leung and Shek (2011a) developed the Chinese Parental Sacrifice for Child's Education Scale. The qualitative findings showed that there are five dimensions, including "striving for financial resources," "time spent on child education," "restructuring of daily routine," "sacrifice of lifestyle and aspiration," and "shielding of worries." According to the conceptual model, the researchers developed an item pool and engaged several experts to comment on the relevance, clarity, and representativeness of the items. Leung and Shek (2011b) further examined this scale in 125 parents. Results supported the reliability of the scale. Factor analysis showed that while there were three factors based on adolescent responses, five dimensions were found for the parent sample. To further understand the dimensionality of the measure, Leung et al. (2016) used confirmatory factor analysis to examine the dimensions and factorial invariance of the Chinese Parental Sacrifice Scale based on the perceptions of Chinese adolescents (N=373) on related paterna and maternal attributes. Results showed support for the five dimensions and factorial invariance across the parental and maternal scales.

Research studies showed that parental sacrifice for a child's education is related to the child's developmental outcomes. In the study involved 432 Chinese single-mother families with financial difficulties, Leung (2017) studied the inter-relationships amongst Chinese cultural beliefs of familism, perceived maternal sacrifice, and developmental outcomes, including adolescent identity, cognitive competence, and a positive future perception. Results showed that Chinese cultural beliefs of familism influenced adolescent developmental outcomes with perceived maternal sacrifice as a mediating factor.

Regarding the relationship between parental sacrifice and life satisfaction in poor adolescents (N=716), Leung and Shek (2020b) showed that while there was full mediation of reciprocal and authoritarian filial piety on the relationship between maternal sacrifice and adolescent life satisfaction, and there were related partial mediation effects between paternal sacrifice and adolescent life satisfaction. Using the same data set, Leung and Shek (2021) reported that perceived sacrifice was stronger in mothers than in fathers. Besides, the primary and interaction effects of perceived paternal sacrifice and maternal sacrifice on the self-identity, self-determination, and self-efficacy of adolescents were reported. While maternal sacrifice was not related to adolescent developmental outcomes under low paternal sacrifice, maternal sacrifice positively influenced adolescent development with high paternal sacrifice in that family.

Using three waves of longitudinal data collected from 1,569 Chinese adolescents analysed by cross-lagged analyses, Leung (2020b) revealed the relationship between maternal sacrifice and filial piety, which was also related to hopelessness; the bidirectional effect of parental sacrifice and adolescent hopelessness was also found. The findings concluded that maternal sacrifice protects adolescent hopelessness via filial piety.

Besides, Leung (2018) studied the relationship between discrepancies in perceived parental sacrifice in parents and adolescents and adolescent developmental outcomes in poor Chinese families (N=275). Results showed that the interaction effects of parental (both paternal and maternal) perceptions and adolescents' perceptions of adolescent resilience and cognitive competence were evident. In particular, when parental sacrifice was high, the families with higher convergent parent-adolescent perceptions of parental sacrifice exhibited high adolescent resilience and cognitive competence.

Research also showed that parental sacrifice for a child's future was related to other family processes. In a study based on 275 poor Chinese parents, Leung and Shek (2015b) reported that positive parental child-specific beliefs (i.e., positive family beliefs), particularly parents' expectations of the future of children, were positively associated with both paternal and maternal sacrifice for children's education. In another study based on 432 Chinese single-mother families undergoing financial difficulties, Leung (2017) studied the inter-relationships among Chinese cultural beliefs of familism, perceived maternal sacrifice, and developmental outcomes, including adolescent identity, cognitive competence, and a positive future perception. The findings revealed that Chinese cultural beliefs of familism influenced adolescent developmental outcomes with perceived maternal sacrifice as a mediating factor.

Overparenting

While overparenting is a recent research topic in Western parenting literature, it is not foreign to Chinese people, as shown by the cultural belief that "if you rear a child for 100 years, you have to worry about him/her for 99 years constantly." To examine this phenomenon, Leung et al. (2018) examined the views of Chinese parents and youths through four focus groups. Results showed eight themes, including close monitoring, parental intrusion, strong emphasis on academic excellence, comparisons with peers, forward problem-solving, overscheduling, over-care of the child, and over-affective involvement. While some of the above concepts resonate with Western concepts, some concepts are unique to Chinese people. Leung and Shek (2018) examined measures of overparenting in Chinese adolescents in 642 university students. They found that the Chinese Paternal Overparenting Scale (CPOS) and Chinese Maternal Overparenting Scale (CMOS) revealed good internal consistency, test-retest reliability, and convergent validity. Factor analyses supported the proposed conceptual model with eight dimensions. Moreover, the research conducted by Leung and Shek (2019a) validated that the eight primary factors in the CPOS and CMOS can be categorized under two secondary factors: "over-demandingness" and "over-responsiveness."

Crucially, it has been identified that over-parenting can influence children's developmental outcomes. For instance, Leung (2020c) examined how perceived parenting affects adolescent well-being and several moderators in a sample of 1,735 secondary school students in Hong Kong. The findings revealed that while paternal overparenting predicted adolescent life satisfaction, maternal overparenting influenced adolescent anxiety and depression. Conflicts between father and child also moderated the linkage between paternal overparenting and adolescent anxiety and depression. Besides, family structure and family dynamics can also influence the parent–child relationship. Using the same data set, Leung et al. (2021) further investigated the linkages between overparenting and adolescent developmental outcomes, as well as several moderators in early adolescents in Hong Kong (N=1,735). The study revealed that there is a positive relationship between parental overparenting and adolescent egocentrism and positive developmental outcomes. Besides, maternal overparenting's influence on egocentrism and positive youth development was moderated by father-child conflict. Family structure and the gender of adolescents can also moderate the influence of parental overparenting. Based on the responses of 1,570 adolescents, Leung (2020a) studied the predictive relationship between parental overparenting and adolescent anxiety based on two waves of longitudinal data, with parent–child conflict as the mediating factor. The study suggested that mother–child conflict was a mediator in the longitudinal relationship between maternal overparenting and adolescent anxiety. At the same time, adolescent anxiety also predicted maternal overparenting via mother–child conflict. The findings highlighted the bidirectional relationship between maternal overparenting and adolescent anxiety, with mother–child conflict over time.

Future research directions

Based on the review of the research on parenting expectations and practice, this paper discusses some future research directions. First, in view of the rich knowledge of parental socialization beliefs in the traditional Family Instruction books, it is suggested that research should be conducted to examine and organize the related materials systematically. In view of the observation that traditional family instruction books resonate with contemporary parenting science, it would be exciting to tease out the essence of positive parenting, which is universal across cultures (Shek et al., 2022).

Second, there are several research gaps we have to address. First, we have to further examine the consequences of parental socialization beliefs and practices on child developmental outcomes. Besides ill-being measures such as depression and anxiety, positive well-being measures such as life meaning and thriving should be used. Second, there are fewer studies examining the antecedents of socialization beliefs and practices. In particular, it is theoretically interesting to understand whether parents would model the beliefs and practices of their parents that are hypothesized by family therapy theories. Third, there is a need to identify the mediating and moderating factors involved in the relationships between beliefs and practices and the outcomes, such as the gender of the parents and adolescent children, as well as psychosocial competence.

Third, regarding the consequences of parental socialization practice, one crucial intervening factor that should be examined is the interpretations of the child. For example, if parental behavioural control is interpreted as restraining the child's autonomy, parent–child conflict would likely take place. On the other hand, if psychological control is seen as a sign of concern, it may not adversely affect the well-being of adolescent children. As highlighted by Smetana (2017), "beliefs about parental authority legitimacy also influence the responses to parenting" (p. 20). Hence, it is essential to examine the interpretations of the children of the parental beliefs and practices.

Fourth, it is vital to carry out longitudinal studies to understand the interplay between parental socialization practice and child developmental outcomes. Without longitudinal studies, the dynamics involved in the family processes and adolescent development are not explicit. However, as Hong Kong people basically endorse the "fast food" culture and it is not uncommon for academics to stick to "quick" publication for tenure and appraisal purposes, there is a need to build up a culture emphasizing the importance of patience and long-term accumulation of research data.

Fifth, as different stakeholders in a family may have different experiences, the involvement of different family members in a study can help to provide diverse perspectives on how family processes are perceived differently. As most of the studies rely on the reports of children, there is a need to include parental views, which can also help to generate a dynamic picture of the interplay among the perception of family processes by different family members. Adopting a systemic perspective would be helpful in examining socialization beliefs in terms of child, parent, and family perspectives. For example, family beliefs about ideal child development would shape parental beliefs, which eventually influence the child's perceptions.

Sixth, as commented by Smetana (2017), it would be helpful to pay more attention to "cultural and contextual variations have led to greater specificity in defining parenting in terms of different parenting dimensions" (p. 19) and "refined understanding of parenting" (p. 22) because different parenting situation may involve various parenting needs and socialization goals. Such contextual variations include gender, economic disadvantage, family intactness, and cultural variations (Shek & Ma, 2016).

Finally, as there are few validated parenting programs in Hong Kong, there is a need to develop culturally appropriate parenting programs covering parental beliefs and expectations and conduct an evaluation of the programs that are being developed. Research on parenting program development, implementation, and evaluation is significant based on the review of family life education and parenting programs in Hong Kong (Chan et al.,

2012; Chan et al., 2017) that highlight the importance of evidence-based programs embracing positive parenting beliefs and practices.

Policy and practical implications

This chapter also highlights some implications for service providers, parents and the general public, as well as policy implications for the Government. First, as revealed in *Di Zui Gui* and *Family Instruction of Master Zhu*, there are many cultural beliefs on parental expectations and socialization goals. Hence, parents and the general public need to understand and reflect on the related "positive" parental socialization beliefs and practices. Besides, although people usually hold the belief that traditional Chinese parental beliefs and practices are outdated and useless, the present analyses of *Di Zui Gui* and *Family Instruction of Master Zhu* showed that some traditional parental beliefs are, in fact, consistent with contemporary parenting science. Hence, it is helpful to consider retaining the related wisdom on the development of children outlined in traditional Chinese family instruction books, such as the need to promote personal virtues and interpersonal harmony. Of course, parents should also appreciate the differentiation of "healthy" versus "unhealthy" parental beliefs and practices and understand the relative strengths and weaknesses of possible consequences of different parental practices based on parenting science (Maccoby & Martin, 1983) on adolescent developmental outcomes.

Another practical implication is to review research on parental socialization beliefs and practices. As shown in the previous section, academics in tertiary institutions undertake most related work in an ad hoc and uncoordinated manner, and there is no known systematic database in Hong Kong. Hence, there is a need for the government to develop a central database, tease out the valuable information to be used by different stakeholders, and identify research, service, and policy gaps.

As the previous section shows, there are many "authority-based" (i.e., not "evidence-based") parenting programs in Hong Kong. Hence, it is essential to highlight the importance of evidence-based parenting and parenting science. With reference to the existence of parenting beliefs and practices, one has to ask what the best parental beliefs and practices for childrearing are. In terms of program effectiveness, there are several types of parenting programs: harmful and ineffective, ineffective, having both positive and negative effects, and promising and effective programs. As such, a clearing house for evidence-based parenting programs in Hong Kong would be helpful in the long run.

With reference to the parenting problems highlighted by Shek and Siu (2019), such as morbid emphasis on academic excellence and lack of holistic understanding of child development, the following practical implication is how to prevent such problems. Based on the public health approach, one practical method is to consider prevention at different stages, including tertiary prevention, secondary prevention, and primary prevention.Besides parenting programs, positive youth development programs that can promote the quality of family life through enhancement of the psychosocial competencies of young people (Shek, 2024; Shek & Dou, 2024) are promising tools to be considered.

The final practical implication is to review and follow up on recommendations for parenting programs in Hong Kong. In a review of family education in Hong Kong, Chan et al. (2012) highlighted several recommendations. Similarly, in their study of parenting in Hong Kong, Chan et al. (2017) also made several recommendations, such as the development of conceptual frameworks on parent education and parenting programs and inter-sectoral collaboration and building up an enriching ecology for parenting.

Conclusion

This chapter examines Chinese socialization beliefs and practices in Hong Kong, which is a Chinese society that is influenced by Western cultures. Regarding the attributes of socialization beliefs and practices in the traditional Chinese culture, our review suggests that moral and interpersonal attributes, as well as emphasis on non-materialistic values, are intrinsic to traditional Chinese cultural beliefs. Concerning socialization beliefs in Hong Kong, traditional socialization beliefs are still strong but gradually evolving, and they are associated with adolescent developmental outcomes. For parental control, Chinese parents in Hong Kong focused on the academic achievement of their children, and they used behavioural control, psychological control, and control based on indigenous Chinese parenting concepts. Studies also showed that different forms of parental control were related to different developmental outcomes. Parental sacrifice and over-parenting were related to adolescent developmental outcomes. We also propose several directions for future research and policy considerations.

References

Chan, Y. C., Chung, P. K., Lee, T. K., Chung, C. P., Yip, H. M., Kong, S. T., & Kam, C. Y. (2012). *Report on the study of family education in Hong Kong*. The Hong Kong Polytechnic University. www.familycouncil.gov.hk/tc/files/research/consultancy_study.pdf.

Chan, Y. C., Leung, M. C., Tsang, K. M., Lu, H. J., & Fok, H. K. (2017). *Report on parenting practices in Hong Kong*. The Government of the Hong Kong Special Administrative Region. www.familycouncil.gov.hk/tc/files/research/Final%20report_study_on_parenting_practices_in_hong_kong.pdf.

Jordan, D. K. (1998). Zhū Bólú's maxims for managing the home. https://pages.ucsd.edu/~dkjordan/chin/chtxts/JuBorlu.html.

Lam, C. M., To, S. M., & Kwong, W. M. (2020). Development and validation of a questionnaire on Chinese parents' beliefs in parental roles and responsibilities. *Applied Research in Quality of Life, 15*, 693–712. https://doi.org/10.1007/s11482-018-9682-4.

Leung, J. T. Y. (2016). Maternal beliefs, adolescent perceived maternal control and psychological competence in poor Chinese female-headed divorced families. *Journal of Child and Family Studies, 25*, 1815–1828. https://doi.org/10.1007/s10826-016-0367-z.

Leung, J. T. Y. (2017). Cultural family beliefs, maternal sacrifice, and adolescent psychological competence in Chinese poor single-mother families. *Social Development, 26*(4), 767–782. https://doi.org/10.1111/sode.12239.

Leung, J. T. Y. (2018). Parent-adolescent discrepancies in perceived parental sacrifice and adolescent developmental outcomes in poor Chinese families. *Journal of Research on Adolescence, 28*(2), 520–536. https://doi.org/10.1111/jora.12356.

Leung, J. T. Y. (2020a). Concerted cultivation and adolescent psychopathology over time-mediation of parent–child conflict. *International Journal of Environmental Research and Public Health, 17*(24), 9173. https://doi.org/10.3390/ijerph17249173.

Leung, J. T. Y. (2020b). Perceived parental sacrifice, filial piety and hopelessness among Chinese adolescents: A cross-lagged panel study. *Journal of Adolescence, 81*, 39–51. https://doi.org/10.1016/j.adolescence.2020.04.005.

Leung, J. T. Y. (2020c). Too much of a good thing: Perceived overparenting and well-being of Chinese adolescents in Hong Kong. *Child Indicators Research, 13*(5), 1791–1809. https://doi.org/10.1007/s12187-020-09720-0.

Leung, J. T. Y. & Shek, D. T. L. (2011a). "All I can do for my child" – development of the Chinese Parental Sacrifice for Child's Education Scale. *International Journal on Disability and Human Development, 10*(3), 201–208. https://doi.org/10.1515/ijdhd.2011.037.

Leung, J. T. Y. & Shek, D. T. L. (2011b). Expecting my child to become "dragon"-development of the Chinese Parental Expectation on Child's Future Scale. *International Journal on Disability and Human Development, 10*(3), 257–265. https://doi.org/10.1515/ijdhd.2011.043.

Leung, J. T. Y., & Shek, D. T. L. (2011c). Validation of the Chinese parental expectation on child's future scale. *International Journal on Disability and Human Development, 10*(3), 267–274. https://doi.org/10.1515/ijdhd.2011.039.

Leung, J. T. Y. & Shek, D. T. L. (2013). Parental beliefs and family functioning in Chinese families experiencing economic disadvantage in Hong Kong. *International Journal on Disability and Human Development, 12*(2). 151–161. https://doi.org/10.1515/ijdhd-2013-0006.

Leung, J. T. Y. & Shek, D. T. L. (2015a). Parental attributions of children's success and failure and family processes in poor Chinese families. *Journal of Child and Family Studies, 24*, 2191–2203. https://doi.org/10.1007/s10826-014-0022-5.

Leung, J. T. Y. & Shek, D. T. L. (2015b). Parental beliefs and parental sacrifice of Chinese parents experiencing economic disadvantage in Hong Kong: Implications for social work. *British Journal of Social Work, 45*(4), 1119–1136. https://doi.org/10.1093/bjsw/bct190.

Leung, J. T. Y. & Shek, D. T. L. (2016). The influence of parental beliefs on the development of Chinese adolescents experiencing economic disadvantage: Maternal control as a mediator. *Journal of Family Issues, 37*(4), 543–573. https://doi.org/10.1177/0192513X13518776.

Leung, J. T. Y. & Shek, D. T. L. (2018). Validation of the perceived Chinese overparenting scale in emerging adults in Hong Kong. *Journal of Child and Family Studies, 27*, 103–117. https://doi.org/10.1007/s10826-017-0880-8.

Leung, J. T. Y., & Shek, D. T. L. (2019a). Hierarchical factor analysis and factorial invariance of the Chinese overparenting scale. *Frontiers in Psychology, 10*, 1873. https://doi.org/10.3389/fpsyg.2019.01873.

Leung, J. T. Y. & Shek, D. T. L. (2019b). The influence of parental expectations and parental control on adolescent well-being in poor Chinese families. *Applied Research in Quality of Life, 14*, 847–865. https://doi.org/10.1007/s11482-017-9540-9.

Leung, J. T. Y. & Shek, D. T. L. (2020a). Parental control and adolescent wellbeing in Chinese adolescents in Hong Kong. *Child Indicators Research, 13*(2), 703–727. https://doi.org/10.1007/s12187-019-09642-6.

Leung, J. T. Y. & Shek, D. T. L. (2020b). Parental sacrifice, filial piety and adolescent life satisfaction in Chinese families experiencing economic disadvantage. *Applied Research in Quality of Life, 15*(1), 259–272. https://doi.org/10.1007/s11482-018-9678-0.

Leung, J. T. Y. & Shek, D. T. L. (2021). Relationships between perceived paternal and maternal sacrifice and developmental outcomes of Chinese adolescents experiencing economic disadvantage. *Applied Research in Quality of Life, 16*, 2371–2386. https://doi.org/10.1007/s11482-020-09821-6.

Leung, J. T. Y., Shek, D. T. L., Fung, A. L. C., & Leung, G. S. M. (2021). Perceived overparenting and developmental outcomes among Chinese adolescents: Do family structure and conflicts matter? *Journal of Social and Personal Relationships, 38*(2), 742–764. https://doi.org/10.1177/0265407520971713.

Leung, J. T. Y., Shek, D. T. L., Kwok, L. M. H., & Cheung, J. H. L. (2022). Actor–partner interdependence of socially prescribed parenting perfectionism and parental control in Chinese families. *Family Process, 62*(2), 722–736. https://doi.org/10.1111/famp.12794.

Leung, J. T. Y., Shek, D. T. L., Kwok, L. M. H., & Yung, E. T. Y. (2022). Marital dissatisfaction, psychological control and parent–child conflict in Chinese families-An actor-partner interdependence model analysis. *Journal of Social and Personal Relationships, 39*(12), 3596–3618. https://doi.org/10.1177/02654075221102634.

Leung, J. T. Y., Shek, D. T. L., & Lin, L. (2017). Mother–child discrepancy in perceived parental control and adolescent filial piety in poor single-mother families. *Journal of Adolescence, 60*, 1–10. https://doi.org/10.1016/j.adolescence.2017.06.006.

Leung, J. T. Y., Shek, D. T. L., & Ma, C. M. S. (2016). Measuring perceived parental sacrifice among adolescents in Hong Kong: confirmatory factor analyses of the Chinese parental sacrifice scale. *Child Indicators Research, 9*(1), 173–192. https://doi.org/10.1007/s12187-015-9313-7.

Leung, J. T. Y., Shek, D. T. L., & Ng, L. S. L. (2018). Over-parenting from the perspectives of Chinese parents and youths. *International Journal of Child and Adolescent Health, 11*(3), 315–325.

Maccoby, E. E. & Martin, J. A. (1983). Socialisation in the context of the family: Parent–child interaction. In P. H. Mussen & E. M. Hetherington (Eds), *Handbook of child psychology: Socialisation, personality, and social development* (pp. 1–101). Wiley.

Pepitone, A. (1994). Beliefs and cultural social psychology. In L. L. Adler & U. P. Gielen (Eds), *Cross-cultural topics in psychology* (pp. 139–152). Praeger.

Ridao, P., López-Verdugo, I., & Reina-Flores, C. (2021). Parental beliefs about childhood and adolescence from a longitudinal perspective. *International Journal of Environmental Research and Public Health, 18*(4), 1760. https://doi.org/10.3390/ijerph18041760.

Shek, D. T. L. (2003). A longitudinal study of parenting and adolescent adjustment in Chinese adolescents with economic disadvantage. *International Journal of Adolescent Medicine and Health, 15*(1), 39–50. https://doi.org/10.1515/IJAMH.2003.15.1.39.

Shek, D. T. L. (2004). Family processes and developmental outcomes in Chinese adolescents. *Journal of Pediatrics, 9,* 316–324. https://citeseerx.ist.psu.edu/document?repid=rep1&type=pdf&doi=5ff78e68ab26993ea6a6272798c1b58e2044444b.

Shek, D. T. L. (2024). Enhancement of psychosocial competence and well-being of chinese high school students under the covid-19 pandemic: Tin ka ping P.A.T.H.S. Project in mainland china. *Applied Research in Quality of Life*. Advance online publication. https://doi.org/10.1007/s11482-024-10350-9

Shek, D. T. L., Chai, C. W. Y., & Dou, D. Y. (2021). Parenting factors and meaning of life among Chinese adolescents: A six-wave longitudinal study. *Journal of Adolescence, 87,* 117–132. https://doi.org/10.1016/j.adolescence.2021.01.004.

Shek, D. T. L., & Chan, L. K. (1999). Hong Kong Chinese parents' perceptions of the ideal child. *The Journal of Psychology, 133*(3), 291–302. https://doi.org/10.1080/00223989909599742.

Shek, D. T. L., & Dou, D. (2024). The reach and impact of a positive youth development program (project P.A.T.H.S.) in china and beyond: Review and reflection. *Applied Research in Quality of Life*. Advance online publication. https://doi.org/10.1007/s11482-024-10364-3

Shek, D. T. L., Kwong, W. M., Zhu, X. Q., & Yang, Z. (2019). Gendered expectation towards sons and daughters in Chinese parents in Hong Kong. *International Journal of Child and Adolescent Health, 12*(4), 357–367.

Shek, D. T. L., Lam, C. M., & Yang, Z. (2019). Division of labor in parenting amongst Chinese parents in Hong Kong. *International Journal of Child and Adolescent Health, 12*(4), 369–378.

Shek, D. T. L., Lam, C. M., & Zhu, X. Q. (2019). Parental expectations amongst Chinese parents in Hong Kong: Profiles and demographic correlates. *International Journal of Child and Adolescent Health, 12*(4), 345–356.

Shek, D. T. L. & Law, M. Y. M. (2019). Parenting in contemporary Hong Kong: Observations and reflections. *International Journal of Child and Adolescent Health, 12*(4), 391–401.

Shek, D. T. L. & Ma, C. M. (2016). A six-year longitudinal study of consumption of pornographic materials in Chinese adolescents in Hong Kong. *Journal of Pediatric and Adolescent Gynecology, 29*(1), S12–S21. https://doi.org/10.1016/j.jpag.2015.10.004.

Shek, D. T. L. & Siu, A. M. H. (2019). "UNHAPPY" environment for adolescent development in Hong Kong. *Journal of Adolescent Health, 64*(6), S1–S4. https://doi.org/10.1016/j.jadohealth.2019.01.007.

Shek, D. T. L., Sun, R., Leung, J. T. Y., & Law, M. (2022). Parenting in contemporary Hong Kong: Observations based on recent research findings. In *Parenting across cultures: Childrearing, motherhood and fatherhood in non-Western cultures* (pp. 149–164). Springer Nature. https://doi.org/10.1007/978-3-031-15359-4_10.

Shek, D. T. L., To, S. M., & Dou, D. Y. (2019). Parental beliefs about parental roles and responsibilities in Chinese parents: Pioneer findings. *International Journal of Child and Adolescent Health, 12*(4), 379–389.

Shek, D. T. L. & Zhu, X. Q. (2019). Paternal and maternal influence on delinquency among early adolescents in Hong Kong. *International Journal of Environmental Research and Public Health, 16*(8), 1338. https://doi.org/10.3390/ijerph16081338.

Shek, D. T. L., Zhu, X. Q., Dou, D. Y., & Chai, W. Y. (2019). Influence of family factors on substance use in early adolescents: A longitudinal study in Hong Kong. *Journal of Psychoactive Drugs, 52*(1), 66–76. https://doi.org/10.1080/02791072.2019.1707333.

Shek, D. T. L., Zhu, X. Q., & Ma, C. M. S. (2018). The influence of parental control and parent–child relational qualities on adolescent internet addiction: A 3-year longitudinal study in Hong Kong. *Frontiers in Psychology, 9*, 642. https://doi.org/10.3389/fpsyg.2018.00642.

Smetana, J. G. (2017). Current research on parenting styles, dimensions, and beliefs. *Current Opinion in Psychology, 15*, 19–25. https://doi.org/10.1016/j.copsyc.2017.02.012.

Wu, C. C. (2022). The effects of Chinese parenting belief on preschoolers' temperament and secure attachment. *Children, 10*(1), 9. https://doi.org/10.3390/children10010009.

Zhang, X. T. (1993). *Zhuzi parental instruction* (Trans.) Shanghai People's Publishing House.

5

PARENTING IN CHANGING SOCIAL AND ECONOMIC CONTEXTS IN ASIAN SOCIETIES

Sumie Okazaki, Xiaolin Ou, and Niobe Way

Introduction

In their introduction to the 2012 special issue of the *New Directions for Youth Development* on youth success and adaptation in times of globalization and economic change, Chen, Christmas-Best, Titzman, and Weichold wrote: "The issue of changing context for individual development is particularly relevant to research and practical work on today's youth given the substantial social and economic changes originating from globalization, economic volatility, and technological development. The macro-level changes cascade down to nearly all aspects of a young person's life, such as education, career, and family and peer relationships" (p. 1). The same macro-level changes that impact adolescents, of course, also shape parenting. Social ecological theory (Bronfenbrenner & Morris, 2006) posits that human development is shaped by interactions among various layers of social ecological contexts, from microsystem (e.g., parent–child relationships, peers) to exosystem (e.g., mass media, parent workplace) to macrosystem (e.g., economic system, political system, culture). However, the linkages and mechanism of influence between parenting in the microsystem and large-scale social and economic changes in the macrosystem remain poorly understood (Yoshikawa, Way, & Chen, 2012).

In this chapter, we contend that major forces of social change in Asia in the past half century, namely economic development and globalization, have brought about significant shifts in how parents in Asia raise their children. Specifically, we trace the value fluctuations between social connectedness and individual autonomy that parents view as most suitable to

DOI: 10.4324/9781003383949-5

their children's future adaptation to the contextual demands of changing societies. Although a comprehensive review of all relevant empirical and theoretical works is beyond the scope of this chapter, we will review the literature on social change and parenting from South Korea, Singapore, and China as they are the most active sites of scholarly attention. We then examine the nature of parental changes in attitudes about social connectedness and individual autonomy using our longitudinal and mixed method data from Nanjing, China. We conclude with practice and policy implications.

Social and Economic Changes in Asia

The rapid social and economic changes that swept Asia in the latter half of the 20th century must be understood in the context of global development that originated in the West. Neoliberalism–generally understood as a set of economic reform policies that privilege deregulated economy, liberalization of trade, and privatization of state-owned businesses, with accompanying political, social, and ethical implications–is a political-economic ideology that was seeded by intellectuals and institutions in post-World War I Europe and the United States (Ganti, 2014) and gained ascendency in the late 1970s following the rising oil prices and economic downturns and taken up by conservative policymakers in the U.S. and the U.K. in the 1980s (Beeson & Islam, 2005). Neoliberalism became a popular concept in anthropology and related disciplines as a frame for the global political and economic structural force, within which particular populations' lives were impacted (Ganti, 2014). Of particular interest were neoliberalism's implications for the self, namely the individual as accruing attributes and skills that enable them to thrive in the market economy. The neoliberal notion of individuals' abilities as sources of future income recast parenting as cultivation of their children's self. That is, parents make "investments" in their children's human capital through their time and money (Foucault, 2008). According to Foucault, the stakes of childrearing under neoliberal knowledge-based economy is shifted from parents simply passing down economic capital to parents' concerted cultivation of their children's human capital.

The rapid economic development of Pacific Asia in the second half of the 20th century in what Kyung-Sup (2010) described as "compressed modernity"—starting initially with post-World War II Japan, followed by the Newly Industrializing Economies of South Korea, Taiwan, Hong Kong, and Singapore, then by the Southeast Asian economies of Thailand, Malaysia, Indonesia, and the Philippines—was dubbed the "Asian economic miracle" (Ozawa, 1994). Notably, the Asian economic miracle had not followed the Western neoliberal model of free market economy but instead had been facilitated by significant state intervention (World Bank, 1993).

While the 1997 Asian financial crisis precipitated the International Monetary Fund (IMF)-mandated economic reforms in Asia with neoliberal underpinnings, Beeson and Islam (2005) argued that many Asian capitalist economies' entrenched political-business institutions may have resisted the full embrace of the neoliberal ideology. For example, China's dramatic economic transition was set in motion in the late 1970s as Deng Xiaoping sought to gradually transition China's economy from the planned economy established under Mao Zedong's Community Party control to a modern market economy through a series of radical economic reforms (Guthrie, 2012). Over the last several decades, China moved from a largely agrarian society of planned economy controlled by state-owned enterprises to a modern society that is increasingly urban, market oriented, and shaped by a mix of state, private, and foreign enterprises now boasting the second largest GDP in the world (Guthrie, 2012). Yet, China's capitalism–and those of Japan, Korea, Singapore, and other Asian nations–is still distinct from Western economies (Beeson & Islam, 2005), and it is these tensions between the autonomous self demanded by Western neoliberalism and the relational self typical in Asian cultures that constitute the challenges of Asian parenting in the context of social and economic changes.

Broad Theories connecting Social Change to Families and Parenting

There have been major theories in behavioral science fields to explain the connections between societal change and individual behavior. Developmental Idealism (DI), a sociological theory proposed by Thornton (2005), is a cultural model that draws a reciprocal causal relationship between modern social structures and modern family behavior. The attributes that are associated with modernity and valued by DI encompass a wide range of domains, including national resources and social structure (e.g., industrial and urban society, wealth and health), social institutions (e.g., free and open markets, democratic social and political institutions), social norms and values (e.g., an emphasis on the individual rather than family and community, freedom, equality, scientific-rational decision making), and individual and family arrangements (e.g., gender egalitarianism, planned and low fertility, high degree of personal autonomy and self-expression) (Thornton, Dorius, & Swindle, 2015). While these DI attributes that are viewed as the desirable end point of development may be Eurocentric in origin, Thornton et al. (2015) argue that globalization has proliferated DI as the global cultural models of modernity. Importantly DI posits causes and consequences of economic development. For example, economic development is considered as causal factors in promotion of democracy, declining fertility, and expansion of education; in turn forces such as democracy, education, planned and low fertility, personal freedom, and gender equality facilitate economic development. It is these causal links in the DI that allow us to theorize that economic development in Asia has had significant consequences to various dimensions of parenting and on family life, including gender roles and childbearing.

Within psychology, Greenfield (2009) proposed a theory of social change and human development, linking societal change with developmental change. Greenfield premised her theory on the general direction of historical social change from *Gemeinschaft* (more rural, poorer, low technology, homogenous communal) sociocultural ecologies to *Gesellschaft* (more urban, richer, high technology, complex, heterogeneous) sociocultural ecologies. Greenfield argued that these social changes cause shifts in cultural values held by people in those environments (from collectivism to individualism), which then influence the learning environment of the developing children in those settings (e.g., shifting from informal socialization at home to more formal schooling; shifting from large families to small families), which in turn result in shifts in human development (shift from strict gender roles and emphasis on familial responsibility to more gender egalitarian roles and individual preferences and achievements).

Silbereisen and Chen (2010) noted that in the U.S. and Europe, changes in parents' work experiences (stemming from economic and social changes) are associated with changes in parenting beliefs and practices such as amount of control and monitoring of their children, expressions of warmth, and parental investment in children's schooling and extracurricular activities. The values promoted in the parents' workplace (e.g., obedience to authority vs. individual initiative) are also thought to influence the values that the parents socialize in their children. China's transition from the planned to market economy has incentivized individual risk taking, competition, and merit-based rewards in workplaces (Guthrie, 2012) that invariably shape parents' beliefs about autonomy and social connectedness (Yoshikawa, Way, & Chen, 2012). In turn, Chinese parents are more likely to instill values and to encourage behavior in their children to equip them with skills and characteristics that the children will need to thrive in the new market economy.

Impact of Social and Economic Changes on Parenting

Scholars of marriage and fertility demography have noted a more rapid trend of later or no marriage and later or no childbearing among families in East Asia than in other parts of the world. East Asian families from societies associated with Confucian ethos of patriarchal family systems (e.g.,

China, Japan, South Korea, Taiwan) have traditionally held strict gender divisions of labor that had obligated women to filial duties. Raymo, Park, Xie, and Yeung (2015) argued that economic development and globalization have exerted pressure on these societies to expand opportunities for women outside of the home (including higher education), yet there have been limited changes in the gendered expectations and obligations to the family for women in East Asia. The combined effect of these forces has resulted in particularly low marriage and low fertility rates in East Asia, according to Raymo et al.

A major consequence of later and lower fertility rates among East Asian women is that each family has fewer children. In the case of China, the state had instituted a One Child Policy (1979–2015), which fundamentally was an economic policy that fueled China's rapid economic ascendance but with grave social consequences such as the elevated sex ratio and a rapidly aging population (Cai & Feng, 2021). In China, the one child policy implementation brought about a rapid drop in fertility rates that had occurred more gradually in other Asian nations, but with similar consequences for parents and children, especially among the higher socioeconomic class families. In families with a single child, the pressure and competition for the child to obtain elite education and higher-paying jobs have become intense (Fong, Yu, & Zhu, 2020).

Intensive mothering, first named by Hays (1996), is a gendered model of child rearing that is "construed as *child-centered, expert-guided, emotionally absorbing, labor-intensive, and financially expensive*" (p. 8, italics in the text). Hays theorized that this ideology of intensive mothering—which posits that women's primary responsibility is to be a self-sacrificing, doting mother who willingly take on the labor of child rearing without social or financial compensation—facilitates not only the maintenance of gender hierarchy but also of capitalism. Intensive mothering reflects the dominant patriarchal ideology of contemporary U.S. and European societies that shapes the experiences not only of White, middle-class mothers from those societies but all mothers, including mothers of color and those from lower socioeconomic backgrounds and those from other cultural contexts (Way, 2024). Minotte (2023) argues that intensive mothering ideology arose out of specific historical contexts, including the economic developments of post-World War II industrial economies that allowed single-wage earner fathers to provide comfortably for the family. In a similar vein, based on extensive ethnography with middle-class and working-class American families, Lareau (2003) described middle-class and upper-class parenting as that of "concerted cultivation" in which parents manage their children's out-of-school schedules around adult- or expert-led extracurricular activities (e.g., music lessons, sports leagues) to cultivate cognitive and noncognitive skills that would later help their children thrive in elite higher education and careers. Some scholars (e.g., Matsuoka, 2019) have argued that in highly standardized education systems in Asia (with high-stakes testing as the primary means of academic advancement), concerted cultivation of middle-class parents takes a different form than those documented in the U.S. Parents in Japan, for example, are more likely to spend time and resources on intensive private tutoring rather than on leisure activities.

Of relevance to our present discussion, the intensification of parenting in whatever form must be understood as integral to the application of neoliberal ideology into family life, in which the individual family (rather than the state) is tasked with the responsibility of their child's economic security. Below, we review the literature pertinent to three examples from Asia–Singapore, South Korea, and China– that demonstrates how Asian parenting is changing to meet the demands of compressed modernity and globalization.

Singapore and risk management parenting

Modern Singapore was established as a British trading post in 1819 and remained as a British colony except during the years of World War II until it gained full independence in 1965. Today it is known as the top-performing education system in the world, with Singaporean students consistently earning the highest scores on the Programme for International Student Assessment (PISA). Blackburn (2016) argued that the nation-state's use of education as an economic development strategy was seeded by the British colonial state, in which examinations and educational credentials were privileged as the drivers of mobility. The British colonial administration had established a stratified educational system in which only the local elite received the most advanced education in the service of the British commercial and administrative interests, according to Blackburn. According to Deng and Gopinathan (2016), the education system that emerged in Singapore in the post-colonial period is centrally planned, meritocratic (based on grades and exam scores), with ability tracking beginning in the primary school. A national system designed to meet the needs of an industrializing economy, there are also extensive post-secondary technical and vocational institutes for those not tracked into elite academic courses. Since 1987 there have been a series of ambitious pedagogical reforms from preschool to higher education to meet the challenges of globalizing economy by de-emphasizing traditional models of pedagogy (i.e., transmission of knowledge and emphasis on grades and exams) and attending to social emotional skills and holistic education. However, because the reforms have not abandoned the sole means of academic advancement through high-stakes testing, focus on high academic performance remains salient.

The tension between fostering an environment for children's psychological wellbeing and facilitating their high academic performance is evident in recent scholarly work about Singaporean parenting. For example, Göransson's (2023) ethnographic fieldwork with Singaporean parents of primary school-aged children suggested that their parenting strategy centered on managing the risk and uncertainty of their children's future. Of note, Singaporean children take the Primary School Leaving Examination (PSLE) at the end of grade 6, and their performance on this exam determines the stream of secondary school they attend ("Express," "Normal (academic)," and "Normal (technical)") and their eventual post-secondary education. Given the extreme high stakes of a single exam at the end of grade 6 that sets the course for Singaporean children, primary school parents expressed heightened anxiety and uncertainty about how much to emphasize or downplay their children's academic achievement. Because primary school children are often too young to be able to manage their academic studies (including additional tutoring and drills outside of school), the parents are convinced that whatever they do will have a direct effect on their children's future.

Bach and Christensen's (2021) ethnographic study in Singapore found similar concerns among parents of preschoolers. The researchers argued that educational reform at the preschool level (toward a child-centered learning through play) has upended the middle-class Singaporean parents' previous parenting strategy of intensive parenting and concerted cultivation. The parents of preschool children narrated their worries about their children's socioemotional skills, sending their children to various extracurricular activities (e.g., chess, football, speech, drama) to increase their confidence, sometimes even sending their children to various forms of therapy and interventions (e.g., anger management) at the suggestion of preschool teachers. And while the government strongly discourages parents of preschoolers from sending their children to supplemental academic enrichment classes and tutors, most parents interviewed for the study acknowledged that they did so because of their concerns about their children's preparedness for the PSLE. Of note, while the parents were as critical as the government of the pervasiveness of private tutoring, each had justified their clandestine engagement in the practice of academic tutors and enrichment classes (yet reluctant to admit this to the researchers and to their preschool teachers). In contemporary Singapore, parenting young children appears to have become mired in a series of contradictory goals and a contest of wills among parents as well as between parents and the policymakers about how to raise children who are prepared for the globalized knowledge economy.

Notably, Singapore as the headquarter sites for various multinational corporations has attracted immigrant families from around Asia. A recent study of highly educated Chinese ex-pat families in Singapore by Yang

(2024) found that the mothers had originally thought they could provide their children with a less stressful, less competitive schooling experience than those in China, and they were also attracted to the bilingual (English and Chinese) educational opportunities. However, the Chinese mothers also soon discovered that as immigrants, their children were largely shut out of the highly ranked primary schools in Singapore because of the priority admissions that local Singaporean children receive. The mothers found themselves engaged in intensive parenting (e.g., shuttling them from one after-school academies and lessons to another) to prepare their young children for a Gifted and Talented program screening that occurred in grade 3. The presence of these academically hyper-competitive Chinese immigrant families appeared to be creating waves of anxiety among local Singaporean parents, who now fear that their children are losing out in academic achievements to the immigrant children.

South Korea and the "English fever"

Following the Korean War, the South Korean economy grew exponentially from the 1960s to 1990s as a result of rapid industrialization, technological advances, and education boom that were driven by aggressive state-sponsored industrial expansion. Under Kim Yongsam's regime (1992–1997), the government embraced a globalization policy (*Segyehwa*) and liberalization of overseas travel, which resulted in English language skills becoming a valued social capital that were seen as increasing Korean competitiveness in the global market. Although English language skills had held a symbolic value in South Korea's modern nation building, the introduction of early English language education in public schools in 1997 contributed to the prioritizing of English mastery among the young students (Shim & Park, 2008).

Although the Korean economy had achieved global status by 1996, the Korean economy was badly damaged by the Asian financial crisis in 1997. Following the IMF bailout, the government embraced a more neoliberal economic policy, with increased emphasis on individual human capital, decreased confidence in Korean public schools, and rising economic anxiety among the citizens sparked by growing social inequality and the IMF crisis in the 1990s and into 2000s, More and more South Korean families began to seek out private, after-school, supplemental education for their children to increase their competitive advantage (Kang & Abelmann, 2011). Of note, the urgency with which South Korean parents sought to have their children gain English language fluency has been dubbed "English fever" (Park, 2009). The private after-school English instruction was increasingly seen as an absolute necessity for children's future economic opportunities, yet it also became exceedingly expensive and unaffordable for many families. For some families, then, pre-college study abroad to English-speaking nations represented a feasible alternative to expensive domestic after-school private education (Park & Abelmann, 2004). In these Korean educational migrant families (dubbed *kirŏgi* or wild geese families because of the long distances members of the families travel seasonally to visit one another), mothers and children often lived in English-speaking countries while the fathers stayed behind in South Korea to work. The cost of maintaining two households plus long-distance travels from Korea to the U.S., Canada, England, Australia, or New Zealand meant that early *kirŏgi* families were of upper-middle class background, with stay-at-home mothers who knew some English and who could devote their time solely to managing their children's education abroad.

As "English fever" reached its fever pitch in the mid-2000s, less affluent Korean parents began to strategize alternate pathways to pre-college study abroad, increasingly turning to non-Western locations with English-language instructions such as Singapore, the Philippines, and Malaysia (Okazaki & Kim, 2018). However, the parenting strategy of less affluent Korean families to engage their children in an early study abroad "on budget" realized that they lacked the necessary social capital for their children to make substantive gains. For example, Kim (2010; 2015) found that the less affluent Korean parents who chose to engage in an early study abroad in Singapore with their children realized too late that the Singaporean public school system was not suitable for immigrant, non-English speaking children. With an academic tracking system starting early in Singaporean primary school and the high-stakes Primary School Leaving Examination, Korean students who were not fluent in English were "demoted" to younger grades, which had a devastating impact on their educational trajectories, with little chance of exiting the vocational track in Singapore or re-entering the competitive Korean system. In another study, Kim and Okazaki (2017) interviewed Korean mothers who had longed to engage in intensive mothering of their children much like their affluent stay-at-home counterparts do by devoting all their time, energy, and resources to manage their children's schooling and extracurricular activities to cultivate their human capital (including diligently collecting information and selecting the optimal time and location for the English-language study opportunities.) However, working full-time and not having access to the stay-at-home mothers' networks, nor having the time to review children's school work, ferry them from one extracurricular lesson to another, and so on, these mothers had found little opportunity to practice these forms of intensive mothering in Korea. The working mother, without much cultural knowledge about managing the early study abroad, often took up the opportunity to go with their children to Singapore, the Philippines, or Malaysia to improve their children's

English skills and for them to fulfill their desire to become more ideal Korean mothers who devotes all their time and energy to her children. Some of the mothers took extended leaves from their jobs to live overseas with their children and manage their daily lives. However, the working mothers also realized that a short-term study abroad in Southeast Asia fell short of their expectations because they lacked the cultural knowledge and the economic capital (e.g., private tutors, tuition for international schools) to translate the experience into social advantages for their children.

While fewer Korean families may be engaging in Early Study Abroad (ESA, or pre-college study abroad), especially to the Western English-speaking countries because of the cost, distance, and the perception of lack of safety, Korean parents continue to seek out alternative ESA opportunities for their children. For example, Koh and Kim's (2024) interviews with Korean mothers who brought their children to Kuala Lumpur for ESA found that their families had performed an internal cost-performance ratio calculations to choose Malaysia. For many, the financial and emotional costs associating with high competition for elite universities in Korea (e.g., well-known after-school academies, high stress and anxiety) led them to choose Malaysia because of its close distance to Korea, high quality of living standards, reputed quality of education, a large number of international schools, slower pace of life, climate, and perceived safety. However, once they arrived in Kuala Lumpur, the Korean mothers quickly discovered that they had underestimated the expenses needed to not only maintain a high standard of living they were accustomed to in Korea but also to cover the tuitions for higher-ranked international schools and for Korean after-school academies for their children. Nevertheless, the mothers believed that they still had made the right decisions for their children, reasoning that their investment in cultivating their children's English skills, their academic credentials, and cosmopolitanism would eventually pay off. In this way, this study echoes the themes of Korean neoliberal self-management and the time and cost-intensive nature of Korean parenthood.

China and gender socialization

As fertility declined rapidly in the past half century, China saw an improvement in gender equality in terms of education and work, both because mothers had less child-rearing burdens with just one child (and therefore could invest more time into her own education and careers) and because singleton daughters without brothers were not disadvantaged in parental allocation of attention, expectation, and resources (Fong et al., 2020). For example, Xu and Yeung's (2013) mixed method study of fathers and their teenaged daughters in Shanghai found that, unlike Confucian ethos that had previously privileged sons, contemporary urban Chinese fathers were highly invested and involved in their daughter's upbringing. Not only did the fathers hold high aspirations for their daughters' education and often took hands-on approaches to their parenting (e.g., coaching them academically, staying up late to accompany them in their studies), the fathers and daughters enjoyed emotional closeness, and the fathers valued communicating with and providing emotional support to their daughters.

While the shift to market economy and one-child policy may have expanded economic opportunities for Chinese girls and women and the involvement of fathers, these new expectations for girls and women emphasize independence, power, and higher status that have traditionally been understood as masculinity norms. Western norms of masculinity, which favor autonomy over relationships and emotional and physical toughness over vulnerability (Way et al, 2014), contrast with Chinese norms of masculinity in which men express their dominance using social prestige and emotional and physical control rather than through physical strength and aggression (Louie, 2015). Way et al. (2018) argue that changing economic and social contexts has increased adherence to Western masculinity norms not just in the U.S. but also in China, despite robust evidence connecting adherence to masculinity norms with poorer socioemotional wellbeing (Gupta et al., 2013, Way et al., 2014, Way et al., 2018 Way, 2024). In fact, there has been a concerted effort by the Chinese government and the media to promote Western masculinity norms of toughness and to criticize men and boys who display feminine qualities (e.g., Song, 2022).

These tensions between autonomy that is associated with Western conceptions of masculinity and relational connection that is associated with Western views of femininity have impacted Chinese parenting in complex ways. For example, Yang, Waters, et al. (2024) examined in a nine-year longitudinal study of Urban Chinese families whether self-reported parental gender beliefs and observed maternal sensitivity at 14 and 24 months of their children's lives could predict the children's self-reported adherence to masculinity norms at age ten. They found that maternal sensitivity to their infants was associated with decreased adherence to Western masculinity norms nine years later for boys only. That is, sensitive parenting in the early years appeared to help Chinese boys resist adhering to norms of stereotypical masculinity (i.e., valuing independence over relationships, stoicism over vulnerability) in their middle childhood. Another study showed that maternal sensitivity at 14 and 24 months was associated with the adolescents' friendship quality at 15 years of age (Yang, Gu, et al., 2024). These findings suggest that despite the pressures of economic development to privilege competition and emotional toughness in contemporary China, emotionally attuned early parenting help their children resist attitudes and behaviors that have been proven to have a negative impact on their social and psychological wellbeing.

Case Study: Parenting in Nanjing, China

To illustrate the influence of a changing social context on parenting practice, a qualitative case study conducted in Nanjing, China is presented here. We contrast the parenting narratives from the two cohorts of Chinese families (the infant cohort and the adolescent cohort) from our mixed-method longitudinal study from Nanjing, China that started in 2006 with over 1,100 families that included both a cohort of parents whose children were born in 2006 and a cohort of parents whose children were born in 1994. Specifically, we compare the narratives of parents of the infant cohort at the ten-year follow-up when the children were around ten to 11 years old in 2016 with the previously published parenting narratives of the adolescent cohort when the children were in grade 7 (mean age = 12.3) in 2006 (Way et al., 2013), focusing on the ways in which the two cohorts of parents' attitudes, expectations, and experiences changed and stayed the same across time. The significance of the twelve-year period from 1994 and 2006 lies in the dramatic changes in Nanjing, China during that period as it moved toward a market economy from a planned economy. An example of such changes is that in 1994 Nanjing had only a very small local airport, few cars and many bicycles and busses, and an old dilapidated train station in which it took up to seven or eight hours to travel to Shanghai from Nanjing; by 2006, it had an international airport that flew directly not only to major cities in Asia but around the world, the streets were jammed with cars, and the train station had been rebuilt to a very large and elegant train station serving many cities and taking only around three hours to travel to Shanghai. The city in other words had become its expansion into the global world with a growing market economy and a decreasing number of parents who worked for the state. Given such differences in the social and economic context between 1994 and 2006 in Nanjing, we expected that there would be similarities given that both cohorts were raising children in an increasingly modern society that was moving toward a market economy with its neoliberal ideology. We also, however, expected differences in the perspectives and attitudes of the parents given that they were raising their children in very different periods of growth and development.

The adolescent cohort consisted of 710 families with grade 7 children (age 12) who were drawn from three different schools in Nanjing. For the purpose of the 2013 study, the mothers' narratives from 24 out of 60 families from the adolescent cohort were randomly selected and mothers' interview data were analyzed (Way et al., 2013). The infant cohort consisted of 381 families whose first-born child were born in 2006 and enrolled in the study with the first parent interviews. The infant cohort interviews were drawn from the ten-year follow-up with 80 families, from which randomly selected 32 parents (16 boys, 16 girls). Interviews with both fathers and mothers were available for this sample and analyzed using thematic coding.

Similarities across cohorts

In the adolescent cohort who were born in 1994, most Chinese mothers suggested in their semi-structured interviews conducted in Mandarin that they wanted their children to be socially skilled, happy, healthy, independent, and to attain good grades. Mothers placed equal or even, at times, a greater emphasis on emotional and social goals than on academic attainment (Way et al., 2013). Mothers also often expressed anxiety about their children not having social skills given that their children were only children and those who could afford it spent a considerable amount of money investing in special programs to help develop their children's social skills. The focus on happiness was also evident in the questions that members of the research team were asked by college students at one of the universities where we gave presentations about our research. Questions included, for example, "Are you happy at what you do as our professor told us that we should be happy at what we do?" Similarly, parents in the infant cohort expressed high expectations for their children to be sociable and friendly yet also independent in a way that they are emotionally self-sufficient.

Happiness

Parents of both cohorts placed a strong emphasis on happiness. Parents from both cohorts repeatedly suggested in their interviews that their children do not need to be at the top of the social hierarchy to be happy, and the parents asserted that they do not necessarily associate "happiness" with "success." For example, in the adolescent cohort, when asked about her future expectations of her daughter, one mother said:

> I don't worry a lot about her studies. I think humans should be happy. I hope that she will be happy. She can grow up happily and be healthy. Regarding her studies, as long as she can keep up, that's enough. I don't have very high requirements for her.
>
> *(Way et al., 2013, p. 65)*

Similarly, when asked about her expectations of her daughter, a mother from the infant cohort responded:

> But we are just an ordinary family. I don't want her to try too hard to reach a higher social status. It might be a lot of effort for her to reach

> somewhere that others easily reach. I don't want her to be too tired. Life should be happy as life is just a few dozen years. And she's a girl, she doesn't need to try as hard as boys.

Also, parents in both studies appeared to be aware of the distinction between a "successful" life and a "happy" life, which was mainly reflected in their attitudes towards their children's academic performance. In the adolescent cohort, one mother mentioned that:

> I believe all parents want their children to go to college, but if you cannot, you have to face reality. To go to college is not the only way. To be healthy physically and mentally is more important. You can be accomplished in other ways...
>
> *(Way et al., 2013. p. 65)*

Similar sentiments were found in the infant cohort parents. For example, one mother spoke of trying to balance her own expectations with her daughter's well-being:

> In the future, you want her to be good, but you don't want her to try too hard or be tired. This is a very controversial thing. I really hope that she goes to a great school and that she can self-learn very well. But then I think about it, whether she has talents in it. If she manages to study well it would be best, but if she's not made for it, it would be painful for me to force her to.

Overall, parents in both studies view socioemotional well-being as one of the most important goals of parenting. They also reported being aware of the potential pressure and stress associated with high expectations for academic success, and both cohorts discussed trying their best to foster happy and healthy children despite the increasing social competition in a rapidly developing economy.

Autonomy

Another theme evident in both cohorts of parents was to raise an autonomous child. In the adolescent cohort, parents tried to foster their children's autonomy by encouraging them to make decisions, be assertive, and think for themselves (Way et al., 2013). For example, in raising a decisive and assertive son, a mother in the adolescent cohort said:

> He has to make the decision himself. I said, "It is your own life, you make the decision and finish it yourself." One day there was an issue

> and he called me. I said, "Actually you can solve it yourself. Why did you have to call mom?" I even said, "You called me and I cannot be there in a second. Couldn't you solve the problem yourself?
>
> *(Way et al., 2013, p. 66)*

Parallel to the sentiment above, a mother in the infant cohort expressed her expectations of her son being independent and self-reliant:

> It's that you don't want him to have too rich a life. Boys should fight for themselves (for good lives) in the future. If you give everything to him now, he would think that I don't have to fight for a better life in the future. You have to tell him, that as a boy you need to fight and you need to have a sense of responsibility.

For both cohorts of parents, being independent and being individually responsible for one's action were both important developmental goals, reflecting once again the effects on parenting of the movement toward a market economy. Parents also evaluated themselves regarding the capability to foster an autonomous child, which they saw as necessary for happiness and success. Mothers, for example, emphasized the importance of "not forcing" a child to do something and for allowing enough autonomy for their children to freely explore without imparting the parents' expectations on them to such a degree that it restricted their freedom. For example, a mother of a girl from the adolescent cohort suggested:

> You cannot try to control her and tell her that she was not allowed to read [a nonacademic book] at all. Of course, even if you do not allow it, she would still do it anyway, but you will have no way to deal with her. Nowadays kids are just like that. I said, "If you really, really want it, I will buy it for you."
>
> *(Way et al., 2013., p. 67)*

Similarly, in the infant cohort, a mother criticized herself for being over-protective about her daughter, which she thought could potentially constrain her daughter's freedom to try new things and to make her own decisions:

> I, as a mother, think I take care of her too much, do too many things for her, and let go too little when I reflect on myself (as a mother). I am very close to being attentive to every detail for her. Anyway, it's that I am very careful, I am very careful in doing anything and I am timid. So I may unconsciously make my daughter lose a lot of opportunities. Because for

> mothering, when I predict that there might be problems or danger, I'd rather not let it happen. Sometimes, I invisibly deprive my daughter of many attempts she could have made.

Overall, raising children who could think for themselves was an important parenting goal across both cohorts as China moved toward a capitalist economy that is premised on the idea that an autonomous self is the only way to be successful.

Social Skills

In both cohorts of parents, being sociable or having social skills and being friendly was an important goal for their children, although many considered such skills from a utilitarian perspective reflective of the Chinese concept of "guanxi" which refers to have the social skills necessary for future career opportunities. In other words, they wanted their children to have friendships for their social and emotional well-being but also maintained their belief in "guanxi" for building future opportunities as well. In the infant cohort, for example, a father suggests that for his son:

> Firstly, making friends can determine, whether he's able to blend in the society quickly and assimilate into the community. How to interact with people. Secondly, the kinds of friends that he makes would be very influential to his development.

This collectivistic notion of "assimilating into the community" reflects the ways both old ways and new ways of thinking intersect as the values of societies change over time. A mother in the adolescent sample expressed her concerns about her son in this way:

> When hanging out with people, he is not actively engaged. If you are someone that he likes or if you have a common language with him, he might be willing to talk, but a stranger, he is not good at dealing with them . . . I think in this society, you have to learn how to communicate with people. You have to get help from other people sometimes, right? . . . Because if you communicate well with people, they will help you. . . . Interpersonal communication is very important. . . It is something that you cannot survive without in your life.
>
> *(Way et al., 2013, p. 64)*

Parents in both cohorts, however, did not, put social skills in opposition to autonomy, believing that both were compatible with the other. As a father from the infant cohort suggested, with regard to his expectations of his daughter:

> In her friendship, I think she has her judgment and we have to respect that. She can be friends with whoever she wants, and that's okay. Of course, we would try to learn about what kind of friends she has because her mother would be more concerned about these. But what do I think? These are all her life experiences. It's impossible that you only make good friends. What if there are other situations in the future? There will always be times when she falls. But when it comes to such situations, it depends on her to see how to deal with it.

While emphasizing the importance of social relationships, the father also tried to give his daughter the freedom to learn how to navigate difficult interpersonal relationships on her own, which aligned with the parenting goal of autonomy.

Differences across cohorts

While parents' pursuit of children's autonomy, happiness, and social skills remained similar across the decade, parents in the infant cohort appeared to have a more confident approach to balancing what appeared to them to be competing parenting goals. In the adolescent cohort, parents were frustrated with having little control over their children as they were uncertain about their parenting practices, and they chose to parent in a permissive style that they believed would lead to happier children and less conflict. For example, a mother in the adolescent cohort discussed struggling with a son who had become difficult:

> I just feel that since this semester, he has become increasingly hard to control. He is not like what he was in the past. ... Now he has his own thoughts. You cannot control him. If you want to ask him to do something, you cannot be too demanding.
>
> *(Way et al., 2013, p. 67)*

Parents in the adolescent cohort expressed less confidence about how to raise a happy child, resulting in modulating their own expectations because they felt that disciplining their children would lead to conflict, unhappiness, and potential mental health issues in their children.

In contrast, while the parents in the infant cohort also acknowledged parenting challenges, their frustration did not come from lacking control of their children. Many parents expressed frustration that they were not able to fully live up to their parenting responsibilities, such as having enough time to spend with their children, patience, and emotional control. They expressed a growing awareness of what was considered to be best practices for raising happy and healthy children but also felt that they sometimes fell short. These types of reflections are typical of parents in a capitalist economy who often work too much not only of putting food on the table but to simply gain more wealth and who thus end up often feeling bad that they do not spend enough time with their children. Parents in the infant cohort who were from wealthier communities than the parents in the adolescent cohort often spoke of hoping to spend more quality time with their children, typical of a "Western way" of parenting in a capitalist economy in which the wealthy can afford to do so. For example, a father from the infant cohort stated:

> I would be bold to say that I am a good son, a good son-in-law, and a good father. At least, broadly speaking, I did everything according to what's considered a good father in China. But if you follow Western ideologies, I am not a good father. I don't spend time with my daughter every day. That's where the difference is.

A mother from the infant cohort also provided an empathetic insight into her interaction with her son:

> I think I have a bad temper, sometimes I feel sorry when I blame him. I always compared him with other kids, but he never compared me with other moms. He said no bad words to me, but I always say things about him like 'You are not well-behaved, I told you to do this but you wouldn't.' I always see his weaknesses, but it seems that from his perspective I am perfect.

The differences in the two cohorts likely reflects not only the changing context with the infant cohort more shaped by Western capitalist ideology than the adolescent cohort given that they were raising their children in a city that was significantly more global. It also reflects the difference in economic means of the two cohorts with the wealthier cohort (the infant cohort) having more options to accommodate to the norms of wealthy Westerners than did the lower-income families that were typical in the adolescent cohort.

Summary

Overall, by comparing the parenting narratives of two cohorts of Chinese parents of preadolescent children, ten years apart, who were striving to raise their children and navigating the dilemma of happiness and success in a changing society, this case study illustrates how the rapidly changing economic and social context even within a short period make a difference in how the parents reflected on their own parenting practices and the understanding of developmental goals and their role in promoting them. However, there were also many similarities in both cohorts. These similarities were likely reflective of the fact that both cohorts in 2006 or 2016 (the year of data collection for the adolescent cohort or the ten-year follow-up for the infant cohort respectively) were experiencing the dramatic growth of a market economy that privileges individual happiness and autonomy over the common good or interdependence. Such changes appeared to be having similar effects on parenting with their focus on their children's happiness and independence. Balancing the two aspects of parenting goals—both autonomy and connectedness—presented a dilemma to the parents in both cohorts. However, their response to such challenges differed, with the parents from the adolescent cohort feeling unsure whether to privilege their children's feelings over parental authority and the parents from the infant cohort diminishing their authority to accommodate to the emotional needs to their children.

Future Directions

Future directions include examining how, in the case of China, the movement back to a more planned economy and a movement away from a capitalist economy will once again change parenting practices with a growing emphasis perhaps on "guanxi" and a decreased emphasis on happiness and autonomy. With the change in policy from a one-child policy to a two and now a three-child policy, the question is how these policy changes will shape not only how many children parents have but also how they raise their children. If a growing number of families choose to have one child even though they could theoretically have three, will the focus on individual happiness and autonomy continue to dominate their parenting as they focus on the success of only one child? Finally, will the parents who were one child themselves raise their children significantly differently than if the parents themselves were not the only child? We have yet to know how much the one-child policy shaped our findings as both cohorts raised their children within a one-child context.

Regarding other Asian contexts, there are many questions that have yet to be asked. For example, globalized economies have precipitated many parents (mothers and fathers) from the Philippines, China, Sri Lanka, and other Asian nations to work overseas for long stretches of time, leaving their children behind to be cared for by one parent or relatives (e.g., Parrenas, 2001, 2008). It is unclear what the consequences are of such long-distance parenting for parent–child relationships and child development. While such long-distance parenting is often portrayed in a negative light through a purely Western perspective, it may be that such parenting allows for more economic opportunities for their children in their futures. Understanding the influence of economic, social, and political changes on the values, attitudes, and practices of parents in Asian contexts and the impact of such changes on their children is not only critical to better understanding Asian families but more importantly, it allows us to understand how such parents adapt to their contexts in ways that promote their children's abilities to thrive let alone survive.

Implications for Practice and Policy

Because contemporary Asia comprises of a wide-ranging pace and forms of economic development and social change, it is not possible to recommend specific practices and policy implications. However, even in our selective review of parenting in the context of societal change in China, South Korea, and Singapore, it is clear that rapid globalization and economic development in the past half century has brought about considerable uncertainty and anxiety among parents in Asia. Of course, parenting worries and anxieties is not specific to Asia, as modern parenting call for cultivating a hegemonic ideal of an autonomous yet interpersonally skilled, cosmopolitan self that seemingly require intensive parenting. Practitioners who work with parents from various Asian locales must be mindful of the pervasive and global push for the neoliberal selfhood while appreciating the particular societal and economic context of each Asian nation. There is no singular form of Asian parenting, but it is also critical that we appreciate the genuine desire of parents from Asia to equip their children with attributes for future thriving that they glean from their particular societal context that are constantly and rapidly changing.

References

Bach, D. & Christensen, S. (2021). Middle-class cultivation out of tune? Challenges to intensive parenting in Singapore. *British Journal of Sociology of Education, 42*(4), 475–489.

Beeson, M. & Islam, I. (2005). Neo-liberalism and East Asia: resisting the Washington consensus. *The Journal of Development Studies, 41*(2), 197–219.

Blackburn, K. (2016). *Education, industrialization and the end of empire in Singapore*. New York: Routledge.

Bronfenbrenner, U. & Morris, P. A. (2006). *The bioecological model of human development. In W. Damon (Series Ed.) & R. M. Lerner (Vol. Ed.), Handbook of child psychology: Theoretical models of human development* (pp. 793–828). New York: Wiley.

Cai, Y., & Feng, W. (2021). The social and sociological consequences of China's one-child policy. *Annual Review of Sociology, 47*(1), 587-606.

Chen, X., Christmas-Best, V., Titzmann, P. F., & Weichold, K. (Eds). (2012). *Youth Success and Adaptation in Times of Globalization and Economic Change: New Directions for Youth Development, Number 135* (Vol. 121). John Wiley & Sons.

Deng, Z., & Gopinathan, S. (2016). PISA and high-performing education systems: Explaining Singapore's education success. *Comparative Education, 52*(4), 449–472.

Fong, V. L., Yu, D., & Zhu, Y. (2020). One Child and More. In *Routledge Handbook of Chinese Culture and Society* (pp. 248–259). Routledge.

Foucault, M. (2008). *The birth of biopolitics: Lectures at the Collège de France, 1978–1979*. (G. Burshell, Trans.). New York: Springer.
Ganti, T. (2014). Neoliberalism. *Annual Review of Anthropology, 43*, 89–104.
Göransson, K. (2023). 'The big crossroad': Parenting, risk and educational transitions in Singapore. *Global Studies of Childhood*, 20436106231201175.
Greenfield, P. M. (2009). Linking social change and developmental change: Shifting pathways of human development. *Developmental Psychology*, 45, 401–418.
Guthrie, D. (2012). *China and globalization: The social, economic and political transformation of Chinese society*. New York: Routledge.
Hays, S. (1996). *The cultural contradictions of motherhood*. Yale University Press.
Kang, J. & Abelmann, N. (2011). The domestication of South Korean pre-college study abroad in the first decade of the millennium. *Journal of Korean Studies, 16*(1), 89–118.
Kim, J. (2010). 'Downed' and stuck in Singapore: Lower/middle class South Korean wild geese (kirogi) children in Singapore. In E. Hannum, H. Park, & Y.G. Butler (Eds.) *Globalization, Changing Demographics, and Educational Challenges in East Asia* (pp. 271–311). Bingley, U.K.: Emerald Group Publishing Limited.
Kim, J. (2015). The "other half" goes abroad: The perils of public schooling in Singapore. In A. Lo, S. Kwon, N. Abelmann, & S. Okazaki (Eds.) *South Korea's Education Exodus: The Life and Times of Study Abroad* (pp. 103–122), Seattle, WA: University of Washington Press.
Kim, J. & Okazaki, S. (2017). Short-term intensive mothering on a budget: Working mothers of Korean children studying abroad in Southeast Asia. *Asian Women, 33*(3), 111–139.
Koh, S. Y. & Kim, T. S. (May, 2024). *Ga-Seong-Bi (cost-performance ratio): South Korean families' speculative educational migration to Kuala Lumpur*. [Paper presentation] 1st International Workshop on Global Korea/Asia Pacific, Transnational Koreans/Asians. Seogwipo, South Korea.
Kyung-Sup C. (2010). The second modern condition? Compressed modernity as internalized reflexive cosmopolitization. *British Journal of Sociology*, 61, 444–464.
Lareau, A. (2003). *Unequal childhoods: Class, race, and family life*. Berkeley, CA: University of California Press.
Louie, K. (2015). *Chinese masculinities in a globalizing world*. New York: Routledge.
Matsuoka, R. (2019). Concerted cultivation developed in a standardized education system. *Social Science Research, 77l,* 161–178.
Minnotte, K. L. (2023). Decentering intensive mothering: More fully accounting for race and class in motherhood norms. *Sociology Compass, 17*(8), e13095.
Okazaki, S. & Kim, J. (2018). Going the distance: Transnational educational migrant families in Korea. In M. R. T. de Guzman, J. Brown, & C. P. Edwards (Eds) *Parenting from afar: The reconfiguration of the family across distance*, (pp. 321–338). New York: Oxford University Press.
Ozawa, T. (1994). Exploring the Asian economic miracle: Politics, economics, society, culture, and history—A review article. *The Journal of Asian Studies, 53*(1), 124–131.
Park, J. K. (2009). "English fever" in South Korea: Its history and symptoms. *English Today, 25*(1), 50–57.
Park, S. J. & Abelmann, N. (2004). Class and cosmopolitan striving: Mothers' management of English education in South Korea. *Anthropological Quarterly, 77*(4), 645–672.
Parreñas, R. S. (2001). Mothering from a distance: Emotions, gender, and intergenerational relations in Filipino transnational families. *Feminist studies, 27*(2), 361–390.

Parreñas, R. S. (2008). Transnational fathering: Gendered conflicts, distant disciplining and emotional gaps. *Journal of ethnic and migration studies, 34*(7), 1057–1072.

Raymo, J. M., Park, H., Xie, Y., & Yeung, W. J. J. (2015). Marriage and family in East Asia: Continuity and change. *Annual review of sociology, 41*, 471–492.

Shim, D. & Park, J. S.-Y. (2008). The language politics of "English fever" in South Korea. *Korea Journal, 48*(2), 136–159.

Silbereisen, R. K., & Chen, X. (Eds.) (2010). *Social change and human development: Concept and results*. Thousand Oaks, CA: Sage.

Song, G. (2022). "Little fresh meat": The politics of sissiness and sissyphobia in contemporary China. *Men and Masculinities, 25*(1), 68–86.

Song, J. (2009). *South Koreans in the debt crisis: The creation of a neoliberal welfare society*. Duke University Press.

Thornton, A. (2005). *Reading history sideways: The fallacy and enduring impact of the developmental paradigm on family life.* Chicago, IL: University of Chicago Press.

Thornton, A., Dorius, S. F., & Swindle, J. (2015). Developmental idealism: The cultural foundations of world development programs. *Sociology of Development, 1*(2), 277–320.

Way, N. (2024). *Rebels with a cause: Reimagining boys, ourselves, and our culture.* Dutton Press.

Way, N., Cressen, J., Bodian, S., Preston, J., Nelson, J., & Hughes, D. (2014). "It might be nice to be a girl... Then you wouldn't have to be emotionless": Boys' resistance to norms of masculinity during adolescence. *Psychology of Men & Masculinity, 15*(3), 241–251.

Way, N., Gilligan, C., Noguera, P., & Ali, Al. (2018). Introduction: The crisis of connection. In N. Way, A. Ali, C. Gilligan, & P. Noguera (Eds). *The crisis of connection: Its roots, consequences, and solutions* (pp. 1–79). New York: New York University Press.

Way, N., Okazaki, S., Zhao, J., Kim, J. J., Chen, X., Yoshikawa, H., ... & Deng, H. (2013). Social and emotional parenting: mothering in a changing Chinese society. *Asian American Journal of Psychology, 4*(1), 61–70.

World Bank (1993). *The East Asian Miracle: Economic Growth and Public Policy*, New York: Oxford University Press.

Xu, Q. & Yeung, W. J. J. (2013). Hoping for a phoenix: Shanghai fathers and their daughters. *Journal of Family Issues, 34*(2), 182–207.

Yang, P. (May, 2024). *Insecurity and migrant parenting: A study of middle-class Chinese immigrants in Singapore.* [Paper Presentation] 1st International Workshop on Global Korea/Asia Pacific, Transnational Koreans/Asians. Seogwipo, South Korea.

Yang, R., Gu, Y., Cui, L., Li, X., Way, N., Yoshikawa, H., Chen, X., Okazaki, S., Zhang, G., Liang, Z., & Waters, T. E. (2024). A cognitive script perspective on how early caregiving experiences inform adolescent peer relationships and loneliness: A 14-year longitudinal study of Chinese families. *Developmental Science*, e13522.

Yang, R., Waters, T. E., Gu, Y., Way, N., Yoshikawa, H., Chen, X., Zhang, G., & Deng, H. (2024). Developmental antecedents of adherence to masculinity norms: A 9-year longitudinal study of urban Chinese families. *Developmental Psychology*.

Yoshikawa, H., Way, N., & Chen, X. (2012). Large-scale economic change and youth development: the case of urban China. *New Directions for Youth Development, 135,* 39–55.

6

CARE-BASED POWER-ASSERTIVE PARENTING IN CHANGING ASIAN SOCIETIES

Xinyin Chen, Jiaxi Zhou, Dan Li, Yan Li, Min Wu, and Jingyao Wang

Research findings and observations indicate that, relative to parents with a Western European background, Asian parents tend to use more adult-centered, forceful, and restrictive strategies in parenting (e.g., "I do not allow my child to question any decisions I make.") to push their children to obtain school and social achievements. This parenting style appears to fit into Baumrind's authoritarian category, which is described as parental use of coercion and emphasis on child obedience in childrearing (Baumrind, 1971). However, the high-power parenting style that Asian parents use is believed to be accompanied by parental concern, care, and high expectations of the child (Chao, 1995), making it different from authoritarian parenting that is often expressed as negative affect and unresponsiveness. Researchers have attempted to understand the distinguishing features of Asian parenting and its role in child development from different perspectives (e.g., Juang et al., 2013; Ho, 1986). Despite the efforts, the meaning and implications of Asian parenting remain largely unclear, perhaps owing to the involvement of multiple social, cultural, and educational factors, such as the traditional belief of filial piety, group-oriented values, social change, and educational practices.

Based on the literature (e.g., Chao, 1994; Cheah et al., 2019; Chen et al., 2019; Tobin et al., 1989), Chen (2023) proposes a perspective focusing on care-based power-assertive parenting (CBPAP) in Asian cultures, which refers to the expression of parental care in power-assertive behavior or parental use of power assertion with care in interactions with children. In this chapter, we first discuss the cultural background and research on Asian parenting. Then, we elaborate on the notion of CBPAP, especially

DOI: 10.4324/9781003383949-6

in terms of how it serves socialization goals in Asian societies. Next, we report two studies in China about the development of CBPAP measures and the results. In addition, we discuss the role of social change in shaping the display and functional meaning of parenting in Asian societies.

It should be noted that although Asians consist of diverse groups, such as Chinese, Koreans, Indians, and Indonesians, the issue of Asian parenting is mostly concerned with socialization beliefs and practices among families with an East Asian cultural background that is predominantly influenced by Confucianism. We focus on the parenting of East Asian, particularly Chinese, parents in this chapter. In addition, the issue has recently received much attention, due to the findings of differences in parenting between Asian and other ethnic groups in North America. Given its cultural origins, it is necessary to discuss Asian parenting from a broad perspective to achieve an in-depth understanding of its nature and significance. Thus, we include a review of the relevant literature and research on parenting of Asian parents in Western and Asian nations.

Cultural Background and Parenting in East Asian Societies

Cultural beliefs and values concerning interpersonal relationships and the organization of the family inevitably play an important role in shaping parenting and its relations with child development (Bornstein 2012; Chen et al., 2019). As an ideological guideline for social activities in East Asian societies, Confucianism emphasizes maintaining social harmony and achieving group wellbeing through establishing social standards and rules. According to Confucian principles, a primary goal of family functioning, including parenting and child education, is to socialize children to learn behaviors and qualities that are conducive to enhancing the social status and welfare of the family. To achieve this goal, the doctrine of filial piety requires children to pledge obedience and reverence to their parents and parents to ensure that children learn socially appropriate behaviors and acquire achievement, as indicated in the famous Three Character Classic "The father (parent) is guilty if the son (child) is not taught." As a result, parents are encouraged to maintain constant pressure on their children to improve their performance and to use power-assertive parenting to facilitate the socialization process (Ho, 1986).

Confucian principles concerning individual behaviors and relationships have had a pervasive influence on family functioning and socialization in many East Asian societies. Most of these societies have undergone substantial changes in the last century that have weakened the influence of traditional values. However, it has been argued that the core of the traditional Asian cultural system may still be reflected in parenting goals, attitudes, and practices in contemporary Asian societies (Chen, 2023).

Researchers have found that parents in East Asian societies tend to display a high level of involvement in children's activities through behavioral control (e.g., direct guiding and monitoring the child's behaviors), psychological control (e.g., comparing the child with others and invoking feelings of shame, guilt, and anxiety), or both (Cheah, et al., 2015). By observing mother-infant interactions in the home setting, for example, Bornstein et al. (2012) found that, whereas European American mothers were more likely than their infants to display responses to social initiations, perhaps in an attempt to foster child independence, Japanese American mothers were more likely than infants to lead and direct interactions. Jose et al. (2000) found that Chinese American parents were more likely than European American parents to make the decisions and tell children to follow without question. Lamborn et al. (2013) noticed that during interviews, Hmong American adolescents frequently talked about their mothers' assertions of authority such as supervision (e.g., "She keeps track of us . . . I have a cell phone, so I either call her and tell her where I'm at, or I'm safe and stuff. Or either she'll call me and ask me where am I, or what am I doing, am I safe and all this stuff." p. 54). Continual and persistent monitoring and direction by parents are particularly evident in learning activities. Ng et al. (2007) found that Chinese parents used more explicit direction to guide children on learning tasks than American parents. Specifically, Chinese parents tended to focus on children's errors during performance, emphasize failure more than success, and structure children's time and learning processes. Similar results were found by other researchers (e.g., Huntsinger et al., 2009).

Authoritarian Parenting and Its Relations with Adjustment Outcomes in Asian Children

There is no doubt that substantial subgroup and individual differences exist among Asian parents, just like parents with other cultural and ethnic backgrounds. It is inappropriate or incorrect to categorize Asian parents as authoritarian in general (Way et al., 2013). Nevertheless, given the traditional cultural endorsement of parental authority in using high control and power assertion in Asian societies, it is not surprising that Asian parents are higher than European American parents on measures of authoritarian parenting style since high control is a major characteristic of this parenting style.

Dornbusch et al. (1987) conducted the first study that systematically examined ethnic differences in authoritarian parenting styles. The researchers collected self-report data on parenting from a large, diverse sample of high school students in the San Francisco Bay Area. Authoritarian parenting was measured using items concerning demanding and unsupportive behaviors (e.g., parents tell youth that parents should not be questioned; show negative emotions in response to youth's poor school performance; use punitive strategies such as reducing youth's allowance or restricting youth's activities). The results showed that Asian American adolescents reported significantly higher levels of authoritarian parenting than European American adolescents. Camras et al. (2012) and Shen et al. (2018) also found that Chinese American middle school students and college students reported more authoritarian parenting (e.g., "My parents use threats as punishment with little or no justification.") than their European American counterparts.

Similar results were found based on parental reports (e.g., Chao, 1994; Su & Hynie, 2011). For example, Chao (1994) found that Chinese American mothers reported a higher level of authoritarian parenting than European American mothers. Wu et al. (2002) found that Chinese mothers had higher scores than European mothers on authoritarian style. The results are consistent with the findings from observations. Chen et al. (2000) found in a Chinese sample that more authoritarian parents used more high-power coercive strategies and fewer equalitarian and inductive strategies such as information exchanges, suggestions, and explanations in their interactions with children.

Despite the group differences on the mean level of authoritarian parenting, research has shown that authoritarian parenting is similarly associated with social, behavioral, academic, and psychological problems in Asian and Western children. In Dornbusch et al.'s study (1987), although Asian American adolescents reported a higher level of authoritarian parenting than European American adolescents, authoritarian parenting was negatively associated with school achievement in both groups. Lee and colleagues (2014) conducted a study concerning neighborhood characteristics, parenting, and behavioral problems in Chinese American families. The results showed that neighborhood Asian concentration (i.e., percentage of residents of Asian descent) was positively associated with authoritarian parenting as reported by parents, which, in turn, was positively associated with parent-rated externalizing and internalizing problems in children. Similar results concerning the positive links between authoritarian parenting and children's behavioral problems have been found in other studies with Asian families in the United States, Europe, and Asia (e.g., Chen et al., 1997; Chen et al., 2000; Kho et al., 2019; Nguyen, 2008). Authoritarian parenting was also associated with children's incompetence in social and cognitive domains (e.g., peer rejection, low self-control) in Asian and non-Asian children (e.g., Pinquart & Kauser, 2018; Shen et al., 2018).

An interesting issue concerning Asian parenting is the so-called "paradox" of the relatively more authoritarian parenting of Asian parents and the higher school achievement of Asian children (compared with their European American counterparts at the group level) (e.g., Chao & Sue, 1996; Dornbusch et al., 1987). The relatively high level of authoritarian parenting and its association with children's incompetence and problems seem to suggest that, as an outcome of this parenting style, Asian children would generally display lower competence and more school and behavioral problems than European American children, which is inconsistent with research findings (e.g., Chao, 2001; Chen & Tse, 2008; Dornbusch et al., 1987; Mullis et al., 2008). Researchers have argued that other factors, such as positive peer influence, may compensate for the negative effects of authoritarian parenting on Asian children's performance (Steinberg et al., 1992). Given the literature on the crucial role of parents in socialization in Asian societies (Ho, 1986), however, it is necessary to explore the meaning of Asian parenting from different perspectives.

Explorations of Asian Parenting

Researchers have argued that traditional Asian parenting is characterized by a mixture of high involvement, directiveness, discipline, concern, and care (e.g., Chao, 1995; Chen et al., 2019; Ho, 1986; Huang & Gove, 2015; Stewart et al., 2002). This argument can be illustrated in Chao's (1994) notion of *chiao shun* (training) or *guan*. According to Chao, *chiao shun* and *guan* have positive connotations because they imply training, care, love, and governing. Chao's view of Asian parenting is important as it indicates that the Western models may not adequately capture potential features of Asian parenting. Nevertheless, ideas suggested in the literature, including those of Chao (1994), about Asian parenting are generally vague and need to be clarified in order to achieve an in-depth understanding of Asian parenting and to conduct further research on its role in child development.

For example, the meanings of *chiao shun* and *guan* that Chao (1994) used are ambiguous. The Chinese phrase of *chiao shun* means educating/teaching (*chiao*) and training/disciplining (*shun*). This term, similar to "education" and "training," may allude to broad aspects of parental attempt to help children in socialization, but it does not specifically indicate what the aspects are. The word *guan* means "looking after" or "taking care of" (or "governing" as pointed out by Tobin et al., 1989), largely focusing on managing, controlling, and involvement. Indeed, whereas the meaning of *guan* in Chinese is complex, it is often used in daily life to refer to monitoring and control over individuals, especially those who display problem behaviors.

The conceptual ambiguity of the terms may contribute to the difficulty in delineating and examining what constitutes Asian parenting and how the components are connected with each other and work together in child development. The issue may be more evidently shown in the measures of *chiao shun* or *guan* that Chao (1994) and others used. The items in Chao's measure tap many parental beliefs and behaviors, such as "Parents must begin training child as soon as ready," "When child continues to disobey you, he/she deserves a spanking," and "Child should be allowed to sleep in mother's bed." Based on Chao's work, Stewart and colleagues (Stewart et al., 1998, 2002) developed a similar child-report measure of training or *guan,* which included items such as "My parents used physical punishment when I misbehaved," "My parents helped me with my studies as much as his/her education allowed," and "Emphasize neatness and organization." These items, drawn from different sources of literature, cover various aspects of childrearing in Asian cultures, such as the nature of the child as inherently good, exposing the child to the adult world, early training, and using examples of other children (Chao, 1994; Chen-Bouck et al., 2019; Gao et al., 2015; Stewart et al., 1998).

Whereas the items in the existing measures may assess some features of parental childrearing attitudes and practices in Asian societies, they do not appear to reflect a coherent parenting construct. For example, it is unclear how allowing a child to sleep in parents' bed is related to emphasizing the importance of hard work or early training. The lack of conceptual clarity is also indicated by low internal consistency and blurry factor structure of the measures and unexpected research results (Chen-Bouck et al., 2019; Gao et al., 2015; Stewart et al., 1998). Chao (1994) did not provide information on the psychometric features of the *guan* or training measure, although internal consistencies (Cronbach's alphas) of other measures in the study were presented. In Stewart et al.'s studies (1998, 2002), items that were regarded as important in reflecting *guan* (e.g., "My parent used physical punishment when I misbehaved," "My parent pointed out good behaviors in others as a model for me.") were deleted in calculating the final score because of their low item-total correlations or factor loadings. The results also showed that parents in Pakistan had higher scores than parents in the United States, who, in turn, had higher scores than parents in Hong Kong on *guan*, which were inconsistent with what one would expect. Moreover, no significant relations between *guan* and parental control were found in samples in Hong Kong, Pakistan, or the United States, raising a question about what construct the *guan* items indicated. Chen-Bouck et al. (2019) speculated that the items in the *guan* measure may involve (1) beliefs about child development and learning; and (2) beliefs about the mother–child relationship, but the analysis failed to confirm the two-factor structure.

Whereas researchers may continue to improve the assessment with refined items for the existing measures or use Western-based measures in the study of Asian parenting, it is necessary to explore the conceptual and measurement issues from a different perspective.

Care-Based Power-Assertive Parenting in Asian Families

As an expansion of the discussions in the field (e.g., Chao, 1994; Cheah et al., 2019; Chen et al., 2019; Ho, 1986; Tobin et al., 1989), Chen (2023) proposes a perspective that explicitly emphasizes two integrated aspects of Asian parenting, care and power assertion, in their contributions to child development, using the construct of care-based power-assertive parenting. CBPAP is defined as parental expressions of care in power-assertive behavior or the use of power assertion with care in childrearing. The goal of CBPAP is to help children develop socially desirable behaviors and attain achievement in group-oriented societies. It differs from the goal of authoritative parenting, which is based on a combination of parental warmth and democratic control, mainly to promote children's independence and autonomy in Western societies (Baumrind, 1971; Maccoby & Martin, 1983).

A major defining feature of CBPAP is its emphasis on parental care, which refers to attentiveness and concern arising from the awareness of responsibility to socialize children to succeed in society. Asian parents' care is typically expressed in forms of guidance and instrumental support for learning appropriate behaviors and educational activities (e.g., "I help and guide the child to develop good habits and be polite," Cheah et al., 2015). Parental care may overlap with but differ from parental warmth that is indicated by outward and direct expression of affection to children to enhance their feelings of security and confidence to explore the environment in Western societies (e.g., Maccoby & Martin, 1983). Asian parents tend to be reluctant to explicitly display affect in parent–child interactions, perhaps owing to the concern that it may weaken their authority in parenting (Cheah et al., 2015; Chen et al., 1998). However, they are willing to express care, especially to help children achieve success. Parental care makes CBPAP different from "tough love" parenting, which focuses on the use of harsh, rigid, and unresponsive strategies that are believed to benefit children in the long run, because providing support and guidance is an important part of parental care. Asian parents often express their care as high levels of involvement, sacrifice, and worry about the child's failure, which may result in the use of power assertion (Chen, 2023).

Parental power assertion indicates the use of rules and discipline to monitor and regulate children's behaviors with parental authority (Xu et al., 2020). Parents in Western societies are often discouraged to use power assertion in childrearing because it is incompatible with the socialization goal to help children develop personal autonomy (Maccoby & Martin, 1983). In Asian societies, however, parental power assertion based on care is regarded as necessary, and inadequate parental power assertion may be viewed as an indication of a lack of parental responsibility and competence (Ho, 1986; Ju et al., 2021). Nevertheless, parents are encouraged to exert power assertion with care for the purpose to help children learn socially acceptable and desirable behaviors and internalize social expectations, and the use of power assertion should not result from hostility, coldness or low responsiveness, or rejection. In short, CBPAP is represented by parental use of power assertion derived from care for children to learn socially valued behaviors in group-oriented Asian societies. As the core element, parental care and associated concern guide parents to use power assertion in childrearing to achieve the socialization goals.

Cultural values of parental care-based power assertion in Asian societies may affect children's attitudes toward parenting practices. Research has indicated that Asian children show less negative reactions to parental use of power assertion than Western children (Chao, 1995; Chao & Aque, 2009; Cheah et al., 2019;). Chao and Aque (2009) found that compared with their European American counterparts, Chinese, Korean, and Filipino American adolescents were less likely to be angry with parental strictness. Cheah and colleagues (2019) found that Asian children and adolescents tended to interpret parental use of power assertion in a positive manner (e.g., "for my own good"). Yu et al. (2019) reported that parental power assertion was associated with more positive outcomes and fewer problems among Asian children from families that maintain traditional group-oriented values. Children's understanding and appreciation of parental care and associated investment and sacrifice are likely to prevent potential harmful effects of power-assertive practices and, at the same time, allow them to benefit from their constructive functions.

In summary, according to Chen (2023, 2024), CBPAP represents a primary parenting style that captures culturally relevant features of socialization in traditional East Asian societies. It is "child-centered," focusing on helping children learn social standards, develop socially valued behaviors, and attain success. Power assertion is used to elicit child compliance largely as a strategy to achieve the socialization goals, often accompanied with the attempt to seek child understanding and cooperation, not with negative attitudes toward the child (e.g., coldness, hostility, rejection, neglect) as in authoritarian parenting. Parental care in CBPAP is derived from a high level of childrearing responsibility, often manifested as parental anxiety, involvement, and sacrifice. CBPAP is likely to contribute to child development in socially relevant domains, such as prosocial behavior and academic achievement, particularly in contexts where traditional group-oriented cultural values are maintained.

Care-Based Power Assertive Parenting and Child Adjustment: Empirical Studies

We conducted two studies of CBPAP and its relations with child adjustment outcomes in China. The studies were conducted in samples with a rural background. Traditional values, including those concerning socialization practices, tend to be maintained to a greater extent and, accordingly, CBPAP may be more representative of parenting in rural contexts than in urban contexts. In the studies, the measures of CBPAP (see Table 6.1) assessed parental attitudes and behaviors indicating the levels of care and power assertion in helping children achieve socialization goals. As suggested in the previous studies of Asian parenting (e.g., Chao & Aque, 2009), parental care largely focused on support for children to learn standards and to strive for achievement whereas parental power assertion mainly captured control, monitoring, and use of rules to regulate children's behaviors. The items tapped, for example, how parents express care by requiring children to learn social standards, have strict rules for children to help them improve their performance, closely monitor and guide children so they will not develop misconduct, criticize children to push them to work harder, and express concerns when children fall behind expectations. The two aspects are integrated in each of the items, so the two aspects are assessed simultaneously. As such, the scores of CBPAP in these measures reflect the overlapping part of care and power assertion, which indicates care using power assertion or power assertion derived from care. The scores differ from the combined scores of items assessing separate aspects or factors of general high power assertion (based on care and non-care) and general high care (using power assertion and non-power assertion).

In the first study, the participants included 1,214 mothers of kindergartens children (515 boys) from rural migrant families in Shanghai, China. The migrant families came from different regions of China. Most of the mothers had an education of high school or lower and worked as unskilled laborers in manual labor sectors in the city. The mothers completed a self-report measure of maternal CBPAP. To control for (and compare with) authoritarian parenting style in the analysis, the mothers also completed a measure of authoritarian parenting (e.g., "I do not allow my child to get angry with me"). We collected data from teachers for the children on social and school performance for the assessment of construct validity of CBPAP measure. The teacher rating measure included subscales of sociability, externalizing problems, internalizing problems, and learning problems.

TABLE 6.1 Items in Parent- and Child-Report Measures of Parental CBPAP

Parent-Report Measure

1. I am strict with my child because I want him/her to become better.
2. I maintain high control over my child to make him/her learn and thrive.
3. I have strict demands for my child because I care about him/her.
4. I criticize my child to push him/her to work harder.
5. I have firm and strict rules for my child for his/her own good.
6. I worry about my child when he/she falls behind others.
7. If parents don't discipline the child, he/she may learn bad behaviors.
8. I believe that criticism makes the child improve.
9. To care about the child, parents should closely monitor and guide him/her so he/she will not develop misconduct or problems.

Child-Report Measure

1. My mother/father is strict with me because he/she wants me to become better.
2. My mother/father maintains high control over me to make me learn and thrive.
3. My mother/father has strict demands for me to learn good behavior because he/she cares about me.
4. My mother/father criticizes me to push me to work harder.
5. My mother/father worries about me when I fall behind others.
6. My mother/father believes that to care about me, he/she should closely monitor and guide me so I will not develop misconduct or problems.
7. My mother/father compares me with others to let me know my shortcomings and make greater effort to improve.

The means of the items in maternal CBPAP ranged from 3.12 to 3.66 with standard deviations ranging from 0.92 to 1.04. The average score of scale was 3.14 with a standard deviation was 0.67. The internal reliability (Cronbach's alpha) was 0.87. We conducted both exploratory and confirmatory factor analyses to assess the structure of the measure. The analyses supported a one-factor model with satisfactory fit. The standardized factor loadings ranged from 0.531 to 0.768. Maternal CBPAP did not differ for boys and girls. Measurement invariance tests supported full metric and full scalar equivalence for the measure across gender and grade. We examined relations between maternal CBPAP and child adjustment. After controlling for child gender and the effects of maternal authoritarian parenting, maternal CBPAP was positively associated with teacher-rated sociability and negatively associated with externalizing problems and internalizing problems, B =.129, -.116, and -.122, SE =.051,.053, and.050, t = 2.548, -2.195, and -2.458, ps <.05. The main effect of maternal CBPAP on teacher-rated learning problems was not significant. We conducted multigroup analyses to test gender and grade differences on the relations in the model. No significant gender or grade differences were found, indicating that the predictive effects of maternal CBPAP on the adjustment variables were consistent across gender and grade levels. Maternal authoritarian parenting was not significantly associated with child adjustment variables.

In the second study, the sample included 710 students (385 boys) in grade 4 in a rural area of China. Most of the parents had a high school education or below. The students completed a self-report measure of CBPAP and a measure of authoritarian parenting separately for their mothers and fathers. The students also completed self-report measures of depression and loneliness. In addition, students were group administered a sociometric nomination measure of peer rejection and acceptance and a peer assessment measure of prosociality. Teachers completed a rating scale for each student, focusing on prosociality, externalizing problems, and internalizing problems. Data on academic achievement and leadership were obtained from school records.

The means of the items ranged from 3.04 to 3.75 and 2.70 to 3.59 (*SDs* ranging from 1.32 to 1.54 and from 1.36 to 1.32) for maternal and paternal CBPAP measures, respectively. The average score of scale was 3.47 (SD = 0.90) for maternal CBPAP and 3.37 (SD = 0.98) for paternal CBPAP. The internal reliability was 0.78 and 0.82 for maternal CBPAP and paternal CB-PAP. Exploratory and confirmatory analyses indicated a one-factor model for child-reported maternal and paternal CBPAP measures with satisfactory fit. Standardized factor loadings ranged from 0.439 to 0.724 for maternal CBPAP, and from 0.460 to 0.766 for paternal CBPAP. Compared to boys (M = 3.58 and 3.55, SD = 0.90 and 0.96), girls reported lower maternal and paternal care-based power-assertive parenting (M = 3.35 and 3.16, SD = 0.87 and 0.96). Measurement invariance tests supported full metric and full scalar equivalence for the measure across gender. Maternal CBPAP was positively associated with academic achievement and leadership and negatively associated with peer rejection, teacher-rated internalizing problems, depression, and loneliness, B =.200, 0.149, -0.113, -0.102, -0.065, and -0.101, SE = 0.044, 0.049, 0.043, 0.046, 0.016, and 0.035, t = 4.500, 3.056, -2.663, -2.214, -4.038, and -2.899, $ps < 0.05$, respectively. Paternal CB-PAP was positively associated with peer-assessed prosociality, teacher-rated prosociality, academic achievement, and leadership and negatively associated with teacher-rated externalizing problems, depression, and loneliness, B = 0.089, 0.129, 0.094, 0.128, -0.087, -0.053, and -0.130, SE = 0.044, 0.043, 0.041, 0.044, 0.041, 0.014, and 0.031, t = 2.025, 3.045, 2.309 2.891, -2.138, -4.662, and -4.133, $ps < 0.05$, respectively. Multigroup invariance tests showed no significant gender differences in the relations between maternal and paternal CBPAP and child adjustment variables, suggesting that the relations were consistent for boys and girls. In this study, parental authoritarian parenting was negatively associated with social and academic competence and positively associated with adjustment problems.

Taken together, the results indicated adequate psychometric qualities of the parent and child measures of CBPAP that were developed in the two studies, including construct validities and internal reliabilities. Parental CBPAP was positively associated with social, school, and psychological adjustment and negatively associated with adjustment problems. The associations between parental CBPAP and children's social and school performance support the argument that the primary goal of CBPAP is to help children develop socially appropriate and desired behaviors that contribute to the wellbeing of the family and other groups (Chen, 2023). The negative associations between parental CBPAP and children's psychological problems, such as loneliness and depression, are also interesting. It has been argued that individual psychological wellbeing has traditionally been neglected in Asian societies because it may not have significant effects on collective functioning (Chen & Liu, 2016). Research has shown that Asian youth in the United States and Asia tend to report more negative self-feelings and affect disturbances than their counterparts with a European background (e.g., Chen & Liu, 2016; Huntsinger & Jose, 2006; Lau et al., 2009). The results of the present studies suggest that parental CBPAP serves to mitigate emotional distress and other psychological problems in children. Apparently, children's understanding and appreciation of parental care ("for my own good," Cheah et al., 2019) underlying the requirements of maintaining behaviors according to social standards (e.g., cooperation-compliance in social interaction, persistence on learning tasks) reduce their negative reactions and perhaps increase their feelings of security.

Implications of Social Change

Developmental theorists and researchers have been interested in the impact of social changes on family organization and socialization (e.g., Elder & Shanahan, 2006; Greenfield, 2009; Silbereisen & Chen, 2010). This issue is relevant to the understanding of Asian parenting, given the ongoing massive movement of populations, technological development, and interaction with Western social and cultural systems in many Asian countries. According to the pluralist-constructivist perspective (Chen, 2015; Kağıtçıbaşı, 2012), the social changes taking place in many developing countries may lead to the coexistence and integration of diverse cultural beliefs and values. Different beliefs and values, such as those about autonomy and connectedness, serve different functions in human development. For example, the urban lifestyles and increased affluence brought on by modernization provide opportunities to pursue individual autonomy and initiative-taking, which may help children achieve personal goals. At the same time, values of social connectedness are useful for individuals to develop interpersonal relationships and support systems (Kağıtçıbaşı, 2012). From this perspective, Western or non-Asian values inevitably influence the socialization attitudes and behaviors of Asian parents. However, these values are unlikely to be adopted completely, but instead may be modified and integrated with the cultural traditions in Asian societies. Kağıtçıbaşı and colleagues (e.g., Kağıtçıbaşı & Ataca, 2005), for example, found that as a result of social change over the past several decades in Turkey, parents were more inclined to encourage independence in children, but the social change did not weaken parental attitudes towards socialization of social interdependence.

From the pluralist-constructivist perspective (Chen, 2015, 2024; Kağıtçıbaşı, 2012), Asian parents may adopt mixed or integrated traditional Asian and Western parenting styles and practices during social changes. Specifically, while maintaining their high involvement in providing guidance for children to learn socially valued behaviors and achieve educational success, parents may pay greater attention to children's socioemotional wellbeing and display higher sensitivity to children's psychological needs. In a study of childrearing attitudes in China, Chen and Chen (2010) found that parents in the 1990s and early 2000s did not differ in their emphasis on school achievement (e.g., "I encourage my child always to do his/her best in academic achievement"). In more recent years, however, parents have reported a higher level of warmth (e.g., "My child and I have warm, good times together," "I comfort my child when he/she is upset or afraid"). Parents may express their warmth through engaging in leisure activities with children for relaxation and fun (e.g., playing, chatting), in which children experience positive feelings and emotions (Zhao & Chen, 2018). Thus, as a result of social change, Asian parents may increasingly use combined care and warmth or include warmth in care in parent–child activities.

With higher parental warmth or sensitivity to children's socioemotional needs, Asian parents may become more careful or more strategic in using power assertion in parenting. Asian parents likely continue to be firm and strict in requiring children to behave and perform according to social standards. However, parents may be more flexible by using other strategies, such as encouragement and inductive reasoning, to allow children to explore their personal interests and develop self-confidence, when parents recognize the importance of these qualities for achieving success in competitive societies. At the same time, parents may adjust their parenting behaviors according to the child's needs, abilities, and characteristics in parent–child interactions. To ensure children perform optimally on academic and other important tasks, parents may exert power assertion in combination with practices they learn from other cultures (e.g., providing structure that links actions and outcomes through clear guidelines and feedback about children's progress in meeting expectations, Grolnick & Pomerantz, 2009).

Therefore, in the context of social and cultural changes, Asian parents are likely to maintain distinctive features of parenting that encompass broad cultural values to facilitate the development of socially appropriate behaviors as well as individual autonomy and psychological wellbeing.

Summary, Issues, and Future Directions

In this chapter, we have discussed parenting goals, beliefs, and practices in Asian, particularly Chinese, societies from the CBPAP perspective, which highlights the aspects of parental care and power assertion in socialization. Recognizing the two aspects of CBPAP and their inherent connection allows us to better understand the nature of Asian parenting and its potential significance for child development. This perspective may also provide a framework for researchers to explore the involvement of Asian cultural contexts in human development. We have also developed measures of CBPAP and presented the initial findings about them in studies of families with a rural Chinese background.

Several issues should be noted. First, the CBPAP perspective focused on a parenting style that represents the integration of parental care and power assertion. It remains to be clarified how the parenting style and each component are expressed in specific parenting behaviors in childrearing or parent–child interactions. For example, because CBPAP mainly serves to help children develop socially appropriate or desired behaviors and to achieve success, it may be more likely to be exhibited in learning settings than in parent–child leisure activities. In learning settings (e.g., helping child on homework), parents may be inclined to use power assertion, such as criticism, when the child fails on tasks (Ng et al., 2007), although it is based on, and driven by, parental care and associated concern and anxiety.

According to the pluralist-constructivist perspective (Chen, 2015, 2024), whereas many traditionally agricultural societies become more urbanized and individualistic, Western industrialized societies may become more accepting of diverse cultures. This may be particularly the case when people realize that the values of diverse cultures, such as those of autonomy and connectedness, complement each other and serve different functions in personal, interpersonal, and group activities (Maccoby, 1998). It will be interesting to examine how Asian cultures, including their socialization beliefs and values, affect the parenting practices of non-Asian parents, especially those who think some aspects of Asian parenting to be beneficial for child education and development.

To facilitate research in this area, we developed parent-report and child-report measures of CBPAP and used them to explore the relations between CBPAP and children's social, school, and psychological adjustment.

The items in the measures focused mainly on parental power assertion, such as strict discipline, with care indicated by the motivation to help children achieve socialization goals. An important feature of the measures is that the two aspects of parental care and power assertion were integrated in each of the items, which makes the measures different from the existing ones in this area with mixed but un-integrated items. Nevertheless, different measures should be developed and different methods should be used to assess CBPAP in the future. For example, it may be an effective strategy to examine CBPAP through observing parent–child interactions in socially relevant activities (e.g., teaching and learning).

The preliminary studies of CBPAP presented in this chapter were conducted in samples of rural or rural-to-urban families in China. It will be important to validate the measures in urban Chinese families. It will also be interesting to examine whether CBPAP can be applied to the characterization of socialization patterns in other East Asian societies, such as Korean, Singapore, and Vietnamese societies, which share the cultural tradition with Chinese society.

The CBPAP perspective asserts that Asian cultural values of parental power assertion based on care promote children's understanding, appreciation, and cooperation in joint socialization (Chen, 2023). Moreover, children's positive interpretations of, and attitudes toward, parental effort are likely to enhance its effects. Researchers should investigate how parental CBPAP and children's interpretations and responses interact in predicting developmental outcomes.

References

Baumrind, D. (1971). Current patterns of parental authority. *Developmental Psychology Monograph, 4*, 1–103.

Bornstein, M. H. (2012). Cultural approaches to parenting. *Parenting: Science and Practice, 12*(2–3), 212–221. doi:10.1080/15295192.2012.683359.

Bornstein, M. H., Cote, L. R., Haynes, O. M., Suwalsky, J. T., & Bakeman, R. (2012). Modalities of infant-mother interaction in Japanese, Japanese American immigrant, and European American dyads. *Child development, 83*(6), 2073–2088. doi:10.1111/j.1467–8624.2012.01822.x.

Camras, L. A., Sun, K., Li, Y., & Wright, M. F. (2012). Do Chinese and American children's interpretations of parenting moderate links between perceived parenting and child adjustment? *Parenting: Science and Practice, 12*(4), 306–327. doi: 10.1080/15295192.2012.709154.

Chao, R. K. (1994). Beyond parental control and authoritarian parenting style: Understanding Chinese parenting through the cultural notion of training. *Child Development, 65*(4), 1111–1119. doi:10.2307/1131308.

Chao, R. K. (1995). Chinese and European American cultural models of the self reflected in mothers' childrearing beliefs. *Ethos, 23*(3), 328–354. doi:10.1525/eth.1995.23.3.02a00030

Chao R. K. (2001). Extending research on the consequences of parenting style for Chinese Americans and European Americans. *Child development, 72*(6), 1832–1843. doi:10.1111/1467–8624.00381

Chao, R. K. & Aque, C. (2009). Interpretations of parental control by Asian immigrant and European American youth. *Journal of family psychology, 23*(3), 342–354. doi:10.1037/a0015828.

Chao, R. & Sue, S. (1996). Chinese parental influences and their children's school success: A paradox in the literature on parenting styles. In S. Lau (Ed.), *Growing up the Chinese way* (pp. 93–120). Hong Kong: The Chinese University Press.

Cheah, C. S. L., Li, J., Zhou, N., Yamamoto, Y., & Leung, C. Y. Y. (2015). Understanding Chinese immigrant and European American mothers' expressions of warmth. *Developmental Psychology, 51*(12), 1802–1811. doi:10.1037/a0039855.

Cheah, C. S. L., Yu, J., Liu, J., & Coplan, R. J. (2019). Children's cognitive appraisal moderates associations between psychologically controlling parenting and children's depressive symptoms. *Journal of adolescence, 76*, 109–119. doi:10.1016/j.adolescence.2019.08.005.

Chen, X. (2015). Exploring the implications of social change for human development: Perspectives, issues, and future directions. *International Journal of Psychology, 50*(1), 56–59. doi:10.1002/ijop.12128.

Chen, X. (2023). *Socialization and Socioemotional Development in Chinese Children* (Elements in Child Development). Cambridge University Press. doi:10.1017/9781009072380.

Chen, X. (2024). Social change and human development in Chinese context: A pluralist-constructivist perspective. *Acta Psychologica Sinica, 56*(7), 977–993. doi:10.3724/SP.J.1041.2024.00977.

Chen, X. & Chen, H. (2010). Children's socioemotional functioning and adjustment in the changing Chinese society. In R. K. Silbereisen & X. Chen (Eds), *Social change and human development: Concepts and results* (pp. 209–226). Sage Publications.

Chen, X., Dong, Q., & Zhou, H. (1997). Authoritative and authoritarian parenting practices and social and school performance in Chinese children. *International Journal of Behavioral Development, 21*(4), 855–873. doi:10.1080/016502597384703.

Chen, X., Fu, R., & Yiu, V. (2019). Culture and parenting. In M. Bornstein (Ed.), *Handbook of parenting* (pp. 448–473). Routledge.

Chen, X., Hastings, P. D., Rubin, K. H. et al. (1998). Child-rearing attitudes and behavioral inhibition in Chinese and Canadian toddlers: A cross-cultural study. *Developmental Psychology, 34*(4), 677–686. doi:10.1037/0012–1649.34.4.677.

Chen, X. & Liu, L. (2016). Culture, peer relationships, and developmental psychopathology. In D. Cicchetti (Ed.). *Developmental psychopathology* (pp. 723–769). Wiley.

Chen, X., Liu, M., Li, B., Cen, G., Chen, H., & Wang, L. (2000). Maternal authoritative and authoritarian attitudes and mother–child interactions and relationships in urban China. *International Journal of Behavioral Development, 24*(1), 119–126. doi:10.1080/016502500383557.

Chen, X. & Tse, H. C.-H. (2008). Social functioning and adjustment in Canadian-born children with Chinese and European backgrounds. *Developmental Psychology, 44*(4), 1184–1189. doi:10.1037/0012–1649.44.4.1184.

Chen-Bouck, L., Patterson, M. M., & Chen, J. (2019). Relations of collectivism socialization goals and training beliefs to Chinese parenting. *Journal of Cross-Cultural Psychology, 50*(3), 396–418. doi:10.1177/0022022118822046.

Dornbusch, S. M., Ritter, P. L., Leiderman, P. H., Roberts, D. F., & Fraleigh, M. J. (1987). The relation of parenting style to adolescent school performance. *Child Development, 58*(5), 1244–1257. doi:10.2307/1130618.

Elder, G. H. Jr. & Shanahan, M. J. (2006). The life course and human development. In W. Damon & R. M. Lerner (Eds), *Handbook of child psychology: Theoretical models of human development* (Vol. 1, pp. 665–715). Wiley.

Gao, Y., Zhang, W., & Fung, A. L. (2015). The associations between parenting styles and proactive and reactive aggression in Hong Kong children and adolescents. International Journal of Psychology, 50(6), 463–471. doi:10.1002/ijop.12104.

Greenfield, P. M. (2009). Linking social change and developmental change: shifting pathways of human development. *Developmental psychology, 45*(2), 401–418. doi:10.1037/a0014726.

Grolnick, W. S. & Pomerantz, E. M. (2009). Issues and challenges in studying parental control: Toward a new conceptualization. *Child Development Perspectives, 3*(3), 165–170. doi:10.1111/j.1750–8606.2009.00099.x.

Ho, D. Y. F. (1986). Chinese pattern of socialization: A critical review. In M. H. Bond (Ed.), *The psychology of the Chinese people* (pp. 1–37). Oxford University Press.

Huang, G. H. C. & Gove, M. (2015). Asian parenting styles and academic achievement: Views from Eastern and Western perspectives. *Education, 135*, 389–397.

Huntsinger, C. S. & Jose, P. E. (2006). A longitudinal investigation of personality and social adjustment among Chinese American and European American adolescents. *Child development, 77*(5), 1309–1324. doi:10.1111/j.1467–8624.2006.00936.x.

Huntsinger, C. S. & Jose, P. E. (2009). Relations among parental acceptance and control and children's social adjustment in Chinese American and European American families. *Journal of Family Psychology, 23*(3), 321–330. doi:10.1037/a0015812.

Jose, P. E., Huntsinger, C. S., Huntsinger, P. R., & Liaw, F.-R. (2000). Parental values and practices relevant to young children's social development in Taiwan and the United States. *Journal of Cross-Cultural Psychology, 31*(6), 677–702. doi:10.1177/0022022100031006002.

Ju, S. G., Chen, X., Chen, L., Zhao, S., & Fegley, S. G. (2021). Relations of maternal power assertion and autonomy support with children's adjustment in Korea. *Journal of Family Psychology, 35*(3), 335–344. doi:10.1037/fam0000720

Juang, L. P., Qin, D. B., & Park, I. J. K. (2013). Deconstructing the myth of the "tiger mother": An introduction to the special issue on tiger parenting, Asian-heritage families, and child/adolescent well-being. *Asian American Journal of Psychology, 4*(1), 1–6. doi:10.1037/a0032136.

Kağıtçıbaşı, C. (2012). Sociocultural change and integrative syntheses in human development: Autonomous-related self and social-cognitive competence. *Child Development Perspectives, 6*, 5–11. doi:10.1111/j.1750–8606.2011.00173.x.

Kağıtçıbaşı, C. & Ataca, B. (2005). Value of children and family change: A three-decade portrait from Turkey. *Applied Psychology: An International Review, 54*(3), 317–337. doi:10.1111/j.1464–0597.2005.00213.x.

Kho, C., Main, A., Chung, S., & Zhou, Q. (2019). Intrusive parenting in Chinese American immigrant families: Relations with cultural orientations and children's adjustment. *Asian American Journal of Psychology, 10*(4), 341–350. doi:10.1037/aap0000165.

Lamborn, S. D., Nguyen, J., & Bocanegra, J. O. (2013). Hmong American adolescents' perceptions of mothers' parenting practices: Support, authority, and intergenerational agreement. *Asian American Journal of Psychology, 4*(1), 50–60. doi:10.1037/a0031045.

Lau, A. S., Fung, J., Wang, S. W., & Kang, S. M. (2009). Explaining elevated social anxiety among Asian Americans: emotional attunement and a cultural double bind. *Cultural diversity & ethnic minority psychology, 15*(1), 77–85. doi:10.1037/a0012819.

Lee, E. H., Zhou, Q., Ly, J., Main, A., Tao, A., & Chen, S. H. (2014). Neighborhood characteristics, parenting styles, and children's behavioral problems in Chinese American immigrant families. Cultural Diversity and Ethnic Minority Psychology, 20(2), 202–212. doi:10.1037/a0034390.

Maccoby, E. E. (1998). *The two sexes: Growing up apart, coming together.* Cambridge: Belknap.

Maccoby, E. E. & Martin, J. A. (1983). Socialization in the context of the family: Parent–child interaction. In P. H. Mussen (Series Ed.) & E. M. Hetherington (Vol. Ed.), *Handbook of child psychology: Socialization, personality, and social development* (4th ed., Vol. 4., pp. 1–101). Wiley.

Mullis, I. V. S., Martin, M. O., & Foy, P. (2008). *TIMSS 2007 international mathematics report: Findings from IEA's Trends in International Mathematics and Science Study at the fourth and eighth grades.* Chestnut Hill, MA: TIMSS & PIRLS International Study Center, Boston College.

Ng, F. F.-Y., Pomerantz, E. M., & Lam, S.-F. (2007). European American and Chinese parents' responses to children's success and failure: Implications for children's responses. *Developmental Psychology, 43*(5), 1239–1255. doi:10.1037/0012-1649.43.5.1239.

Nguyen P. V. (2008). Perceptions of Vietnamese fathers' acculturation levels, parenting styles, and mental health outcomes in Vietnamese American adolescent immigrants. *Social work, 53*(4), 337–346. doi:10.1093/sw/53.4.337

Pinquart, M. & Kauser, R. (2018). Do the associations of parenting styles with behavior problems and academic achievement vary by culture? Results from a meta-analysis. *Cultural diversity & ethnic minority psychology, 24*(1), 75–100. doi:10.1037/cdp0000149.

Rohner, R. P. & Lansford, J. E. (2017). Deep structure of the human affectional system: Introduction to interpersonal acceptance–rejection theory. *Journal of Family Theory & Review, 9*(4), 426–440. doi:10.1111/jftr.12219.

Shen, J. J., Cheah, C. S. L., & Yu, J. (2018). Asian American and European American emerging adults' perceived parenting styles and self-regulation ability. *Asian American Journal of Psychology, 9*(2), 140–148. doi:10.1037/aap0000099.

Silbereisen, R. K., & Chen, X. (2010). *Social change and human development: Concepts and results.* London: Sage Publications.

Steinberg, L., Lamborn, S. D., Dornbusch, S. M., & Darling, N. (1992). Impact of parenting practices on adolescent achievement: authoritative parenting, school involvement, and encouragement to succeed. *Child development, 63*(5), 1266–1281. doi:10.1111/j.1467-8624.1992.tb01694.x.

Stewart, S. M. & McBride-Chang, C. (2000). Influences on children's sharing in a multicultural setting. *Journal of Cross-Cultural Psychology, 31*(3), 333–348. doi: 10.1177/0022022100031003003.

Stewart, S. M., Rao, N., Bond, M. H. et al. (1998). Chinese dimensions of parenting: Broadening western predictors and outcomes. *International Journal of Psychology, 33*(5), 345–358. doi:10.1080/002075998400231.

Su, C. & Hynie, M. (2011). Effects of life stress, social support, and cultural norms on parenting styles among Mainland Chinese, European Canadian, and Chinese Canadian immigrant mothers. *Journal of Cross-Cultural Psychology, 42*, 944–962. doi:10.1177/0022022110381124.

Tobin, J. J., Wu, D. Y. H., & Davidson, D. H. (1989). *Preschool in three cultures*. New Yale University Press.

Way, N., Okazaki, S., Zhao, J., Kim, J. J., Chen, X., Yoshikawa, H.,... Deng, H. (2013). Social and emotional parenting: Mothering in a changing Chinese society. *Asian American Journal of Psychology, 4*, 61–70.

Wu, P., Robinson, C. C., Yang, C., Hart, C. H., Olsen, S. F., Porter, C. L., Jin, S., Wo, J., & Wu, X. (2002). Similarities and differences in mothers' parenting of preschoolers in China and the United States. *International Journal of Behavioral Development, 26*(6), 481–491. doi:10.1080/01650250143000436.

Xu, X., Zhao, S., Yiu, W.Y.V., Li, D., Liu, J., Liu, S., & Chen, X. (2020). Relations between maternal power-assertive parenting and adjustment in Chinese children: A longitudinal study. *International Journal of Psychology, 55*(2), 154–162. doi:10.1002/ijop.12570.

Yu, J., Cheah, C. S., Hart, C. H., Yang, C., & Olsen, J. A. (2019). Longitudinal effects of maternal love withdrawal and guilt induction on Chinese American preschoolers' bullying aggressive behavior. *Development and Psychopathology, 31*(4), 1467–1475. doi:10.1017/S0954579418001049.

Zhao, S. & Chen, X. (2018). Maternal involvement in children's leisure activities in rural China: Relations with adjustment outcomes. *Journal of Family Psychology, 32*(1), 71–80. doi:10.1037/fam0000347.

Zhou, Q., Eisenberg, N., Wang, Y., & Reiser, M. (2004). Chinese children's effortful control and dispositional anger/frustration: Relations to parenting styles and children's social functioning. *Developmental Psychology, 40*(3), 352–366. doi:10.1037/0012–1649.40.3.352.

7

ASIAN PARENTING AND EMOTIONAL DEVELOPMENT IN A MULTI-LEVEL ANALYSIS FRAMEWORK

Qi Wang and Yang Yang

Parents have the best hope for their children to grow up to be happy and good individuals. They wish for their children to lead and enjoy a meaningful life, become pillars of their community and society, persevere through adversities, and be kind and understanding of others. Parenting practices to facilitate children's emotional development often reflect these goals and play a key role in children's psychosocial competence and well-being later on (Cole & Tan, 2007; Denham et al., 2007; Eisenberg, 2020; Yang & Wang, 2019). Importantly, parenting practices are shaped by cultural beliefs and expectations regarding what constitutes emotional competence in a particular cultural community. Research has revealed marked variations across cultures in how people perceive, appraise, experience, express, describe, and regulate emotions (e.g., Kitayama et al., 2000; Mauss & Butler, 2010; Tsai, 2007; Wang, 2006). It is a critical developmental task for children to develop emotional competence specific to their cultural community. Thus, to understand emotional socialization and development, one must take into consideration the role of culture. We focus in this chapter on parenting and children's emotional development in the Asian cultural context. We discuss relevant research through a multi-level analysis framework to reveal the dynamic influences of culture on emotional socialization and development in Asian families (Wang, 2018, 2023).

The Multi-level Analysis Framework

Emotional development can be viewed as an active process of cultural learning in which children interact with parents in the context of culture

DOI: 10.4324/9781003383949-7

in acquiring emotional competence (Halberstadt & Lozada, 2011; Yang & Wang, 2019). Through everyday activities and practices, parents—consciously or unwittingly—convey to their children cultural norms and expectations about the appropriate ways of experiencing, understanding, expressing, and regulating emotions. Children in turn internalize these norms and expectations into their own emotional cognition and behavior and further achieve emotional competence and psychosocial adjustment in their cultural community (Eisenberg, 2020; Halberstadt & Lozada, 2011; Miller-Slough & Dunsmore 2016; Raval & Walker, 2019; Yang & Wang, 2019).

The multi-level analysis framework provides an important way to understand the dynamic interplay between the parent, the child, and the larger societal-cultural environment in shaping the trajectory of emotional development and functioning. Wang first proposed this framework for the study of culture and cognitive development (Wang, 2018), and then applied it to understand emotional socialization and development in cultural context (Wang, 2023). According to the multi-level analysis framework, family socialization and cultural learning take place simultaneously at different levels via which culture exert its influences. Five levels of analysis are highlighted, each corresponding to specific characteristics of culture (see Figure 7.1).

First of all, at the group level of analysis, culture is viewed as a multifaceted, dynamic system that comprises many factors or elements that permeate everyday settings and interactions (Bruner, 1990; Valsiner, 2001). It provides an overarching framework that guides parenting and children's development. Thus, one critical task at this level of analysis is to identify meaningful cultural factors such as beliefs and norms that condition parental practices and child outcomes pertaining to emotion. This allows researchers to make informed hypotheses and design studies to examine the characteristics of emotional socialization and development in a cultural group, or to compare emotional socialization and development between groups.

The dyadic level of analysis emphasizes culture as a *process* of symbolic mediation, where parents and other socialization agents transmit to children cultural beliefs, norms, and expectations and, in turn, shape emotional development in culturally prescribed ways (LeVine & LeVine, 2016; Rogoff, 2003). One critical task at this level of analysis is to identify parental emotional socialization goals and practices (e.g., reasoning, modeling, responding, and so on) in cultural communities. Researchers can then examine how these practices contribute to child outcomes of interest, and whether these practices give rise to cultural similarities or differences in children's emotional competence.

The individual level of analysis highlights the active role of the individual in their cultural learning process, which further gives rise to individual variations in cultural attitudes and identification (Coll & Marks, 2009; Hermans, 2001). One critical task at this level of analysis is to recognize and measure individual variations in parents' adoption of cultural beliefs and practices pertinent to emotional socialization, and to further examine how such individual variations in turn contribute to differences in children's emotional competence within and between cultural groups.

The situation level of analysis emphasizes culture as a dynamic construct embodied within the person and is sensitive to contextual influences (Hong et al., 2000). In any given setting (e.g., home, school, grocery store), culturally prescribed modes of thinking interact with situational demands (i.e., how one should behave in that setting) in shaping psychological experience and behavior. Thus, a critical task at this level is to identify situational characteristics (e.g., with whom the child is interacting and what language the child is speaking) in specific settings that interact with cultural frameworks (e.g., interdependence) and in turn shape parental practices and child outcomes.

Finally, the temporal level of analysis highlights the transitory and ever-changing nature of culture (Greenfield, 2018; Varnum & Grossmann, 2017). It reflects a historical perspective where emotional development is viewed as unfolding under the multitude of influences of culture that itself evolves with societal transformations. A critical task at this level is to identify and examine the impact of societal factors (e.g., family policies, technological breakthrough, economic growth, migration) that transform parental emotional socialization goals and practices and in turn influence children's emotional development at a particular historical moment in time and place.

In sum, the multi-level analysis framework provides both a conceptual and a methodological guide for examining socialization practices and child development in cultural context (Wang, 2018, 2023). It has been applied to understand and study different aspects of human development across the lifespan (e.g., X. Chen, 2018; Greenfield, 2018; Wang & Kushnir, 2019). In the rest of the chapter, we examine empirical research on Asian parenting and children's emotional development through the multi-level analysis framework. The review is intended to be selective rather than exhaustive given the limited space; and the analysis aims to illustrate the dynamic and adaptative nature of emotion socialization in Asian-heritage families that facilitates the development of emotional competence specific to Asian cultural communities.

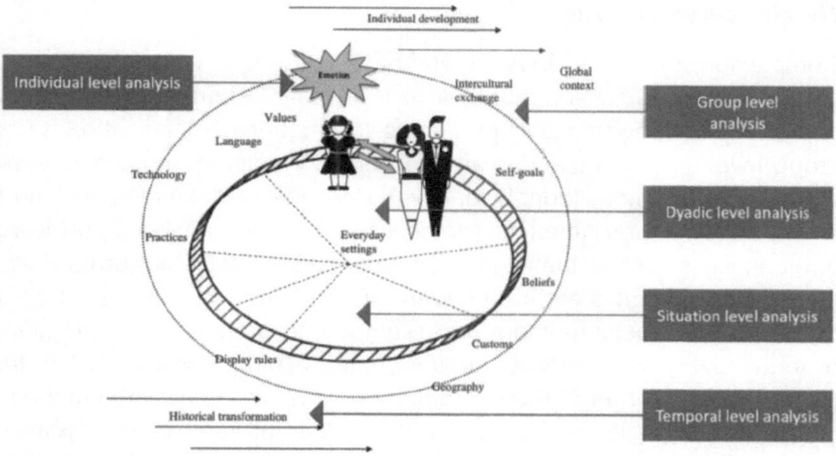

FIGURE 7.1 A multi-level analysis framework for emotional socialization and development in cultural context. From Wang (2023) with permission.

Asian Parenting of Emotional Socialization

Parenting practices pertaining to emotional socialization are conditioned in multilayers of cultural influences. Among the diverse Asian communities, there is a generally shared cultural emphasis on interdependence, social harmony, and group interest and, accordingly, the expectation for strict emotion control, which is considered essential for maintaining close relationships and group cohesion (Potter, 1988; Wang, 2006). This expectation for emotion control—both mentally and behaviourally—reflects the Asian cultural beliefs that emotion, especially negative emotion, can interfere with appropriate behavior and is thus destructive or even dangerous to the existing social order. It is therefore conducive for individuals to maintain moderation in all matters of the heart, as prescribed by Confucian teachings. Free expression of emotions or open discussion of one's feelings is often frowned upon and discouraged.

Within the larger cultural system, parenting can influence children's emotional development through a variety of ways (Eisenberg, 2020; Yang & Wang, 2019). Empirical research on Asian families has examined parental beliefs pertaining to emotion and emotion control, parents' own emotion expressivity, parent–child conversation about emotions, and parents' reactions to child emotions, all of which are deeply shaped by Asian cultural values and socialization goals (e.g., M. Chan et al., 2023; Son & Doan, 2023; Vu et al., 2023; Zhu & Dunsmore, 2023). The research has further revealed the influence of culture as a dynamic process taking place at multiple levels.

The group-level analysis

Comparisons of families in Asian and other cultures as well as subcultural groups within Asian communities have revealed similarities and differences in parenting practices pertaining to emotional socialization at the group level. For instance, Korean and Korean immigrant mothers endorse emotion control more strongly than do European American mothers (Son & Doan, 2023). Indian American mothers and Chinese mothers report lower emotional expressivity than European American mothers (McCord & Raval, 2016). These findings are in line with the different expectations for emotion control for social harmony versus emotion expression as an indication of individuality in respective cultural contexts (Yang & Wang, 2019). Importantly, the relation of these parenting practices to children's emotional competence may depend on the specific cultural context. For instance, whereas European Americans mothers' positive expressivity is associated with adaptive child outcomes and their negative expressivity is unrelated to child outcomes, Indonesian mothers' positive expressivity is unrelated to child outcomes and their negative-submissive emotion expressivity is associated with child behavior problems and poor social competence (Eisenberg et al., 2001; McCord & Raval, 2016).

In a similar vein, Asian parents are more likely to minimize children's negative emotions and less likely to encourage children's emotional expression than Western parents (Karkhanis & Winsler, 2016; Teo et al., 2017). For example, Indian mothers report using more "non-supportive," such as punitive, minimizing, scolding, and dismissing, reactions to their children's negative emotions than American mothers (Karkhanis & Winsler, 2016; Teo et al., 2017), and Korean and Asian American parents endorse more emotion suppression and shaming in response to their children's emotions (Louie et al., 2013). Chinese immigrant mothers also report more non-supportive responses to children's negative emotions than European American mothers, although the two groups use similar levels of supportive strategies (Doan & Song, 2022; Yang et al., 2020). Even for positive emotions, Chinese immigrant mothers report using more emotion dampening reactions than European American mothers (Song et al., 2019). Within India, mothers from a more traditional region report using more minimizing and punitive reactions to children's negative emotions than mothers from suburban areas (Raval & Martini, 2009). Asian parents' minimizing and other reactions to children's negative emotions may reflect their intention to encourage emotion control in children as well as their folk belief that negative emotions are inevitable and therefore should not be dowelled upon (Fishman et al., 2014).

The impact of these practices on children's emotional development appears to be complex. Research has shown that maternal supportive reactions to children's emotional expression positively predict children's emotional understanding and social functioning in Chinese and Korean families (W. T. Kim & J. L. Kim, 2012; Yang et al., 2020), and maternal non-supportive or punitive reactions negatively predicts Indian and Chinese children's psychological adjustment (Tao et al., 2010, 2017), findings similar as in Western children (Eisenberg et al., 1999; Fabes et al., 2002). However, given that parental non-supportive reactions to children's emotions are more common or considered more acceptable in Asian families, the negative effect of such practices, if any, seems attenuated, when compared with Western families. For example, non-supportive parental reactions are unrelated to emotional understanding and regulation in Indian and Chinese immigrant children, but negatively associated with emotional competence in European American children (Doan & Song, 2022; McCord & Raval, 2016; Song et al., 2019; Yang et al., 2020). Whereas parental control through suppressing and shaming children's emotions is associated with more expressions of anger and exuberance in a challenging situation among European American preschoolers, it is unrelated to emotion expressivity among Asian American and Korean children (Louie et al., 2013). The findings highlight the functional meaning of parenting practices as embedded in specific cultural contexts in shaping developmental outcomes.

The dyadic-level analysis

Many studies of Asian parenting directly examine the interaction between parents and children at the dyadic level. For example, Liu and colleagues (2013) observed European American and Chinese immigrant mothers' emotional expressivity during face-to-face interactions with their four-month-old infants. They found that European American mothers displayed more positive affect and less neutral or negative affect than did Chinese immigrant mothers who recently immigrated to the U.S. Similarly, Song and colleagues (2016) observed that during free play with their preschool-aged children, European American mothers displayed more positive facial and vocal expressions and fewer negative vocal expressions than did first-generation Chinese immigrant mothers. These findings may reflect the Asian cultural attitudes towards negative emotions as an inevitable, natural part of life and, accordingly, compared with Western cultures, Asian cultures place a less emphasis on experiencing positive emotions at all times (Heine & Hamamura, 2007; Oishi, 2002; Wang, 2013). Interestingly, whereas maternal facial expression of positive emotions was associated with emotional understanding in European American children, maternal vocal expression of positive emotions was associated with emotional understanding in Chinese immigrant children (Song et al., 2016). This may contribute to the greater sensitivity to emotional vocal cues in Chinese than European American children (Yang et al., 2021).

Parental positivity, sensitivity, and warmth during dyadic interactions with their children have been shown to be associated with many positive child outcomes in emotional adjustment and competence (Delgadillo et al., 2021; Quach et al., 2015; Tsotsi et al., 2020). For example, Delgadillo and colleagues (2021) examined positive emotional exchanges in mother–child dyads in relation to the children's physiological response (i.e., respiratory sinus arrhythmia; RSA) during a distressing situation. Singaporean mothers and their preschool-aged children participated in a "Laughing Task" in which their positive emotional exchanges were measured, and children's RSA was continuously monitored in an emotionally frustrating task. It was found that mothers' greater positive emotional responses to children were associated with children's RSA at baseline and in recovery from frustration. In other words, positive emotion responsivity from mothers may protect children from distress and facilitate emotion regulation in challenging situations.

Research on emotional discourse in the family is another example for the dyadic level of analysis. In line with their cultural emphasis on emotion control and the expectation for being attuned to others' feelings without being told (Wang, 2003, 2006), Asian and Asian immigrant parents discuss emotion infrequently with their children during family conversations. Different from Western parents who frequently talk about the causes and consequences of emotions with their children to help children express themselves and understand emotions, Asian parents instead tend to emphasize to children emotion display rules, sensitivity to others' emotions, and proper behavioural conduct (S. M. Chan et al., 2009; Doan & Wang, 2010; Wang, 2001, 2013; Wang & Fivush, 2005). In one study, for example, Doan and Wang (2010) observed mother–child dyads during a joint story-telling task in European American and Chinese immigrant families. Mothers' discussions of internal states and external behaviors during the conversation were coded, and their three-year-old children's emotion knowledge was assessed. European American mothers referred more frequently to internal thoughts and emotions than did Chinese mothers, who commented more frequently on behaviors during the storytelling. Furthermore, across both groups, maternal internal states language was positively associated with children's emotion knowledge, whereas their references to behaviors were negatively related to children's emotion knowledge. A follow-up study with the sample showed that maternal internal states language continued to facilitate Chinese children's emotion knowledge longitudinally (Doan et al., 2019). Similarly, Japanese and Chinese mothers' discussion of emotions during storytelling and memory sharing with their preschool-aged children is positively associated with children's emotional understanding (Watanabe, 2015) and positive self-views (Song & Wang, 2020). Thus, although Asian parents tend not to frequently engage their children in emotional discourse, such conversations appear to facilitate children's emotional competence, consistent with the general literature (Denham et al., 2007; Gottman et al., 1997).

The individual-level analysis

Parental emotion socialization practices further reflect the degree of cultural identification and internalization by the parents. Thus, at the individual level, Chinese immigrant parents in the U.S. who identify more with American culture exhibit greater emotion expressivity, whereas those who identify more with Chinese culture exhibit lower emotion expressivity (S. Chen et al., 2015). Similarly, when discussing emotion with their children, immigrant mothers' Chinese cultural orientation is associated with fewer emotion questions and explanations and lower quality of emotion talk in general, whereas their American cultural orientation is associated with more frequent use of positive emotion words and emotion explanations (Tao et al., 2013).

Importantly, the individual level of analysis can be combined with other levels of analysis in the research design, which contributes to our understanding of the dynamic interplay between parental cultural values and goals, socialization practices, and child outcomes in the larger cultural context. For example, in a cross-cultural longitudinal study, Koh and Wang (2021) utilized a combination of individual, dyadic, and group levels of analysis to examine the longitudinal relation between mother–child reminiscing of emotionally negative events and children's socioemotional development in European American and Chinese American families. Mothers discussed with their four-and-a-half-year-old children a negative event, and children's externalizing problems, internalizing problems, and other outcomes were assessed at age seven. Cultural differences emerged at the group and dyadic levels: Whereas European American mother–child pairs most commonly discussed negative events concerning injuries and medical procedures that focused on the child, Chinese American mother–child pairs most commonly discussed events concerning conflicts with siblings or peers that focused on social relations. During the conversations, Chinese American mothers were more likely than European American mothers to use negative emotion terms, and Chinese American children were more likely than their European American peers to talk about moral rules and behavioural expectations (e.g., *"Children should listen to their parents"*). European American children, on the other hand, were more likely than Chinese American children to discuss their own emotions. At the individual level, maternal use of negative emotional terms and maternal explanation of children's emotions were related to fewer externalizing and internalizing problems in children, independent of culture. Culture also moderated the link between some maternal practices and child outcomes, such as maternal use of negative emotional terms was related to fewer depressive symptoms in Chinese, but not European, American children. These findings underscore the importance of family emotional reminiscing for children's long-term emotional competence and well-being and the role of culture in shaping the process.

In a more recent study, Vu and colleagues (2023) examined first-generation Chinese immigrant mothers' cultural values and emotion socialization practices in relation to their children's emotional expressivity, which combined individual and dyadic levels of analysis. The study focused on parenting strategies such as emotion dismissing and moral and behavioural socialization that facilitate emotional restraint and social harmony in traditional Chinese families, in contrast to strategies such as emotion coaching to support and encourage children's emotional expressivity in White American families. The researchers observed in two consecutive home sessions how school-age children reacted to disappointment with anger and sadness and how mothers in turn responded to their children's negative emotions. Mothers also reported their Asian cultural values and parenting style. It was found that maternal cultural values moderated the impact of maternal practices on as well as maternal reactions to child emotional expression. Whereas emotion coaching led to more anger and sadness among children whose mothers strongly endorsed Asian cultural values, it eased anger and sadness for children whose mothers endorsed less traditional Asian values. In turn, children's anger and sadness evoked more moral and behavioural socialization responses from mothers who strongly endorsed Asian values, but more emotion coaching from mothers who endorsed less Asian values. It appears that emotion coaching is only effective for reducing child negative emotions in more Americanized Chinese immigrant families, and that parents respond to children's emotions in accordance with their cultural values. Thus, parental cultural value orientations at the individual level shape the emotional transactions between parent–child dyads and in turn the effectiveness and consequences of emotion socialization practices.

The situation-level analysis

Parenting practices often reflect the characteristics of the social setting in which emotion is experienced and expressed in line with the situational demands and cultural expectations. Thus, at the situation level of analysis, studies have examined within-individual variations in emotional practices and behaviors across different contexts or tasks. For example, whereas Chinese mothers and children do not make frequent references to the child's emotions when sharing personal memories, they talk frequently about story characters' emotions during book-reading or storytelling, consistent with the cultural expectation for downplaying one's own emotions on the one hand and attending to others' feelings on the other (Wang, 2013; Wang & Leichtman, 2000).

Studies with bilingual and bicultural Asian individuals often utilize the situation level of analysis to examine the impact of speaking different languages - being associated with different cultural value systems and expectations - on emotional experiences. For example, East-Asian Canadians exhibit an affective pattern resembling that of Westerners (i.e., their positive and negative affect are inversely associated) when they have recently interacted with a Western peer or spoken a non-Asian language; however, the same individuals exhibit an affective pattern resembling that of East Asians (i.e., no inverse association between positive and negative affect) when they have recently interacted with an Asian peer or spoken an Asian language (Perunovic et al., 2007). Research has also examined code-switching (i.e., alternate between different languages) during emotionally charged parent–child interactions to trace the dynamic association between emotional state and language use over time. In one study (Williams et al., 2020), Chinese American parents and children were asked to work together on a dyadic emotion-inducing puzzle box task. The bilingual parents' language use and code-switching as well as their emotional states as indexed by facial expressions were recorded. Negative emotion predicted subsequent code-switching, particularly from English to Chinese. In contrast, positive emotion predicted less code-switching from English to Chinese. These findings are consistent with the observation that individuals behave more in line with their cultural heritage (e.g., speaking their native language in this case) when experiencing negative affect (Ashton-James et al., 2009). Given that negative affect bound people to cultural norms, one may expect that bilingual Asian parents to speak more frequently Asian languages and endorse more strongly traditional Asian values such as interdependence in a negative emotional state such as when disciplining their children.

Another suite of research utilizing the situation level of analysis is the studies of parent–child discussion of positive versus negative emotional experiences (Wang, 2001; Fivush & Wang, 2005). For example, Fivush and Wang (2005) examined European American and Chinese mother–child dyads discussing a highly positive and a highly negative event. Mothers discussed with their three-year-olds at home one of the best things that had ever happened to the child and one of the worst things that had ever happened to the child. At the situation level, different patterns of emotional discourse emerged given the different purposes of discussing positive (e.g., to facilitate positive self-views and parent–child bonding) and negative emotions (e.g., to help children cope). Mother–child dyads in both cultures frequently dwelled on the child's emotional experience when discussing the positive event, conversations that may help the child reexperience a positive past self and further create a shared perspective between mother and child. In contrast, mother–child dyads refereed to a great variety of emotions and engaged in more negotiations about the child's emotion when discussing the negative event, whereby mother and child worked hard to explain and resolve the negative affect. In addition, at the group level, Chinese dyads used more negative emotion words than did European American dyads, which may reflect Chinese mothers' greater concern with instilling in their children appropriate expression and regulation of aversive affect. In contrast, European American dyads more frequently negotiated about the child's emotion than did Chinese dyads, which may reflect European American mothers' greater inclination to ensure children's authenticity of their own emotional experiences.

The temporal-level analysis

Research on Asian parenting and child's emotional development has taken into consideration the impact of cultural change on values and practices. One approach at the temporal level of analysis is to study different generations of immigrant families in the host culture who conceivably experience different levels of acculturation. For example, Liu and colleagues (2013) observed that when engaging in face-to-face interactions with their four-month-old infants, second-generation Chinese immigrant mothers or those who had lived in the U.S. for over ten years showed similar patterns of emotional expressivity as European American mothers, whereas Chinese immigrant mothers who recently immigrated to the U.S. differed significantly from European American mothers in their emotional expressivity. Similarly, when sharing memories or telling stories with their school-aged children, Chinese immigrant mothers who had lived in the U.S. for a long period of time discuss internal states equally frequently as

European American mothers (Yang et al., 2017) and engage in more emotional discourse than those who immigrated more recently (Curits et al., 2020), which reflects the influence of acculturation on parenting. Within the family, whereas Korean immigrant mothers uphold Asian cultural beliefs and endorse emotion control more strongly than European American mothers, Korean immigrant children exhibit similar emotional expressivity as their European American peers (Son & Doan, 2023).

Another approach to examine parenting in changing cultural contexts is to study Asian families in their home culture and those in the host culture. For example, Wang (2013) compared emotional discourse between first generation Chinese immigrant mothers in the U.S. and Chinese mothers in China and their three-year-old children. Mothers and children shared memories and read a storybook together. Chinese immigrant mothers exhibited more traditional Chinese parenting in their emotion talk: They focused less on their children's emotions and less frequently explained the causes or consequences of emotions while referring more frequently to others' emotions, when compared with Chinese mothers in China who exhibited a more Western pattern of emotion talk with their children. Wang suggested that first generation Chinese immigrant mothers may actively preserve traditional Chinese cultural values and ethnic identity, which in turn influences their parenting practices (Doan & Wang, 2010; B. Kim, 2009). In contrast, mothers in China, especially those living in modern cities like Beijing, are shifting their cultural values and the associated socialization goals and practices in the context of modernization, Western influences, and the one-child policy (X. Chen, 2000; Wang et al., 1998).

Perhaps the most direct approach at the temporal level of analysis is to understand the transformation of cultural values and the associated parenting practices and child outcomes. An example of this approach comes from X. Chen's work (2018), which demonstrates that cultural meanings ascribed to particular emotional characteristics such as shyness and self-control may change over time with societal-level transformations. This in turn can influence how people evaluate and respond to such characteristics and related behaviors in children, which further determines the expression and manifestation of the characteristics and the consequences for children's psychosocial adjustment. In Chinese and many other Asian cultures, shyness and self-control are traditionally viewed as a positive virtue given that personal restraint of desires and behaviors in social situations is considered crucial for group harmony and wellbeing. Accordingly, parenting practices tend to encourage such characteristics from early ages, and children who exhibit shyness have better adjustment as they grow older. However, with the drastic economic and social changes taking place in urban China in recent decades, the cultural meaning of shyness has transformed to have increasingly a negative connotation. As a result, shyness is encountered with peer rejection and psychological difficulties among urban adolescents, although in rural regions where traditional values are largely maintained, shyness is still associated with social approval and acceptance as well as adjustment in various domains (X. Chen, 2018). Studying different cohorts or populations differentially affected by societal changes can thus reveal the impact of Asian cultural beliefs as evolving constructs on parenting and child development.

Children's Emotional Development

Apart from studies of Asian parenting practices and their relation to child emotional competence, studies that focus on Asian children's emotional development have also revealed the dynamic influences of culture at multiple levels (See Yang & Wang, 2019, for a more comprehensive review). For example, at the group level, Chinese toddlers demonstrate greater self-control abilities and more compliant behaviors than Canadian toddlers (X. Chen et al., 2006), and Chinese preschoolers ascribe less intense emotional reactions across a variety of emotion situations than their European American peers (Wang, 2003). Furthermore, Korean and Asian American children express sadness, happiness, and anger less frequently than European American children in emotion-eliciting tasks (Louie et al., 2013, 2015), and Japanese preschoolers express anger less frequently than their American peers in response to conflict and distress (Zahn-Waxler et al., 1996). These findings suggest that Asian children have internalized at early ages Asian cultural norms of emotion suppression and self-regulation for maintaining social harmony.

At the dyadic level, Asian children increasingly demonstrate emotion control and regulation consistent with their cultural norms and expectations when interacting with parents and others. The patterns of parent–child dyadic influence become increasingly bidirectional with age, where not only parents instil values and expectations in children but also children's characteristics and behaviors shape parents' attitudes and practices towards children (X. Chen, 2018; Wang, 2018). A positive cycle of influences can be formed as a result, as shown in a large-scale longitudinal study in China where parental involvement through communicating and spending time with adolescent children increased children's support-seeking and facilitated a close parent–child relationship, which in turn contributed to children's socio-emotional adjustment (Li et al., 2023). Furthermore, friendship and positive peer relations have been found to be an important protective factor for children's emotional adaptation during life challenges, such as among the left-behind children in rural China (Zhao et al., 2015).

At the individual level, Chinese immigrant children who are more Westernized (e.g., greater English proficiency and lengthier residence in the host culture) are more emotionally expressive and display less shy behavior in peer interactions (X. Chen & Tse, 2008). Furthermore, emotional characteristics in alignment with cultural expectations are associated with psychological adjustment in children, whereas those inconsistent with cultural expectations are associated with maladjustment. For example, Louie and colleagues (2015) observed that emotion expressivity, a characteristic discouraged in Asian cultures, was negatively associated with teacher-rated social competence in Asian American and Korean children. Also, the expressions of sadness and happiness were positively associated with antisocial behaviors in Korean children, and the expression of anger was negatively associated with peer acceptance and prosocial behaviors in Asian American children. In contrast, these relations were absent in European American children. Yang and Wang (2023) found that whereas emotion knowledge predicted fewer internalizing problems in Chinese American school-aged children, it predicted fewer externalizing problems in European American children. In other words, although emotion knowledge facilitates children's psychosocial adjustment in both cultures, it is particularly beneficial for children to cope with issues more prevalent in their respective cultural contexts.

At the situation level, Asian children express different emotions depending on the situation and audience. For example, South Korean children, in line with their cultural expectation for sensitivity to the hierarchy and authority, reported more prosocial and fewer aggressive emotional reactions than Dutch children in negative emotional situations with the presence of the father, whereas there was no cultural difference in children's emotional reactions in situations with the presence of a peer (Novin et al., 2010). Also, although Asian children generally experience and express emotions less frequently or less intensely than Western children (Louie et al., 2013, 2015; Zahn-Waxler et al., 1996), Japanese toddlers are observed to experience more shame and less pride than American toddlers (Furukawa, 2005), and Chinese preschoolers are more likely than their European American peers to perceive anger in situations where social trust and harmony are violated (Wang, 2003), in line with the Asian cultural emphasis on self-reflection and interdependence.

At the temporal level, the patterns of children's emotional development reflect cultural transformations in society at large and within one's immediate environment at the micro level. For example, over the preschool years, Chinese American children show less understanding of emotion situations than European American children across different tasks. These cultural differences in children's emotion knowledge reflect different parental emotion socialization goals and practices early on: Whereas European American mothers frequently discuss and explain emotions to facilitate children's emotional understanding, Chinese mothers focus on moral lessons in their emotional discourse with children to convey behavioural expectations (Doan & Wang, 2010; Wang, 2008; Wang et al., 2006). However, Chinese American children show faster improvement in emotion knowledge than European American children across the early school years and by age eight they achieve the same level of emotion knowledge as their European American peers (Yang & Wang, 2016, 2023). This shift in the developmental trajectory of Chinese American children's emotional understanding reflects the influence of acculturation as children become increasingly integrated into the mainstream American culture. Thus, as Asian immigrant children transition from home to school and the society at large, they are exposed to different cultural values and practices and in turn develop emotional competence in the specific cultural context.

Looking Ahead

The multi-level analysis framework provides an important guide to understand and study parenting and child development in the cultural context (Wang, 2018, 2023). Our analysis of Asian parenting and children's emotional development through this framework demonstrates the complex and dynamic process in which emotional socialization and development take place at the intersection of the micro-context of family and the macro-context of culture. It further reveals the adaptative nature of Asian parenting practices that facilitate through various pathways the development of emotional competence in line with Asian cultural values of interdependence, social harmony, sensitivity to others' feelings and needs, and self-restraint. Asian children play active roles in their cultural learning by interacting with parents and other socialization agents and internalizing, albeit selectively, Asian cultural beliefs about emotion and how it should be experienced, expressed, and regulated. They further develop emotional competence in conjunction with the cultural characteristics of the specific environment in which they grow.

Examining the literature through the multi-level analysis framework also allows us to identify issues and gaps in current research on Asian parenting and children's emotional development. In particular, most work on Asian parenting to date has utilized parental self-reports or reports provided by older children. Such measures of parenting practices, although important for understanding the "perceived" parenting in the eyes of parents themselves or as viewed by children, should not be equated with the "actual" parenting practices in daily life. More rigorous research is required to study Asian parenting in action. Furthermore, many Asian cultural communities are vastly underrepresented in current research; studying family socialization and child development in such communities would be a primary task in future research. In addition, more research utilizing the situation level of analysis is needed to reveal the complexity of Asian parenting and child development in everyday settings. Finally, in our fast-changing society, a historical perspective at the temporal level of analysis is crucial for understanding the impact of societal transformations such as political reforms, economic growth, and technological breakthrough on cultural values and childrearing practices and in turn child development.

References

Ashton-James, C. E., Maddux, W. W., Galinsky, A. D., & Chartrand, T. L. (2009). Who I am depends on how I feel: The role of affect in the expression of culture. *Psychological Science, 20*(3), 340–346. https://doi.org/10.1111/j.1467-9280.2009.02299.x.

Bruner, J. (1990). *Acts of meaning*. Cambridge, MA: Harvard University Press.

Chan, M., Teng, D., Teng, Y. P. T., & Zhou, Q. (2023). Parent emotion talk with preschoolers from low-income Mexican American and Chinese American families: Links to sociocultural factors. *Social Development, 32*(2), 481–500. https://doi.org/10.1111/sode.12656.

Chan, S. M., Bowes, J., & Wyver, S. (2009). Parenting style as a context for emotion socialization. *Early Education and Development. 20*(4), 631–656. doi:10.1080/10409280802541973.

Chen, S. H., Zhou, Q., Main, A., & Lee, E. H. (2015). Chinese American immigrant parents' emotional expression in the family: Relations with parents' cultural orientations and children's emotion-related regulation. *Cultural Diversity & Ethnic Minority Psychology, 21*(4), 619–629. doi:10.1037/cdp0000013.

Chen, X. (2000). Growing up in a collectivist culture: Socialization and socioemotional development in Chinese children. In H. Comunion & V. Gielen (Eds), *International perspectives on human development* (pp. 331–353). Padua: Cadam Publishers.

Chen, X. (2018). Culture, temperament, and social and psychological adjustment. *Developmental Review, 50*(Part A), 42–53. doi:10.1016/j.dr.2018.03.004.

Chen, X., DeSouza, A. T., Chen, H., & Wang, L. (2006). Reticent behavior and experiences in peer interactions in Chinese and Canadian children. *Developmental Psychology, 42*(4), 656–665. doi:10.1037/0012–1649.42.4.656.

Chen, X. & Tse, H. C. (2008). Social functioning and adjustment in Canadian-born children with Chinese and European backgrounds. *Developmental Psychology, 44*, 1184–1189.

Cole, P. M. & Tan, P. Z. (2007). Emotion socialization from a cultural perspective. In *Handbook of socialization: Theory and research* (pp. 516–542).

Coll, C. G & Marks, A. K. (2009). *Immigrant stories: Ethnicity and academics in middle childhood.* Oxford: Oxford University Press.

Curtis, K., Zhou, Q., & Tao, A. (2020). Emotion Talk in Chinese American Immigrant Families and Longitudinal Links to Children's Socioemotional Competence. *Developmental Psychology, 56*(3), 475–488. https://doi.org/10.1037/dev0000806.

Delgadillo, D., Boparai, S., Pressman, S. D., Goldstein, A., Bureau, J. F., Schmiedel, S.,... & Borelli, J. L. (2021). Maternal expressions of positive emotion for children predicts children's respiratory sinus arrhythmia surrounding stress. *Developmental Psychobiology*, *63*(5), 1225–1240. https://doi.org/10.1002/dev.22082.

Denham, S., Bassett, H., & Wyatt, T. (2007). The socialization of emotional competence. In J. Grusec & P. Hastings (Eds), *Handbook of Socialization: Theory and Research* (pp. 614–637). New York: Guilford Press.

Doan, S. N., Lee, H.Y., & Wang, Q. (2019). Maternal mental state language is associated with trajectories of Chinese immigrant children's emotion situation knowledge. *International Journal of Behavioral Development, 43*(1), 43–52. https://doi.org/10.1177/0165025418783271.

Doan, S. N. & Wang, Q. (2010). Maternal discussions of mental states and behaviors: relations to emotion situation knowledge in European American and immigrant Chinese children. *Child Development, 81*(5), 1490–1503. doi:10.1111/j.1467–8624.2010.01487.x.

Doan, S. N. & Song, Q. (2022) Culture, Emotion Socialization and Children's Inhibitory Control, *Journal of Cognition and Development, 23*(5), 591–607, doi:10.1080/15248372.2022.2072847.

Eisenberg, N. (2020). Findings, issues, and new directions for research on emotion socialization. *Developmental Psychology, 56*(3), 664–670. https://doi.org/10.1037/dev0000906.

Eisenberg, N., Fabes, R. A., Shepard, S. A., Guthrie, I. K., Murphy, B. C., & Reiser, M. (1999). Parental reactions to children's negative emotions: Longitudinal relations to quality of children's social functioning. *Child Development, 70*(2), 513–534. doi:10.1111/1467–8624.00037.

Eisenberg, N., Liew, J., & Pidada, S. U. (2001). The relations of parental emotional expressivity with quality of Indonesian children's social functioning. *Emotion, 1*(2), 116–136.

Fabes, R. A., Poulin, R. E., Eisenberg, N., & Madden-Derdich, D. A. (2002). The Coping with Children's Negative Emotions Scale (CCNES): Psychometric properties and relations with children's emotional competence. *Marriage & Family Review*. doi:10.1300/J002v34n03_05.

Fishman, J. L., Raval, V. V., Daga, S. S., & Raj, S. P. (2014). Meta-emotion philosophy among Asian Indian immigrant mothers in the United States. *Qualitative Health Research, 24*(7), 875–889. doi:10.1177/1049732314537403.

Fivush, R. & Wang, Q. (2005). Emotion talk in mother–child conversations of the shared past: The effects of culture, gender, and event valence. *Journal of Cognition and Development, 6, 4,* 489–506. doi:10.1207/s15327647jcd0604_3.

Gottman, J., Katz, L., & Hooven, C. (1997). *Meta-emotion: How families communicate emotionally*. Mahwah, NJ: Lawrence Erlbaum.

Greenfield, P. M. (2018). Studying social change, culture, and human development: A theoretical framework and methodological guidelines. *Developmental Review, 50*(Part A), 16–30. https://doi.org/10.1016/j.dr.2018.05.003.

Halberstadt, A. G. & Lozada, F. T. (2011). Emotion development in infancy through the lens of culture. *Emotion Review*, *3*(2), 158–168. https://doi.org/10.1177/1754073910387946.

Heine, S. J. & Hamamura, T. (2007). In search of East Asian self-enhancement. *Personality and Social Psychology Review, 11*(1), 4–27. https://doi.org/10.1177/1088868306294587.

Hermans, H. M. (2001). The dialogical self: Toward a theory of personal and cultural positioning. *Culture & Psychology, 7*, 243–281. doi:10.1177/1354067X0173001.

Hong, Y., Morris, M. W., Chiu, C., & Benet-Martinez, V. (2000). Multicultural minds: A dynamic constructivist approach to culture and cognition. *American Psychologist, 55*, 709–720. doi: 10.1037//0003–066X.55.7.709.

Karkhanis, D. G. & Winsler, A. (2016). Temperament, gender, and cultural differences in maternal emotion socialization of anxiety, somatization, and anger. *Psychological Studies, 61*(3), 137–158. doi:10.1007/s12646-016-0360-z.

Kim, B. K. (2009). Acculturation and enculturation of Asian Americans: A primer. In N. Tewari & A. N. Alvarez (Eds), *Asian American psychology: Current perspectives* (pp. 97–112). New York: Routledge/Taylor & Francis Group.

Kim, W. T. & Kim, J. L. (2012). The effects of parental attitude toward young children's emotional expression on their emotional intelligence and playfulness. *Journal of Yeolin Education, 20*, 71–92.

Kitayama, S., Markus, H. R., & Kurokawa, M. (2000) Culture, emotion, and well-being: Good feelings in Japan and the United States. *Cognition and Emotion, 14(1)*, 93–124. doi:10.1080/026999300379003.

Koh, J. B. M. & Wang, Q. (2021). Mother–child reminiscing about emotionally negative events and children's long-term mental health. Frontiers in Psychology. doi:10.3389/fpsyg.2021.632799.

Lee, H. R. & Chung, O. B. (2002). Children's emotional intelligence: Relationships with parental attitudes. *Korean Journal of Child Studies, 23*, 17–35.

LeVine, R. A & LeVine, S. (2016). *Do parents matter?: why Japanese babies sleep soundly, Mexican siblings don't fight, and American families should just relax.* New York: Public Affairs.

Li, Q., Cao, Z., & Zhao, D. (2023). Home-based parental involvement and early adolescents' socio-emotional adjustment at middle school in China: A longitudinal exploration of mediating mechanisms. *Journal of Child and Family Studies, 32*(7), 2153–2163. https://doi-org.libproxy.nie.edu.sg/10.1007/s10826-023-02594-0.

Liu, C. H., Yang, Y., Fang, S., Snidman, N., & Tronick, E. (2013). Maternal regulating behaviors through face-to-face play in first- and second-generation Chinese American and European American mothers of infants. *Research in Human Development, 10*(4), 289–307. doi:10.1080/15427609.2013.846042.

Louie, J. Y., Oh, B. J., & Lau, A. S. (2013). Cultural differences in the links between parental control and children's emotional expressivity. *Cultural Diversity and Ethnic Minority Psychology, 19*(4), 424–434. doi:10.1037/a0032820.

Louie, J. Y., Wang, S., Fung, J., & Lau, A. (2015). Children's emotional expressivity and teacher perceptions of social competence. *International Journal of Behavioral Development, 39*(6), 497–507. doi:10.1177/0165025414548775.

Mauss, I. B. & Butler, E. A. (2010). Cultural context moderates the relationship between emotion control values and cardiovascular challenge versus threat responses. *Biological Psychology, 84*(3), 521–530. doi:10.1016/j.biopsycho.2009.09.010.

McCord, B. L. & Raval, V. V. (2016). Asian Indian immigrant and White American maternal emotion socialization and child socio-emotional functioning. *Journal of Child and Family Studies, 25*(2), 464–474. doi:10.1007/s10826-015-0227-2.

Miller-Slough, R. L. & Dunsmore, J. C. (2016). Parent and Friend Emotion Socialization in Adolescence: Associations with Psychological Adjustment. *Adolescent Research Review, 1*(4), 287–305. https://doi.org/10.1007/s40894-016-0026-z.

Novin, S., Rieffe, C., & Mo, T. J. H. (2010). The role of situational goals and audience on self-reported emotion experience and expression: Dutch and South Korean children compared. *Infant and Child Development, 19*(4), 406–421. doi:10.1002/icd.671.

Oishi, S. (2002). The experiencing and remembering of well-being: A cross-cultural analysis. *Personality and Social Psychology Bulletin 28,* 1398–1406. doi:10.1177/014616702236871.

Perunovic, W.Q., Heller, D., & Rafaeli, E. (2007). Within-person changes in the structure of emotion: the role of cultural identification and language. *Psychological Science, 18*(7), 607–613. doi: 10.1111/j.1467–9280.2007.01947.x.

Potter, S. H. (1988). The cultural construction of emotion in rural Chinese social life. *Ethos, 16, 2,* 181–208.

Quach, A. S., Epstein, N. B., Riley, P. J., Falconier, M. K., & Fang, X. (2015). Effects of parental warmth and academic pressure on anxiety and depression symptoms in Chinese adolescents. *Journal of Child and Family Studies, 24,* 106–116. https://doi.org/10.1007/s10826-013-9818-y.

Raval, V. V. & Martini, T. S. (2009). Maternal socialization of children's anger, sadness, and physical pain in two communities in Gujarat, India. *International Journal of Behavioral Development.* doi:10.1177/0165025408098022.

Raval, V. V. & Walker, B. L. (2019). Unpacking 'culture': Caregiver socialization of emotion and child functioning in diverse families. *Developmental Review, 51,* 146–174. https://doi.org/10.1016/j.dr.2018.11.001.

Rogoff, B. (2003). *The cultural nature of human development.* Oxford: Oxford University Press.

Son, H. & Doan, S. N. (2023). Cultural differences in maternal emotion control values and children's expressive flexibility. *Social Development, 32*(2), 501–516. https://doi.org/10.1111/sode.12670.

Song, Q. & Wang, Q. (2020). Mother–child reminiscing about peer experiences in European American and Chinese immigrant families: The impact on children's relational self-concepts. *Asian American Journal of Psychology, 11*(1), 40–48. https://doi.org/10.1037/aap0000162.

Song, Q., Yang, Y., Doan, S. N., & Wang, Q. (2019). Savoring or dampening? Maternal reactions to children's positive emotions in cultural contexts. *Culture and Brain, 7,* 172–189. https://doi.org/10.1007/s40167-019-00080-3.

Song, Q., Yang, Y., & Wang, Q. (2016, August). Maternal socialization of facial and vocal expression of emotions and children's emotion knowledge: A cross-cultural investigation. Poster session presented at 23rd International Congress of the International Association for Cross-Cultural Psychology (IACCP), Nagoya, Japan.

Tao, A., Zhou, Q., Lau, N., & Liu, H. (2013). Chinese American immigrant mothers' discussion of emotion with children. *Journal of Cross-Cultural Psychology, 44*(3), 478–501. doi:10.1177/0022022112453318.

Tao, A., Zhou, Q., & Wang, Y. (2010). Parental reactions to children's negative emotions: Prospective relations to Chinese children's psychological adjustment. *Journal of Family Psychology, 24*(2), 135–144. doi:10.1037/a0018974.

Teo, B. H., Raval, V. V., & Jansari, A. (2017). Emerging adults' reports of maternal emotion socialization and their adjustment across cultures. *Journal of Applied Developmental Psychology, 52,* 59–68. doi:10.1016/J.APPDEV.2017.06.009.

Tsai, J. L. (2007). Ideal affect: Cultural causes and behavioral consequences. *Perspectives on Psychological Science, 2*(3), 242–259. doi:10.1111/j.1745–6916.2007.00043.x.

Tsotsi, S., Borelli, J. L., Abdulla, N. B., Tan, H. M., Sim, L. W., Sanmugam, S.,... & Rifkin-Graboi, A. (2020). Maternal sensitivity during infancy and the regulation of startle in preschoolers. *Attachment & Human Development, 22*(2), 207–224. https://doi.org/10.1080/14616734.2018.1542737.

Valsiner, J. (2001). Process structure of semiotic mediation in human development. *Human Development, 44,* 84–97.

Varnum, M. E. W. & Grossmann, I. (2017). Cultural change: The how and the why. *Perspectives on Psychological Science, 12,* 956–972. doi:10.1177/1745691617699971.

Vu, K. T. T., Cheah, C. S. L., & Halberstadt, A. G. (2023). Cultural Values Moderate Bidirectional Associations between Chinese Immigrant Mothers' Emotion Socialization and Children's Anger and Sadness. *Social Development.*

Wang, Q. (2001). 'Did you have fun?' American and Chinese mother–child conversations about shared emotional experiences. *Cognitive Development, 16*(2), 693–715. doi:10.1016/S0885–2014(01)00055-7.

Wang, Q. (2003). Emotion situation knowledge in American and Chinese preschool children and adults. *Cognition & Emotion, 17*(5), 725–746. doi:10.1080/02699930302285.

Wang, Q. (2006). Developing emotion knowledge in cultural contexts. *International Society for the Study of Behavioral Development Newsletter, 1*(49), 8–12.

Wang, Q. (2008). Emotion knowledge and autobiographical memory across the preschool years: A cross-cultural longitudinal investigation. *Cognition, 108*(1), 117–135. doi:10.1016/j.cognition.2008.02.002.

Wang, Q. (2013). Chinese socialization and emotion talk between mothers and children in native and immigrant Chinese families. *Asian American Journal of Psychology, 4*(3), 185–192. doi:10.1037/a0030868.

Wang, Q. (2018). Studying cognitive development in cultural context: A multi-level analysis approach. *Developmental Review, 50,* 54–64. doi:10.1016/j.dr.2018.03.002.

Wang, Q. (2023). Emotion socialization in cultural context: Lessons from Asian-heritage families. *Social Development, 32*(2), 517–526. https://doi.org/10.1111/sode.12658

Wang, Q., & Fivush, R. (2005). Mother–child conversations of emotionally salient events: exploring the functions of emotional reminiscing in European-American and Chinese families. *Social Development, 14*(3), 473–495. doi:10.1111/j.1467–9507.2005.00312.x.

Wang, Q., Hutt, R., Kulkofsky, S., McDermott, M., & Wei, R. (2006). Emotion situation knowledge and autobiographical memory in Chinese, immigrant Chinese, and European American 3-year-olds. *Journal of Cognition and Development, 7*(1), 95–118. doi:10.1207/s15327647jcd0701_5.

Wang, Q. & Kushnir, T. (2019). Cultural pathways in cognitive development [Special issue]. *Cognitive Development.* www.sciencedirect.com/journal/cognitive-development/special-issue/10FK9210FB0.

Wang, Q. & Leichtman, M. D. (2000). Same beginnings, different stories: A comparison of American and Chinese children's narratives. *Child Development, 71*(5), 1329–1346. doi:10.1111/1467–8624.00231.

Wang, Q., Leichtman, M. D., & White. S. H. (1998). Childhood memory and self-description: The impact of growing up an only child. *Cognition, 69,* 73–103. doi:10.1016/S0010–0277(98)00061-4.

Watanabe, N. (2015). *Parental socialization of emotion in Japan: Contribution to preschoolers' emotion knowledge*. George Mason University.

Williams, A., Srinivasan, M., Liu, C., Lee, P., & Zhou, Q. (2020). Why do bilinguals code-switch when emotional? Insights from immigrant parent–child interactions. *Emotion, 20*(5), 830–841. doi: 10.1037/emo0000568.

Yang, Y., Koh, J. B. M., & Wang, Q. (2017, April). Discussion of internal states and behaviors in mother–child reminiscing: The longitudinal relations to children's emotion knowledge in European American and Chinese immigrant families. In A. Halberstadt (Chair) & W. Friedlmeier (Co-chair), Socialization of emotion regulation: Goals and practices around the world. Paper symposium conducted at the biennial meeting of the Society for Research in Child Development, Austin, TX.

Yang, Y., Song, Q., Doan, S. N., & Wang, Q. (2020). Maternal reactions to children's negative emotions: Relations to children's socio-emotional development among European American and Chinese immigrant children. *Transcultural Psychiatry, 57*(3), 408–420. https://doi.org/10.1177/1363461520905997.

Yang, Y. & Wang, Q. (2016). The relation of emotion knowledge to coping in European American and Chinese immigrant children. *Journal of Child and Family Studies, 25*(2), 452–463. doi:10.1007/s10826-015-0224–5.

Yang, Y., Wang, L., & Wang, Q. (2021). Take your word or tone for it? European American and Chinese children's attention to emotional cues in speech. *Child Development, 92*(3), 844–852. doi: 10.1111/cdev.13576.

Yang, Y. & Wang, Q. (2016). The relation of emotion knowledge to coping in European American and Chinese immigrant children. *Journal of Child and Family Studies, 25*(2), 452–463. https://doi.org/10.1007/s10826-015-0224-5.

Yang, Y. & Wang, Q. (2019). Culture in emotional development. In V. LoBue, K. Perez-Edgar, & K. Buss (Eds), *The Handbook of Emotional Development* (pp. 569–594). Springer.

Yang, Y. & Wang, Q. (2023). Longitudinal relations of emotion knowledge to psychosocial adjustment in European and Chinese American school-age children. *Social Development, 32*(4), 1149–1167. https://doi.org/10.1111/sode.12679.

Zahn-Waxler, C., Friedman, R. J., Cole, P. M., Mizuta, I., & Hiruma, N. (1996). Japanese and United States preschool children's responses to conflict and distress. *Child Development, 67*(5), 2462–2477. doi:10.1111/j.1467–8624.1996.tb01868.x.

Zhao, J., Liu, X., & Wang, M. (2015). Parent–child cohesion, friend companionship and left-behind children's emotional adaptation in rural China. *Child abuse & neglect, 48,* 190–199. https://doi.org/10.1016/j.chiabu.2015.07.005.

Zhu, D. & Dunsmore, J. C. (2023). Family functioning and emotion socialization in Chinese two-parent Households: A person-centered approach. *Social Development.*

8

PARENTAL EMOTION-RELATED SOCIALIZATION IN ASIAN FAMILIES

Qing Zhou and Megan Chan

Acknowledgment

The authors' work on this chapter has been supported by a grant from the Eunice Kennedy Shriver National Institute of Child Health and Human Development to Qing Zhou (R01HD091154) and a National Science Foundation Graduate Research Fellowship to Megan Chan. The authors wish to thank Nancy Eisenberg and Sharlene Wolchik for their guidance on early development of ideas and the graduate and undergraduate students at the UC-Berkeley Culture and Family Study Lab for their contributions to the research mentioned in the chapter.

The experience of parenthood is full of emotions. From the moment a child is born (or even before the newborn's arrival), parents (or expectant parents) are constantly immersed in abundance of emotional experiences of their own, their spouses/partners, other family members, and of course, their child(ren). Although emotion is typically considered a by-product of parenting (for parents) and growing up (for children) in Asian cultures, in which collective/family/interpersonal goals often take higher priority than individual needs and desires, emerging research in the last decade on emotion socialization in Asian-heritage families around the world has revealed a different picture: emotion plays a critical role in shaping parenting and parent–child relationship, parents' psychological wellbeing, and interparental and family relationships in Asian-heritage families. More importantly, parental emotion-related socialization behaviors (ERSBs) have emerged as one of the most salient parenting domains that is consequential for children's mental health and socioemotional development. In this chapter, we briefly review the concepts, dimensions, and measurements of ERSBs and their theorized roles in children's socioemotional development. Next, we discuss socio-cultural factors that can shape the forms, norms, and functions of parental emotion socialization in Asian families. We then provide

DOI: 10.4324/9781003383949-8

a selective review of empirical studies examining three types of parental ERSBs in Asian-heritage families: parental reactions to children's emotions, parental expressions of emotion, and parental emotion talk. We conclude with a discussion of future research directions and implications for parenting interventions for Asian families.

Parental Emotion-Related Socialization Behaviors: Constructs, Measurement, and Theory

Parental emotion-related socialization behaviors (ERSBs) are defined as parenting behaviors that "influence a child's learning (or lack thereof) regarding the experience, expression, and regulation of emotion and emotion-related behaviors" (Eisenberg, Spinrad, & Cumberland, 1998, p. 317). In contrast, global parenting style (e.g., authoritative, authoritarian, or permissive parenting) is defined as "a constellation of attitudes toward the child that are communicated to the child and create an emotional climate in which parents' behaviors are expressed" (Darling & Steinberg, 1993, p. 493). Thus, ERSBs are domain-specific parenting practices that "are expected to affect the child's emotional experience, learning of content, and emotion-related behavior in a manner consistent with socializers' beliefs, values, and goals about emotion and its relation to individual functioning and adaptation in society" (Eisenberg, Spinrad, & Cumberland, 1998, p. 317).

While there are many forms of ERSBs, developmental researchers have primarily focused on three types of ERSBs: parental reactions to children's emotions, parental expression of emotions, and parental emotion talk or emotion discussion (Eisenberg, Cumberland, & Spinrad, 1998). Parental reactions to children's emotions can be assessed using parent self-reported questionnaires (e.g., Coping with Children's Negative Emotions Scale/CCNES, Fabes et al., 2002) and observational coding of parental behaviors during parent–child interaction tasks (e.g., Vu et al., 2023). Commonly assessed types of parental responses include problem-focused responses, emotion-focused responses (e.g., comforting), encouragement of emotion expression, minimizing reactions, and parents' own distress reactions (Fabes et al., 2002). Although much research has focused on parental responses to children's negative emotions, Song et al. (2019) adapted the CCNES to assess parental reactions to children's positive emotions.

Parental expression of emotions can be assessed using two approaches: self-reported parent questionnaires (e.g., Self-Expressiveness in the Family Questionnaire/SEFQ, Halberstadt et al., 1995), and observational coding of parents' facial, body, or verbal expression of emotions during parent–child interactions (e.g., S. H. Chen et al., 2015). It is important to note that self-reported measures such as the SEFQ differ from observational measures not only by the methods of assessment, but also by the contexts in which emotions are expressed (e.g., the general family context vs. a specific parent–child interaction situation). Moreover, the SEFQ reflects trait-level variations in parents' emotional expressivity, whereas observational coding of parent–child interactions tends to capture situation-level emotion expressions. Thus, the degree of convergence between self-report and observed measures of parental emotion expression or other parenting behaviors tended to be low (e.g., S. H. Chen et al., 2015; Herbers et al., 2017).

Parental emotion talk is commonly assessed using observational measures of parent–child verbal interactions. Shared book reading tasks, which are typically used to examine narrative development, have been adapted to assess parent–child emotion talk (e.g., Chan et al., 2023a, 2023b; Huang & Kan, 2021). Emotion talk can also be assessed using dyadic reminiscing tasks (e.g., discussing a past emotional event, Wang, 2001), storytelling tasks (e.g., making up a story involving a specific emotion episode, Cervantes, 2002), or parent–child interactive play tasks (e.g., Lorenzo, Bahrick, & Bagner, 2023). Transcripts of parent–child conversations can be coded for frequencies of parents' and children's use of emotion labels or mental state languages, emotion questions, explanations about the causes and consequences of emotions, linking emotions to past experiences, as well as the overall quality or elaborateness of emotion talk (e.g., Chan et al., 2023a; Tao et al., 2013; Wang, 2001).

According to the heuristic model proposed by Eisenberg, Cumberland, and Spinrad (1998), ERSBs are theorized to shape multiple socioemotional processes in children and adolescents, including children's experience of emotion, expression of emotion, emotion-related regulation, and understanding of emotion or emotion knowledge. There are multiple socialization mechanisms through which ERSBs shape children's emotion-related regulatory skills (Morris et al., 2007). These mechanisms include: a) modeling and social learning (e.g., parents who use more problem-focused reactions to children's negative emotions might be modeling problem-solving coping for children), b) direct teaching and coaching (e.g., parents who provide explanations for causes and consequences of emotions are also teaching children emotion knowledge), and c) influencing children's emotional arousal (e.g., parents' frequent expressions of negative-dominant emotions can evoke children's negative arousal and make it challenging for children to self-regulate their emotions).

Emotion Socialization in Asian Parents: Cultural Considerations

By definition, a key goal of ERSBs is to socialize children to experience, express (or not express), and regulate emotion and emotion-related behaviors in accordance with cultural display rules and emotion values (Eisenberg, Cumberland, & Spinrad, 1998). Therefore, when studying ERSBs among Asian families, it is important consider the cultural values, norms, and display rules related to the specific ERSBs. Cross-cultural research has revealed both universality and cultural differences in emotion display rules (Matsumoto et al., 2008). As for universality, individuals of both individualistic cultures (e.g., the United States, Canada, Australia, Denmark) and collective cultures (e.g., Indonesia, Malaysia, South Korea, and China) endorsed greater emotion expressions towards in-group members than out-group members. As for cultural variations, members of individualistic cultures generally endorsed higher levels of emotion expression than those from collective cultures (Matsumoto et al., 2008). Cultural variations were also found in expressions of specific emotions. For example, members from individualistic cultures endorsed higher expressions of fear, happiness, and surprise towards in-group members than those from collective cultures (Matsumoto et al., 2008).

There are also cultural variations in individuals' emotion regulatory strategies. Consistent with the perspective that open expressions of emotion may disrupt social harmony, individuals with Asian heritage tended to suppress their emotions more frequently than those with European heritage (e.g., Gross & John, 2003; Soto et al., 2011). Correspondingly, the adverse mental and physical health consequences of habitual emotion suppression are attenuated among individuals of Asian heritage compared to those with European heritage (e.g., Butler, Lee, & Gross, 2007; Tsai et al., 2017), suggesting that cultural norms might shape the adaptive functions of specific emotion regulatory strategies.

In addition to cultural differences in general emotion expression or emotion regulation, there are cultural variations in the valuing and expressions of positive emotions. According to the affect valuation theory (Tsai, Knutson, & Fung, 2006), individuals of East Asian cultures tend to value low-arousal positive affect (e.g., calm, peaceful, relaxed) more than high-arousal positive affect (e.g., excited, enthusiastic, elated), whereas individuals of European American cultures value high-arousal positive affect more than low-arousal positive affect. Consistent with this theory, Chinese American and Hong Kong Chinese adults valued low-arousal positive affect more than did European American adults (Tsai et al., 2006). Moreover, consistent with the East Asian cultural emphasis on balanced and moderated emotional experiences (Peng et al., 2006), individuals of Asian heritage were more likely to have a balanced view of appropriateness of feeling positive and negative emotions (Senft et al., 2022). In contrast, individuals of European heritage viewed positive emotions as appropriate and negative emotions as neutral to feel, whereas individuals of Latino heritage were the least tolerant of negative emotions (Senft et al., 2022).

Especially relevant to parental ERSBs, Tan et al. (2023) examined cross-cultural differences and similarities in parents' beliefs about children's emotions between Chinese and U.S. mothers with school-age children. Using the Parents' Beliefs About Children's Emotions questionnaire (Halberstadt et al., 2013), they found that Chinese mothers more strongly believed in the negative consequences of excessive positive emotions, children's use of emotion to manipulate others, and that children should deal with their emotions on their own. In contrast, U.S. mothers more strongly believed in the value/acceptance of anger. The two groups held similar beliefs about how much children can control their emotions. Cultural group differences were also found in the association between mothers' emotion beliefs and their self-reported emotion socialization practices: Chinese mothers with stronger beliefs in the negative consequences of positive emotions, children's use of emotions to manipulate others, and children's ability to control emotions reported higher use of emotion coaching, whereas these emotion beliefs were unrelated to emotion coaching among U.S. mothers. These findings suggest that Chinese mothers may view training/teaching children how to control their emotions in culturally appropriate ways as a key focus of emotion coaching (Tan et al., 2023).

Verbal communications of emotion (e.g., emotion talk) also depend on language. By estimating emotion semantics across a sample of 2,474 spoken languages, a linguistic study found evidence of both universal structure and cultural variation in emotion "colexification"—the phenomenon in which languages name semantically related concepts using the same word (Jackson et al., 2019). While all language families differentiate emotions primarily based on valence and physiological activation, emotion concepts have different patterns of association in different language families. For example, while "anxiety" was closely related to "fear" among Tai-Kadai languages, it was more related to "grief" and "regret" amongst Austroasiatic languages (Jackson et al., 2019). Different languages also vary in the amount of emotion words – words that directly refer to specific affective states (Pavlenko, 2008). While there are more than 2,000 emotion words in English (Wallace & Carson, 1973), a linguistic study only estimated about 953 emotion words in Mandarin Chinese (Ng, Cui, & Cavallaro, 2019). Interestingly, there are more negative emotion words than positive emotion words in Mandarin Chinese (Ng et al., 2019). Moreover, cognitive linguistic researchers theorized that the English and Chinese languages differ in their conceptualizations of embodied emotions (Zhou et al., 2022). In Chinese language, emotion concepts are closely linked to bodily sensations of emotion states. Correspondingly, Chinese speakers may be biased toward being more receptive, reflective, and adaptive in linguistic expressions of emotion. In contrast, the English language places bodily reactions as expression of the embodiment of emotions and are subject to overarching control by the brain (and mind). Thus, native English speakers may be biased toward being more reactive, proactive, and interactive in linguistic expressions of emotion (Zhou et al., 2022).

In summary, cross-cultural research and cognitive and linguistic research have revealed both divergences and universality in experiences and expressions of emotion states between Asian and Western cultures and languages. It is important to consider these perspectives when examining the characteristics and socialization functions of ERSBs in Asian-heritage families.

Parental Reactions to Children's Emotions in Asian Families

Researchers have translated and adapted the instruments for parental reactions to children's emotions and evaluated their psychometric properties in Asian heritage families. In a two-wave longitudinal study of urban middle-class Chinese families with school-age children, Tao et al. (2010) adapted the CCNES for Chinese-speaking parents and collected validity data on parenting styles (by parent report) and children's psychological adjustment (by parent, teacher, child, or peer report). Consistent with findings from Western samples, problem- and emotion-focused reactions and encouragement of expression were positively correlated with authoritative parenting and negatively correlated with authoritarian parenting. These three responses are commonly grouped together as "supportive" parental responses. By contrast, punitive and minimizing reactions were positively correlated with authoritarian parenting, and/or negatively correlated with authoritative parenting. These two responses tend to be grouped together as "unsupportive" parental responses. While some cross-cultural consistencies in the relations between CCNES and children adjustment were found (i.e., supportive responses predicted better psychological adjustment and unsupportive responses predicted worse psychological adjustment over time), cultural differences were also observed. Specifically, neither encouragement of emotion expression nor minimizing responses were associated with children's psychological adjustment in Chinese children, divergent from the findings in Western samples. Tao et al. (2010) speculated that given cultural variations in valuing of emotion expression, the socialization functions of encouragement (or minimizing) of emotion expression likely depend on the goal and context of parenting: the parental response with the goal of supporting and validating (vs. dismissing or punishing) children's emotions that occurs in the context of a warm and supportive (vs. harsh and coercive) parenting can be beneficial (vs. detrimental) for children's adjustment. Indeed, in a sample of Chinese immigrant mothers with school-age children, Vu et al. (2021) found that mothers' greater Asian cultural values buffered the negative effects of their emotion dismissing reactions on children's anger and sadness responses during a disappointment task.

Raval et al. (2018) adapted the CCNES for Chinese and Indian families by adding culturally salient responses to children's emotions (e.g., explanation-oriented responses, scolding, and not talking to the child for a brief period for Indian families, and child training for Chinese families). In a cross-cultural study of urban, middle-class families with middle school-age children in India and China, Raval et al. (2018) examined the factor structure of CCNES and tested their links to parental socialization goals (mother report) and children's emotion regulation (child report) and behavioral problems (mother report). Consistent with the hypotheses, they found that emotion-focused, problem-focused, child training, and explanation-oriented responses loaded on the factor of supportive responses, whereas punitive responses, scolding, and not talking loaded on the factor of nonsupportive responses. Inconsistent with the hypotheses, they found that expressive encouragement loaded on the unsupportive factor, and minimizing responses loaded positively on both factors. Consistent with Tao et al. (2010), neither expressive encouragement nor minimizing were associated with any child outcomes (Raval et al., 2018). Altan-Aytun et al. (2013) evaluated the CCNES in a sample of mothers of preschoolers in urban, middle-class Turkish families. They found that problem-focused, emotion-focused, and encouragement of emotion expression were positively correlated with each other, consistent with the conceptual grouping of supportive responses. In contrast, minimizing and punitive responses were positively correlated, consistent with the conceptual grouping of nonsupportive responses.

Wang and colleagues (Shi, Fan, & Wang, 2024) performed cultural analysis of parental minimizing reactions to adolescents' negative emotions through the lens of Chinese culture and distinguished two types of minimizing reactions commonly displayed by urban Chinese parents: a) devaluing/invalidating the significance of adolescents' emotions (e.g., telling the child they are making too big a deal out of it) and b) discounting the seriousness of the cause of children's emotions (e.g., telling the child that things are as bad as they seem). In two samples of urban Chinese adolescents, they found evidence that adolescents' perceived maternal devaluing/invalidating and discounting/mitigating reactions were two distinct factors and showed different relations to adolescents' socioemotional functioning (Shi et al., 2024).

While prior studies focused primarily on mothers, researchers have begun to examine fathers' reactions to children's emotions. For example,

Wang et al. (2019) used a person-centered approach to identify latent profiles of Chinese fathers' responses to adolescents' negative emotions in a school-based sample of 743 adolescents in urban China. In line with the Chinese cultural expectations of fathers as the role model within the family to practice the value of emotion control, they identified four profiles: a supportive profile (34.1 percent) of fathers who displayed high levels of warmth/responsiveness and expressive encouragement and low levels of punitive and minimizing reactions, a balanced profile (44.2 percent) displaying moderate levels of supportive and nonsupportive responses, a disengaged profile displaying low levels supportive and nonsupportive responses (14.9%), and a harsh profile with high levels of nonsupportive responses and low levels of supportive responses (6.8%). Chinese adolescents with supportive and balanced fathers were more likely to use cognitive reappraisal, an emotion regulatory strategy associated with better psychological adjustment (Wang et al., 2019). In another sample of 195 Chinese school-age children and their mothers and fathers, Han et al., (2015) tested the concurrent associations among mothers' and fathers' emotion regulation, maternal and paternal reactions to children's negative emotions, and children's emotion regulation. They found that maternal and paternal supportive reactions to children's negative emotions mediated the links between maternal and paternal emotion regulation and children's emotion regulation. Moreover, the link between parents' supportive reactions and children's emotion regulation was moderated by emotion regulation of the co-caregiver, such that having a well-regulated co-parent can amplify the benefit of parental supportive emotion socialization on children's emotion regulation.

Song et al. (2019) modified the scenarios in CCNES to assess how parents react to children's positive emotions (e.g., happiness, excitement, proud, and desire). In a cross-cultural study of 117 school-age children of European American (EA) and Chinese American (CA) mothers, Song et al. (2019) grouped maternal responses to children's positive emotions into two categories based on theory and factor analysis: savoring responses (expressive encouragement and problem-focused reactions), and dampening responses (punitive, emotion-focused, and minimizing reactions). Compared to EA mothers, CA mothers scored higher on dampening responses, although the two groups did not differ on savoring responses. While maternal savoring reactions were associated with children's better emotional adjustment, the relation between dampening reactions and child adjustment was moderated by culture group. Specifically, dampening was marginally associated with children's lower emotion knowledge in the EA group (but not in the CA group). The findings provided further evidence that the socialization function of parental reactions depends on the cultural context.

Parental Emotion Expression in Asian Families

Consistent with cultural psychology perspectives on cultural variations in emotion expression, researchers found cultural group differences in parental emotion expression. In two studies of Mainland Chinese mothers, CA mothers, and EA mothers with preschool-age children, Camras and colleagues (Camras et al., 2005, 2008) found that Mainland Chinese and CA mothers self-reported more positive emotional expressions in the family (using the SEFQ measure) than EA mothers. Interestingly, CA mothers scored between EA and Mainland Chinese mothers, although they did not consistently differ from Mainland Chinese mothers, indicating the potential influence of acculturation. No significant differences were found for expression of negative emotion, and no child-gender differences were found. Chen et al. (2011) further investigated the socialization function of parental emotion expression in Chinese families. In the same longitudinal sample of urban Chinese families with school-age children as Tao et al. (2010), Chinese parents' (mostly mothers') self-reported negative-dominant expressivity (e.g., anger, frustration, contempt) predicted children's higher externalizing problems (measured by parent-, teacher-, and peer-ratings) after controlling for prior externalizing problems (Chen et al., 2011). Concurrent relations were also found between parental expressivity and global parenting styles: positive expressivity was associated with higher authoritative parenting, whereas negative-dominant expressivity and negative-submissive expressivity (e.g., embarrassment, disappointment, crying) were associated with higher authoritarian parenting (Chen et al., 2011).

To test the hypothesis that acculturation (i.e., changes that happen as a result of contact with different cultures, Gibson, 2001) shapes parental emotion expression in immigrant families, Chen et al. (2015) investigated the links between degrees of Chinese (heritage) cultural orientation and American (host) cultural orientation and parental emotion expression in a longitudinal study of Chinese American families with first- and second-generation school-age children. They measured parental expression using parent-reported SEFQ and observed emotional expressions in a parent–child problem-solving task. Interestingly, they found the associations between cultural orientations and parental emotion expression varied by both the domains of cultural orientations and the components/measures of emotion expression. Specifically, cultural orientations (in domains of language proficiency and media use) were primarily associated with self-reported expressivity, such that higher American orientations were associated with higher self-reported expressivity, whereas higher Chinese orientation was associated with lower self-reported expressivity. By contrast, cultural orientations were mostly unrelated to observed parental emotion expression, although with one exception: higher American orientation (in the domain of social interactions with American friends) was associated with greater observed positive affect. The findings suggest that acculturation might shape parental emotion expression in complex processes: while language proficiency and media use may influence emotion expression through emotion values, social interactions with members of other culture(s) may influence emotion expression through social learning (e.g., observation).

In one of the first studies examining fathers' emotion expression in Asian families, Li and Li (2018) used an observational approach to study the dynamic relations between fathers' and their school-age children's emotional expressivity during a real-time father-child problem-solving interaction in a sample of 85 urban Chinese families. Fathers' and children's verbal, facial, and behavioral expression were separately coded at every 5-second interval on a 3-point scale (1 = positive, 0 = neutral, −1 = negative). The time-series data allowed researchers to examine within- and between-person variations in Chinese fathers' emotional expressivity, as well as the dynamic and bidirectional relations between fathers' and children's emotional expressivity. Li and Li (2018) found that at the within-individual level, fathers' and children's emotional expressivity changed as a function of each other concurrently but not subsequently. At the between-individual level, both initial levels and later changes in fathers' emotional expressivity were associated with fathers' perceptions of children's emotion regulation, and initial level of fathers' emotional expressivity was also associated with their emotion-related beliefs. In sum, contrary to the traditional gender role expectation of Chinese fathers as being "strict," "tough," and refraining from openly expressing emotions (especially positive emotions), considerable heterogeneity was found in contemporary Chinese fathers' emotional expressivity (including positive expressivity). Chinese fathers expressed a range of emotions when interacting with their children, and they adjusted their emotional expressivity based on children's emotion regulation.

Parent–Child Emotion Talk in Asian Families

In a series of papers, Q. Wang and colleagues examined cultural variations in mother–child conversations of emotionally salient events using an emotion reminiscing task. Compared to European American dyads, Chinese dyads used more negative words overall but engaged in fewer negotiations of emotion (Fivush & Wang, 2005). Wang and Fivush (2005) coded each conversation turn based on its narrative style, self/social content, and emotional content. They found qualitative differences in the narrative style and content of conversations between cultural groups: European American mothers initiated more interactive and elaborative conversations that focused on the child's roles and predilections in the study, and they employed a "cognitive approach" when discussing emotion-related content by providing explanations for the cause of emotions. In contrast, Chinese American mothers took a directive role by asking and repeating memory questions and focusing on social interaction, and they used a "behavioral approach" to emotion regulation by emphasizing negative consequences of children's behaviors. Interestingly, Wang (2013) compared emotion talk styles between immigrant Chinese families in the U.S. and native Chinese families in Beijing using an emotion reminiscing task and a storytelling task. Immigrant Chinese mothers appeared more "Chinese" in their emotion talk: they attributed fewer emotions to their children during reminiscing but ascribed more emotions to the story protagonist during storytelling, and they provided fewer explanations of emotions in both tasks compared to native Chinese mothers, who displayed a more Western pattern of emotion talk. Wang (2013) attributed the subgroup difference to increasing influences of Western ideology in urban China and strong desires to preserve traditional Chinese values among Chinese immigrant families.

Tao et al. (2013) examined within-cultural variations in mother–child emotion talk in Chinese American immigrant families with school-age children using a shared book-reading task. They found that the first-generation Chinese immigrant mothers with higher Chinese orientation asked fewer emotion question, provided fewer emotion explanations, and overall displayed less elaborative emotion talk compared to those with lower Chinese orientation. The above relations were found after controlling for socioeconomic status, mother's age, child age, gender, generation status, and the length, elaborateness, and language of storytelling. Using longitudinal follow-up data from the same sample, Curtis et al. (2020) examined the implications of parental emotion talk to children's socioemotional development. They found that the latent factor of parental emotion talk was prospectively related to children's higher effortful control controlling for stability, and that higher effortful control was concurrently related to children's higher sympathy and more socially appropriate behaviors. The findings provided support for the socioemotional benefits of emotion talk for Chinese immigrant children.

Chan et al. (2023a, 2023b, 2024) examined parental emotion talk with preschoolers from low-income families across three cultural groups: Chinese immigrant and Mexican immigrant families in the U.S., and Chinese-heritage families in Taiwan. They found that Chinese immigrant parents used fewer emotion explanations and engaged in less elaborate emotion talk than Mexican immigrant parents and Taiwanese parents. Furthermore, socioeconomic factors (parental education and income) were positively associated with quantity and quality of emotion talk, and parents' heritage culture orientation was associated with more elaborate emotion talk among immigrant families (Chan et al., 2023a). Consistent with Curtis et al. (2020), some socioemotional benefits of emotion talk were found such that parents' greater use of positive emotion words were associated with fewer externalizing problems in children, and parents' more elaborate emotion talk was associated with children's more open expressions of negative emotions during a frustration task (Chan et al., 2023b, 2024).

Using an innovative parent–child affirmation discussion task, Williams et al. (2024) conducted qualitative analyses of parents' verbal expressions of love and affection to children in a sample of 110 Chinese American immigrant families with school-age children (age = 7–11 years). They identified three types of parental verbal expressions of love: training (parental control motivated by love), relational affection (affirmation of the parent–child or family relationships and roles), and validation (acceptance of children's independent expressions of self). Frequencies of parental use of training and validation were positively associated with child-rated parent–child attachment security. The findings demonstrated that Chinese American immigrant families draw on both Chinese (heritage) and American (host) cultural scripts to express love and care to children (Williams et al., 2024).

Emerging Directions and Implications for Parenting Interventions for Asian Families

As we conclude this literature review, we have observed a few encouraging trends in the research on ERSBs in Asian families. First, researchers are increasingly utilizing more rigorous research designs and methods, such as the use of longitudinal study to examine changes in ERSBs and the directional relations between ERSBs and child outcomes, as well as the use of multi-method (e.g., questionnaire, behavioral observation, ecologically momentary assessment) assessments. Second, more researchers began to study ERSBs in Asian fathers, a population largely ignored by earlier literature. Third, while earlier studies often sampled two-parents, middle-class families, recent studies began to study ERSBs in demographically and socioeconomically more diverse samples (e.g., Chinese families with left-behind children, Wang et al., 2021). Fourth, studies examining sociocultural influences on ERSBs have increasingly utilized different research designs to operationalize "culture," including cross-cultural comparative studies, within-cultural studies of migrant and immigrant families, and studies examining cohort differences in parenting in a changing historical context (e.g., X. Chen et al., 2021).

This line of research has implications for designing and adapting parenting interventions for Asian families. Importantly, emerging findings from this field has provided theoretical justifications for ERSBs as a key target of parenting interventions for Asian-heritage families. Indeed, in a randomized controlled trial of 104 low- to middle-SES families with preschool-age children in Hong Kong, Chan et al. (2021) evaluated the intervention effects of *Turning to Kids*, an evidence-based parenting program developed in Western populations targeting emotion coaching, on Chinese parenting, parental reactions to children's emotion, parenting stress and parental emotion regulation, and children's emotion regulation. Compared to the waitlist control group, the intervention group reported reduced punitive parenting and parenting stress at both post-intervention and six-week follow-up. Moreover, the intervention group displayed improvements in parents' use of expressive encouragement and children's emotion regulation at six-week follow-up. Furthermore, Fabrizio et al. (2015) developed a culturally appropriate, brief, preventive interaction program for Hong Kong Chinese families, *Effective Parenting Programme* (EPP), by partnering with local community. The EPP is a cognitive-behavioral therapy-based intervention targeting parents' emotion management strategies and parent–child relationship. In a randomized controlled trial of a community sample of 412 Hong Kong middle- and low-income mothers with school-age children, the EPP group (compared to an informational control group) demonstrated improvements in mothers' use of adaptive emotion management strategies during parent–child interactions, lower negative affect and greater positive affect, and improved psychological wellbeing and perceived family harmony at three-, six-, and 12- month follow up (Fabrizio et al., 2015). Together, these two studies have provided promising evidence that targeting parental ERSBs is an effective intervention pathway to strengthen parent–child relationship, improve family functioning, and promote children's socioemotional competence and wellbeing in Asian families.

References

Altan-Aytun, Ö., Yagmurlu, B., & Yavuz, H. M. (2013). Turkish mothers' coping with children's negative emotions: A brief report. *Journal of Child and Family Studies, 22,* 437–443.

Butler, E. A., Lee, T. L., & Gross, J. J. (2007). Emotion regulation and culture: Are the social consequences of emotion suppression culture-specific? *Emotion, 7*(1), 30.

Camras, L. A., Chen, Y., Bakeman, R., Norris, K., & Cain, T.R. (2005). Emotional expression in Chinese, Chinese American, adopted Chinese and European American children. *Emotion, 6*(1), 103–114.

Camras, L. A., Kolmodin, K., & Chen, Y. (2008). Mothers' self-reported emotional expression in Mainland Chinese, Chinese American and European American families. *International Journal of Behavioral Development, 32*(5), 459–463.

Cervantes, C. A. (2002). Explanatory emotion talk in Mexican immigrant and Mexican American families. *Hispanic Journal of Behavioral Sciences, 24*(2), 138–163.

Chan, M., Taw, M., Eisenberg, N., & Zhou, Q. (2024). *Relations between parental emotion talk and preschoolers' emotion expression and regulatory behaviors in low-income Chinese American and Mexican American families.* Unpublished manuscript.

Chan, M., Teng, D., Teng, Y. P. T., & Zhou, Q. (2023a). Parent emotion talk with preschoolers from low-income Mexican American and Chinese American families: Links to sociocultural factors. *Social Development, 32*(2), 481–500.

Chan, M., Williams, A. I., Teng, Y. P. T., & Zhou, Q. (2023b). Links between parent–child emotion talk and preschoolers' socioemotional behaviors in Chinese-heritage families. *Early Education and Development, 34*(2), 366–386.

Chan, R. F. Y., Qiu, C., & Shum, K. K. M. (2021). Tuning in to kids: A randomized controlled trial of an emotion coaching parenting program for Chinese parents in Hong Kong. *Developmental Psychology, 57*(11), 1796.

Chen, S. H., Zhou, Q., Eisenberg, N., Valiente, C., & Wang, Y. (2011). Parental expressivity and parenting styles in Chinese families: Prospective and unique relations to children's psychological adjustment. *Parenting, 11*(4), 288–307.

Chen, S. H., Zhou, Q., Main, A., & Lee, E. H. (2015). Chinese American immigrant parents' emotional expression in the family: Relations with parents' cultural orientations and children's emotion-related regulation. *Cultural Diversity and Ethnic Minority Psychology, 21*(4), 619.

Chen, X., Chen, X., Zhao, S., Way, N., Yoshikawa, H., Zhang, G., Deng, H., Cao, R., Chen, H., & Li, D. (2021). Autonomy- and connectedness-oriented behaviors of toddlers and mothers at different historical times in urban China. *Developmental Psychology, 57*(8), 1254–1260.

Curtis, K., Zhou, Q., & Tao, A. (2020). Emotion talk in Chinese American immigrant families and longitudinal links to children's socioemotional competence. *Developmental Psychology, 56*(3), 475–488.

Darling, N. & Steinberg, L. (1993). Parenting style as context: An integrative model. *Psychological Bulletin, 113,* 487–496.

Eisenberg, N., Cumberland, A., & Spinrad, T. L. (1998). Parental socialization of emotion. *Psychological Inquiry*, *9*(4), 241–273.

Eisenberg, N., Spinrad, T. L., & Cumberland, A. (1998). The socialization of emotion: Reply to commentaries. *Psychological Inquiry*, *9*(4), 317–333.

Fabes, R. A., Poulin, R. E., Eisenberg, N., & Madden-Derdich, D. A. (2002). The Coping with Children's Negative Emotions Scale (CCNES): Psychometric properties and relations with children's emotional competence. *Marriage & Family Review, 34,* 285–310.

Fabrizio, C. S., Lam, T. H., Hirschmann, M. R., Pang, I., Yu, N. X., Wang, X., & Stewart, S. M. (2015). Parental emotional management benefits family relationships: A randomized controlled trial in Hong Kong, China. *Behaviour Research and Therapy, 71,* 115–124.

Fivush, R. & Wang, Q. (2005) Emotion talk in mother–child conversations of the shared past: The effects of culture, gender, and event valence, *Journal of Cognition and Development, 6*(4), 489–50.

Gibson, M. A. (2001). Immigrant adaptation and patterns of acculturation. *Human Development, 44,* 19–23.

Gross, J. J. & John, O. P. (2003). Individual differences in two emotion regulation processes: Implications for affect, relationships, and well-being. *Journal of Personality and Social Psychology, 85*(2), 348.

Halberstadt, A. G., Cassidy, J., Stifer, C. A., Parke, R. D., & Fox, N. A. (1995). Self-expressiveness within the family context: Psychometric support for a new measure. *Psychological Assessment, 7,* 93–103.

Halberstadt, A. G., Dunsmore, J. C., Bryant Jr., A., Parker, A. E., Beale, K. S., & Thompson, J. A. (2013). Development and validation of the parents' beliefs about children's emotions questionnaire. *Psychological Assessment, 25*(4), 1195–1210.

Han, Z. R., Qian, J., Gao, M., & Dong, J. (2015). Emotion socialization mechanisms linking Chinese fathers', mothers', and children's emotion regulation: A moderated mediation model. *Journal of Child and Family Studies, 24,* 3570–3579.

Herbers, J. E., Garcia, E. B., & Obradović, J. (2017). Parenting assessed by observation versus parent-report: Moderation by parent distress and family socioeconomic status. *Journal of Child and Family Studies, 26,* 3339–3350.

Huang, S. & Kan, P. F. (2021). Chinese American immigrant parents' socialization of emotions in bilingual bicultural preschool children. *Frontiers in Psychology, 12,* 642417.

Jackson, J. C., Watts, J., Henry, T. R., List, J. M., Forkel, R., Mucha, P. J.,... & Lindquist, K. A. (2019). Emotion semantics show both cultural variation and universal structure. *Science, 366*(6472), 1517–1522.

Li, D. & Li, X. (2019). Within-and between-individual variation in fathers' emotional expressivity in Chinese families: Contributions of children's emotional expressivity and fathers' emotion-related beliefs and perceptions. *Social Development, 28*(4), 960–978.

Lorenzo, N. E., Bahrick, L. E., & Bagner, D. M. (2023). Examining the trajectory of parent emotion talk in mothers of toddlers: A predominantly Latine sample. *Infant Behavior and Development, 70,* 101801.

Matsumoto, D., Yoo, S. H., & Fontaine, J., et al. (2008). Mapping expressive differences around the world: The relationship between emotional display rules and individualism versus collectivism. *Journal of Cross-Cultural Psychology, 39*(1), 55–74.

Morris, A. S., Silk, J. S., Steinberg, L., Myers, S. S., & Robinson, L. R. (2007). The role of the family context in the development of emotion regulation. *Social Development, 16*(2), 361–388.

Ng, B. C., Cui, C., & Cavallaro, F. (2019) The annotated lexicon of Chinese emotion words, *Word, 65*(2), 73–92.

Pavlenko, A. (2008). Emotion and emotion-laden words in the bilingual lexicon. *Bilingualism: Language and Cognition 11*(2), 147–64.

Peng, K., Spencer-Rodgers, J., & Nian, Z. (2006). Naïve dialecticism and the Tao of Chinese thought. In U. Kim, K.-S. Yang, & K.-K. Hwang (Eds), *Indigenous and cultural psychology: Understanding people in context* (pp. 247–262).

Raval, V. V., Li, X., Deo, N., & Hu, J. (2018). Reports of maternal socialization goals, emotion socialization behaviors, and child functioning in China and India. *Journal of Family Psychology, 32*(1), 81.

Senft, N., Doucerain, M. M., Campos, B., Shiota, M. N., & Chentsova-Dutton, Y. E. (2023). Within-and between-group heterogeneity in cultural models of emotion among people of European, Asian, and Latino heritage in the United States. *Emotion, 23*(1), 1.

Shi, Z., Fan, L., & Wang, Q. (2024). Scrutinizing parental minimization reactions to adolescents' negative emotions through the lens of Chinese culture. *Journal of Research on Adolescence*. https://doi.org/10.1111/jora.12918.

Song, Q., Yang, Y., Doan, S. N., & Wang, Q. (2019). Savoring or dampening? Maternal reactions to children's positive emotions in cultural contexts. *Culture and Brain, 7*, 172–189.

Soto, J. A., Perez, C. R., Kim, Y. H., Lee, E. A., & Minnick, M. R. (2011). Is expressive suppression always associated with poorer psychological functioning? A cross-cultural comparison between European Americans and Hong Kong Chinese. *Emotion, 11*(6), 1450.

Tan, L., Smith, C. L., & Dunsmore, J. C. (2023). Validation of a Chinese translation of the Parents' Beliefs About Children's Emotions questionnaire and measurement invariance across Chinese and US mothers. *Current Psychology, 42*(16), 13486–13496.

Tao, A., Zhou, Q., Lau, N., & Liu, H. (2013). Chinese American immigrant mothers' discussion of emotion with children: Relations to cultural orientations. *Journal of Cross-Cultural Psychology, 44*(3), 478–501.

Tao, A., Zhou, Q., & Wang, Y. (2010). Parental reactions to children's negative emotions: prospective relations to Chinese children's psychological adjustment. *Journal of Family Psychology, 24*(2), 135–144.

of emotion with children: Relations to cultural orientations. *Journal of Cross-Cultural Psychology, 44*(3), 478–501.

Tsai, J. L., Knutson, B., & Fung, H. H. (2006). Cultural variation in affect valuation. *Journal of Personality and Social Psychology, 90*(2), 288–307.

Tsai, W., Nguyen, D. J., Weiss, B., Ngo, V., & Lau, A. S. (2017). Cultural differences in the reciprocal relations between emotion suppression coping, depressive symptoms and interpersonal functioning among adolescents. *Journal of Abnormal Child Psychology, 45*(4), 657–669.

Vu, K. T., Cheah, C. S., & Halberstadt, A. G. (2023). Chinese immigrant child and maternal reactions to disappointment: Cultural fit impacts the bidirectional associations. *Social Development, 32*(2), 445–462.

Wallace, A. F. & Carson, M. T. (1973). Sharing and diversity in emotion terminology. *Ethos,* 1–29.

Wang, M., Liang, Y., Zhou, N., & Zou, H. (2019). Chinese fathers' emotion socialization profiles and adolescents' emotion regulation. *Personality and Individual Differences, 137*, 33–38.

Wang, Q. (2001). "Did you have fun?": American and Chinese mother–child conversations about shared emotional experiences. *Cognitive Development, 16*(2), 693–715.

Wang, Q. (2013). Chinese socialization and emotion talk between mothers and children in native and immigrant Chinese families. *Asian American Journal of Psychology, 4*(3), 185.

Wang, Q. & Fivush, R. (2005). Mother–child conversations of emotionally salient events: exploring the functions of emotional reminiscing in European-American and Chinese families. *Social Development, 14*(3), 473–495.

Wang, Y., Liu, W., Wang, W., Lin, S., Lin, D., & Wang, H. (2021). Left-behind children's social adjustment and relationship with parental coping with children's negative emotions during the COVID-19 pandemic in China. *International Journal of Psychology, 56*(4), 512–521.

Williams, A. I., Liu, C., Zhou, Q., Wu, J., Meng, L., Deng, X. F., & Chen, S. H. (2024). Parental expressions of love in Chinese American immigrant families: Implications for children's attachment security. *Developmental Science, 27(6), e13549*. https://doi.org/10.1111/desc.13549.

Zhou, P., Critchley, H., Nagai, Y., & Wang, C. (2022). Divergent conceptualization of embodied emotions in the English and Chinese languages. *Brain Sciences, 12*(7), 911.

9

FATHERS IN ASIAN FAMILIES

(Changing) Contexts of Traditions, Cultures, and Religions

Xuan Li, Yeon-Jin Kim, and Ziarat Hossain

Parenting research used to focus heavily on mothers, who are assumed to be the primary figure in childrearing and family functioning. The current fathering and fatherhood scholarship, burgeoning since the 1970s (Lamb, 2000), is grounded in WEIRD (western, educated, industrialized, rich, democratic) societies and in so doing have generated the most empirical evidence and theories that set the norm for later research. Notwithstanding Asia's representation of the world's population and its vast economic, language, cultural, and religious diversity, socioculturally sensitive inquiries on fathering and fatherhood in Asian contexts remain disappointingly scarce. Although notable research has been conducted on fathers in many Asian societies including Bangladesh (e.g., Hossain & Atencio, 2017; Jesmin & Seward, 2011), China (e.g., Li, 2020a), India (e.g., Chaudhury, 2013), Japan (e.g., Hertog et al, 2021), Malaysia (e.g., Hossain & Madon, 2021), and South Korea (Kim, 2022), existing studies tend to be segregated by national borders. Whereas single-country studies can unpack nationally specific contexts of fathering and produce valuable locally relevant knowledge, they exclude the possibility of identifying themes and patterns across borders that may lead to theoretical innovations regarding fathering and fatherhood.

Guided by Bronfenbrenner's (1977) ecological systems theory that recognizes the embeddedness of individuals and families in broader sociocultural contexts and by the intersectional perspective that emphasizes within-group diversity and meaningful cross-group comparisons of seemingly divergent groups (Cole, 2009), this chapter addresses the literature gap by examining fathers in multiple Asian societies. Although an

DOI: 10.4324/9781003383949-9

exhaustive coverage of all factors related to fathering and fatherhood in all Asian societies would be unrealistic, we surveyed fathers' roles and practices in three major sets of Asian societies with different cultural traditions and modernization status and pathways, namely China, South Korea, and Bangladesh, India, and Malaysia. By discussing similarities and discrepancies in fathering and fatherhood in these contexts, we attempt to shed light on how knowledge about Asian fathers will contribute to global research on fathering and fatherhood.

Before presenting specific cases, we would like to draw attention to several contextual factors that are particularly relevant to fathering and fatherhood in Asia. First, Asian societies differ dramatically in general socioeconomic development, inequality, and welfare, ranging from developing countries where substantial fractions of the population still suffer from poverty (such as India and China) to developed economies with functional family welfare schemes, including paternity leave (such as Japan and Korea). These socioeconomic climates impose varying levels of financial stress, insecurity, and perceived deprivation and hope for Asian fathers to actualize their role as providers and caregivers. Second, unlike Euro-American societies where the nuclear family is normative, extended family members (such as grandparents, uncles, and aunts) are highly involved in childrearing in Asia families (Dommaraju & Wong, 2022). The regular presence of non-parental familial caregivers regulates the quantity and quality of father involvement and situates the father's roles in a complicated web of family relationships. Third, fatherhood in Asian societies is shaped by the dynamic interplay of traditional value systems and modern ideals about family life, gender roles, and parent–child relations. Whereas several Asian traditional value systems accord fathers with high prestige, modernization, political ideology, and the changing status of women redefine social expectations for paternal roles in varying ways. The regionally specific manifestations of such common patterns will be elaborated in the sections below.

Fathers in Chinese Societies

Neo-Confucian traditions

Chinese fathers' roles in child development and family functioning are heavily influenced by neo-Confucian ideals and practices that center around patriarchy, patrilocality, and patrilineality. A man's social identity is defined by his position in his paternal lineage, and his value is estimated through his contribution to the continuation and glorification of his paternal family name. Childbearing is the enactment of one's masculine filial duties to one's parents and ancestors and is a necessary marker for socially recognized manhood (Greenhalgh, 2015). In practice, as young couples typically resided with the groom's parents, fathers' parental roles often coexist with their filial roles, both allowing fathers to resort to grandparents as a childcare resource and requiring them to consider grandparents in everyday financial and care arrangements.

Nested in the intergenerational family, the father's and the mother's roles are complementary and hierarchical: The father is responsible for accruing financial and social capital for the family whereas the mother manages housework, child- and eldercare, and family relationships. Nevertheless, although the father is expected to remain distant from hands-on care work, he has the power to make important decisions such as those concerning his children's education, work, and marriage arrangements. The father should also educate and discipline his children and role-model desirable behaviors by dint of his moral and intellectual superiority as a man. To fulfill such expectations, good fathers are supposed to restrain their affection and act in a strict, stern way to strengthen their authority. Towards sons, in particular, fathers are expected to demonstrate culturally desired masculinity through a strong reservation of emotions, including positive emotions (Li, 2020a).

Variations and social changes

Historical and social science research on Chinese families suggests that some traditional values have an enduring impact on modern Chinese fathers, such as the importance of childbearing (Greenhalgh, 2015) and fathers' roles in children's education (Cao & Lin, 2018; Lau, 2016). However, one must be cautious to infer from traditional fatherhood "culture" when describing and interpreting the "conduct" of contemporary Chinese fathers. Even in pre-modern China, several notable literary figures have expressed their care towards their children and mourned their deaths, whereas others left traces of their attentiveness to their children's everyday care and valuation of emotional intimacy with their children, especially daughters (Lu, 2010). Admittedly, little is known about the extent to which Confucian family ethics were practiced beyond the elite literati class. It is therefore critical to note both the ideological doctrine about fatherhood as well as the behavioral deviation in reality.

Chinese fatherhood ideals have also been changing throughout China's complicated modernization processes. In particular, Chinese fathers' intergenerational power over their children has been consistently challenged by the self-critical "New Cultural Movement" in the early 20th century, the socialist revolution which officially overturned patriarchal power in the mid-20th-century, and the fertility decline since the 1970s. Meanwhile,

Chinese fathers' gender privilege is only partially shaken by China's early feminist movements, the socialist gender reform, and global cultural imports since China's rejoining of the global market in the late 1970s (Li, 2020a). These multitude of political, cultural, and economic changes created a context for fathers that mixes persisting traditions and contemporary characteristics. Urban Chinese fathers in the 1990s and 2000s already expressed awareness of involvement in childcare (Liu, 1995; Zhang & Xu, 2008). A recent interview-based study suggested that urban middle-class Chinese fathers embrace caring masculinity and emphasize their roles in providing routine care and companionship to their children, although provision and gender role modeling remain important for some (Wang & Keizer, 2024).

Today's Chinese fathers, like mothers, face competing demands from the globalizing intensive parenthood culture and the ever-greedier neoliberal economy. To cultivate modern citizens that would thrive in fierce competition, Chinese fathers are encouraged to assume individual responsibilities in supporting children's socioemotional development (Tan, 2020) through abundant interaction, autonomy-granting, and nurturance, and are expected to instil their sons' and daughters' "masculine" skills and traits such as STEM capacities, bravery, and perseverance (Li et al., 2024). Yet the retreating state welfare, reversing official gender ideology, and exploitative workplaces leave Chinese fathers with little motivation or resources to engage in family life: The spiraling childrearing costs push fathers to work more, and the absence of an effectively enforced paternity leave excludes fathers from early childcare. As a result, even new generations of middle-class fathers are poorly prepared for parenthood, and their rural counterparts often suffer from the emotional turmoil of parting from their children in pursuit of breadwinning fatherhood (Choi & Peng, 2016). As of 2020, 11.2 percent of Chinese children under 18 years old live with their mothers only, and 16.7 percent with neither parents (UNICEF, 2020), amounting to 27.9 percent of Chinese children living without fathers.

Father involvement in childrearing

Despite the absence of nationally representative data on father involvement, existing evidence suggests that Chinese fathers' involvement remains limited. Findings from a stratified sample of 30,000 respondents suggested that mothers are primarily responsible for daily care among 76.1 percent of families with minors (i.e., children 0–17 years), and mothers are the day-time caregiver of 63.7 percent of all 0–3 children (Fourth Survey on Women's Social Status, 2020). Notably, in approximately two-thirds of all families with minors, mothers also shoulder the main responsibility for homework monitoring and sending children to and from school, tasks that are culturally deemed "masculine." That is, even without accounting for grandparental support in childcare, Chinese fathers fall short in their share of childcare. In another telling survey among urban and rural families with 0-to-6-years-olds across five Chinese provinces, fewer fathers took charge of their children's daily meal arrangements and clothing than grandparents (China National Center for Children, 2017). Similarly, data from the Taiwan Education Panel Survey which includes over 8,000 families with adolescents indicated that fathers also fall behind the mothers in their education involvement (Hsu et al., 2011).

But there are also signs of positive change. The Fourth Survey on Women's Social Status cited above pointed out that, among formally employed women under 35 years of age, 81.2 percent of their partners have taken some paternity leave and 70.8 percent have taken more than seven days off, although the proportion of these fathers account for among all fathers is unclear. Ni and colleagues' (2024) survey among urban Chinese families during the COVID-19 pandemic found that the lockdown situation created opportunities for middle-class fathers to increase their participation in childrearing. In an interesting analysis of two waves of data collected in 2004 and 2011 among young parents with children under six, Zhao (2018) found a slight increase in men's participation in childcare over time, from 11.2 hours per week to 15.9 hours per week (versus 27.6 and 26.4 hours per week, among the mothers).

Today's Chinese fathers appear to have denounced the neo-Confucian expectation that requires them to be the strict and stern disciplinarian, at least attitudinally. Although a recent meta-analysis found Chinese fathers to be less warm, responsive, and supportive than mothers in the eyes of their adolescent children (Dou et al., 2020), numerous qualitative and quantitative studies consistently found that Chinese fathers embrace emotional intimacy with their children. Li's (2020b) interviews with urban and rural Chinese families provided rich accounts of diverse culturally colored ways in which Chinese fathers demonstrate warmth towards their school-age children, such as by cooking their children's favorite dishes or providing help with schoolwork. In fact, several studies found the tradition-reversing pattern of "strict mother, warm father" in Mainland China, Taiwan, and Hong Kong (Dou et al., 2020; Huang et al., 2024; Xie & Li; 2019). This newly emerging trend may signify both a genuine pursuit of Chinese fathers towards greater equality and intimacy with their children, and fathers' marginal role in everyday childrearing which limits their frequency to discipline the child. Whatever the reason, fathers' warm, supportive parenting is repeatedly found to benefit their children's academic and socioemotional development in China, like in other Asian and non-Asian societies (e.g., Liu et al., 2021; Su et al., 2019; Zhang et al., 2021).

At the same time, the quality of Chinese fathers' involvement is worrisome. Several studies found that rural Chinese children living with their father only (with a migrant mother) fared the worst in physical and mental health and academic development, not only compared to children living with both parents but also compared to those living with a mother only (with a migrant father) (Li & Zang, 2010; Zhao et al., 2014; Xu et al., 2019). In fact, father migration benefits children's adjustment, through maternal support, whereas mirroring benefits of paternal support in cases of mother migration were not found (Chen et al., 2019). Such discrepancies may indicate a lower quality of care and parenting provided by stay-behind fathers compared to stay-behind mothers. These findings may also be attributable to the normativeness of father migration in China where stay-behind fatherhood is often confounded with other family adversities that undermine optimal child development.

Taken together, fathers in Chinese societies are inclined to form less hierarchical and more intimate relationships with their children, but continue to adhere to traditional expectations of their secondary position in everyday caregiving. Amidst fierce global economic competition, increased expectations for father involvement remain unsupported by public policy or workplace culture. This makes it difficult for even privileged urban Chinese men to fulfill their aspirations to become involved parents, let alone rural fathers who face the hard choice between breadwinning and participating in their children's lives. Meanwhile, more evidence is needed on changes in father involvement across the lifespan, including into their children's adulthood. How Chinese fathers re-evaluate and navigate their multiple family roles as adult sons, husbands, and parents is also a theoretically interesting question.

Fathers in Korea

Confucian legacies and beyond

Confucianism, which emphasizes the importance of individuals' relation to others within the family, community, and state (Nuyen, 2009), was officially accepted as the state ideology in Korea during the Joseon Dynasty (1392–1910) and served as the foundation of Korean fatherhood. Education was a primary responsibility for traditional Korean fathers, particularly among those of higher social status (Cho, 2011), as it was crucial for both the child's individual development and well-being and the family's social status, wealth, and reputation (see Kim & Lee, 2014). In the late Joseon Dynasty,

Korean fathers under high patriarchy were expected to earn authority by refraining from emotional expressions (Cho, 2011). Although class distinctions in fatherhood in historical Korea have not been thoroughly examined, Confucian paternal roles were likely valued the most among the upper and ruling classes, with others loosely following suit (see Chang, 2001).

The degree to which the legacy of Confucian fatherhood has endured until today is open to debate. On the one hand, elements of Confucian philosophy appear to have persisted despite significant historical events in the 20th century, such as colonization (1910–45), the Korean War (1950–53), and industrialization (approximately 1960s–1980s). Some Korean fathers continue to aspire to become authoritative to set an example within the family (e.g., Kwon & Roy, 2007). In Kim and Lee's (2014) study, highly educated Korean men in their 30s expressed a strong preference for being affable fathers, but this aspiration was not accompanied by increased involvement in childcare practices. Instead, these fathers appeared to pursue affection and kindness as an adapted strategy to guide their children's success—like they would in Confucian fatherhood. Furthermore, the forming of and parenting in seemingly "nuclear" families in Korea continues to be closely linked to extended families' cultural and socioeconomic standing. For instance, young married couples still expect support from their parents for finance and childcare (Lee, 2022). Korean men increasingly choose to remain single, not driven by individualization but rather by growing insecurity in their role as providers, which continues to operate as a yardstick of men's competence as male family members since industrialization (Kim, 2013). As such, Korean fatherhood can arguably be characterized as "modified Confucian fatherhood" (Kim & Lee, 2014) that cannot be fully understood through the lens of the "new fatherhood" from Western societies.

On the other hand, some researchers have reported a clear shift in Korean fathering and fatherhood, particularly among middle-class fathers. For instance, Kwon and Roy (2007) found that working-class Korean fathers tend to align themselves with Confucian ideals, viewing their role as a spiritual leader and teacher of good character, while middle-class fathers place greater emphasis on the caring aspects of fathering, such as being playful, sensitive, and friend-like. Similarly, based on a survey of 900 families and 35 interview cases, Kim et al. (2008) concluded that contemporary Korean fathers' understanding of fatherhood is multidimensional, encompassing emotional, social, and moral aspects.

The mixed findings regarding the transition of Korean fatherhood mirror the compressed and rapid societal changes in Korea, including a significant shift in the labor market, owing to industrialization, globalization, and the financial crisis of the late 20th century, which did not allow an indigenous cultural shift to emerge and mature (Chang, 2001). Some Korean sociologists have identified the core of these postmodern shifts in Korean society as being "the family-oriented individualization" (Kim, 2013) and "post-patriarchy" (Lee, 2022). These notions commonly suggest that Korea, similar to Western societies, has undergone a process of individualization that allows people to increasingly value individual autonomy and needs. However, the transition still features aspects of familism—their choices concerning marriage and parenting are still closely linked to their extended families' cultural and socioeconomic standing. Furthermore, Korea today is facing intricate challenges of having the world's lowest fertility rate and adapting its societal systems to address this demographic crisis.

Father involvement in childrearing: Policy and paradox in practice

Coupled with the demographic crisis, one important aspect of the changing context for fathering is the Korean government's initiative to encourage fathers' involvement in childcare, including fathering programs, fathers' self-help communities, paid leave policies such as paternity leave and parental leave, and flexible work arrangements (FWAs) (for more details of each type of policy, see Kim, 2022). While the first and second types of support are relatively new, the paid leave policies have a longer history and have shown greater advancement over the last two decades. As of 2023, Korean fathers are entitled to ten days of paternity leave, one year of earmarked parental leave, and one year of FWAs.

The impetus provided by shifts in public policy appears to be effective in changing Korean fathers' attitudes and behavior: Korean fathers' uptake of parental leave, a touchstone of how widely involved fatherhood is accepted within a society, has seen a remarkable rise in recent years. Men constituted only 2 percent of leave takers in 2002, but 24.1 percent in 2021 (Statistics Korea, 2022a). As observed in Western-based empirical studies, Korean fathers who have taken parental leave and experienced a period of intensive childcare alone also tend to exhibit positive changes in their attitudes and behaviors (Choi et al., 2019; Kim & Kim, 2015; Kim & Kwon, 2015). These fathers appeared to broaden their childcare involvement from play-centered to mundane activities, shift their primary focus from work to family, and embrace their identities as a carer, rather than a provider (Kim & Kwon, 2015; Kim & Kim, 2015).

Nevertheless, studies on father involvement and fathering practices have consistently confirmed the paradoxical nature of contemporary Korean fathers' transition (Kim, 2022; Kim et al., 2008; Kwon & Roy, 2008). Their actions do not always align with their attitudes and the improvement in fathers' relative involvement remains limited. For instance, despite the notable progress, only 4.1 percent of Korean fathers eligible for paternity leave took their leave in 2021, versus 65.2 percent among eligible mothers (Statistics Korea, 2022a). Sin et al. (2014) compared the time fathers spent on childcare in 1999 with that of 2009 and found that the time fathers put into childcare had grown from 21 percent to 33 percent. This was a notable increase, but still nowhere near the 80 percent of time spent on childcare by mothers. According to the Time Use Survey conducted by Statistics Korea (2020) every five years, in 2019, fathers took care of children younger than ten for one hour per day, while mothers did so for three hours.

Father involvement in Korea also appears different from that of mothers, not only in the quantity of time but also in the quality of practices. For instance, Choi et al. (2016) reported that mothers are usually more involved in children's daily activities, such as helping them with their homework and dropping and picking the kids up from school. Fathers, on the other hand, are more involved in recreational activities, such as playing with the kids. Time use data suggested, too, that on average, mothers spend twice as much time on mundane childcare activities as fathers (Moon, 2016). In addition, fathers are also more passive in collecting information about childcare and their children's education. Specifically, while both fathers and mothers tend to get information from their parents and acquaintances, mothers go a step further, engaging in active, in-depth research online (Moon, 2016).

Challenges for navigating the future

The gap between Korean fathers' behaviors and ideals may be attributed to several key challenges, one of which is a lack of role models and the consequent confusion about the benchmark of good parenthood (Kim, 2022). A social media analysis conducted by the Korean Ministry of Health and Welfare in 2017 reveals that, while fathers' searches for hands-on childcare information such as "meals," "nap," "pram," and "powdered formula" doubled within two years, their most frequently used search keywords were "don't know" and "difficult" (Ministry of Health and Welfare, 2017). An analysis of 34 empirical studies from 2000 to 2022 revealed a noticeable contrast between children's and fathers' perception of paternal roles (Lee & Lim, 2023): Whereas fathers rarely perceived themselves negatively, about one-third of children perceived their fathers negatively as being scary, authoritative, poorly involved, neglected, and unconcerned, reflecting potential inaccuracy in fathers' self-evaluation.

Second, a limited network has also constrained Korean fathers' transition. Lee (2023) notes that fathers often experience exclusion from online communities, which are predominantly occupied by mothers or men who do not express interest in the caregiver role. Given that fathers who are highly engaged in their children's lives tend to look to peer parents as role models (Masciadrelli et al., 2006), the paucity of an available network can, in turn, lead to a lack of role models for highly engaged fathers, perpetuating a vicious cycle.

Furthermore, fathers remain a last resort (Kim & Kim, 2020; Lee, 2022; Yang et al., 2021). Several studies examining paternal experiences on parental leave noted that the primary motivation for fathers to take parental leave was circumstantial (i.e., not having available alternative caregivers, primarily other female family members) rather than ideological (Yang et al., 2021). Fathers' own mothers or mothers-in-law occasionally acted as gatekeepers preventing them from taking parental leave (see Jeoung & Bae, 2022; Kim & Kim, 2020). This suggests that despite the recent shift in attitudes of young couples towards egalitarianism, traditional gender norms are still likely to permeate through extended family.

Fourth, despite consecutive parental leave policy reforms, Korea's current leave policies have strict eligibility criteria that require a minimum of 180 days of employment insurance membership. This condition, in turn, is closely tied to the current structure of the Korean labor market and has both directly and indirectly driven the fatherhood transition to be led predominantly by middle-class fathers. At August 2022 non-regular workers (44.3 percent of whom are men) comprise about 37.5 percent of the employed population in Korea (Statistics Korea, 2022b). Among them, 46.0 percent did not have employment insurance, which only 7.8 percent of regular workers did not have. This indicates that a significant number of fathers are excluded from the opportunity of taking parental leave policies from the beginning.

In addition, the Korean labor market remains unconducive to fathers' caregiving. Fathers who expressed a desire to take parental leave directly or indirectly experienced implicit or explicit judgment from higher-ups and colleagues, as well as disadvantages in performance assessment and promotion (Hong, 2018; Kim & Kwon, 2015). This is further compounded by smaller workplaces, where it is more difficult even for women, let alone men, to take parental leave (Ministry of Gender Equality and Family, 2022). Considering the well-evidenced positive impacts of fathers taking parental leave on father-child relationships and couple relationships (Choi et al., 2019; Kim & Kwon, 2015; Petts & Knoester, 2020; Petts et al., 2020), unfavorable work environments in Korea arguably act as an institutional crossing-gate for fathers to realize their fatherhood ideals.

Overall, while middle-class and highly educated fathers are the primary beneficiaries of government support, leading the contemporary fatherhood transition in Korea, the above challenges are not exclusive to them but affect all fathers. This not only suggests unequal experiences of fatherhood among adult men, but also unequal childhood quality among children. Recent studies from both national and international contexts have increasingly shown the positive effects of fathers' involvement on children's physical, emotional, and cognitive development. The dichotomous transition of contemporary fatherhood in Korea is hence worth paying close attention to, given the potential disadvantages that the children of underprivileged fathers may encounter and its ripple effects in the near and distant future.

Fathers in Bangladeshi, Indian, and Malaysian Societies

> *Zakhan tomi ashechile bhabe/Kedechile tomi eka, heshechilo shabe/*
> *Eman jibon tomi korohe ghatan/Tomer bidaie zano kade tribhuban*
>
> (unknown author, nd)

According to this Bengali proverb, a newborn announces her/his arrival with a cry but the family members, especially the parents, welcome the baby with a smile, telling him/her to build a successful life so that s/he can die smiling while the world cries. This proverb highlights fathers' and mothers' life-long caring roles and responsibilities in ensuring their children's growth, well-being, and productivity in South Asian and Malaysian contexts.

Fathers' roles: Religious beliefs and value systems

In Bangladesh, India, and Malaysia, fathers' roles in the family are shaped through the sex and age hierarchies according to Hindu and Islamic principles. In Hinduism, both motherhood and fatherhood are celebrated social identities and signify elevated family status. Among the four stages of Hindu life, a man becomes a father in the second stage of life called Grihastha (householder), an event signifying responsible adulthood, whereas unmarried or childless men have a very difficult journey to become respectable social leaders. The influential religious scripture *Bhagavad Gita* illustrates that a Hindu father must provide for the family, impart moral knowledge to his son, and help him become a responsible, spiritual adult (see Chaudhary, 2013). As such, an "ideal father" provides for his children and safeguards his children's well-being (Sriram & Navalkar, 2012), especially by arranging marriages and paying dowry for his children together with the mother and aided by elders.

The Hindu *Laws of Manu* (Manusmriti) assign men's and women's family status and roles and impose caste-segregated social interactions in society. Although Hindu philosophy accords women as *Shakti* or power, the *Laws of Manu* promote men's absolute authority in the family and relegate women to second-class citizens in society (Roopnarine & Gol-Guven, 2015). Accordingly, men provide, make decisions, and act as the family patriarch; women are saddled with childcare and household responsibilities and are expected to be loyal and devoted to their husbands (pativrata), at the cost of their well-being if needed (commonly called Sita Syndrome) regardless of their economic contributions to the family. Sons are preferred in Hindu families as they can perform funeral rituals for the deceased parents. Such patriarchal beliefs, together with the cultural scripts of maternal importance and the availability of other female caregivers who could act as alloparents, inhibit fathers' involvement in childcare (Roopnarine & Gol-Guven, 2015). Like their Chinese and Korean counterparts, Indian fathers' emotional distance toward their children also leads them to be less involved (Chaudhury, 2013).

In Muslim families, the *Qur'an* and *Hadith* (Prophet Muhammad's sayings and deeds) are followed regarding men's and women's family roles. Contrary to stereotypes, *Qur'an* and *Hadith* support women's education, rights, and leadership roles in society, and urge parents to treat sons and daughters equally, as also commonly expected in Western families (Hossain & Juhari, 2015). For Muslims, fatherhood is rooted in the marital relationship because premarital sexual relationships are prohibited. Islamic rules also underline the significance of a warm, caring interparental relationship, mothers' and fathers' joint decision-making in family affairs, and their mutual responsibilities in raising children and teaching them religious duties by doing good deeds. The *Hadith* further teaches Muslim fathers to be loving, warm, and gentle with their children, who are born as pure souls. In essence, an ideal Muslim father is expected to be judicious, kind, engaged, and playful, to dine and play with their children, and to invest in children's education and health (Hossain & Juhari, 2015).

Yet fathers' roles in Malaysian, Bangladeshi, and Indian Muslim families are complicated by the interaction between Islamic belief structures and *Adat*, a customary value system that defines acceptable social interactions, behavioral etiquette, and sex relations. Like Islamic values, *Adat* fosters positive parental engagement with children, children's resilience and respect for the family, and collective community responsibilities and moral rules of personal and social conduct (Abdullah et al., 2010). Specifically for fathers, *Adat* prescribes Muslim fathers with a chief objective of facilitating positive child development such as filial piety (e.g., loyalty to and respect for the family) and good moral character (e.g., kindness, respect). However, unlike Islam which promotes egalitarianism, *Adat* tolerates social rules upholding fathers' provisioning and patriarchal authority in the family and society, especially in Malaysia (Karim, 1992). The intersectionality of *Adat* and Islamic law results in mothers' and fathers' differentiated and unequal family roles and statuses. In Bangladeshi families, fathers are expected to be the providers and protectors whereas mothers are responsible for childcare and other household chores (Hossain & Atencio, 2017; Hossain & Juhari, 2015).

Despite divergent religions, Bangladeshi, Indian, and Malaysian families share a collectivistic sociocultural lifestyle as a vital framework for father-child interactions. Not only do fathers socialize children to develop interdependent identities that highlight family well-being over individual gain, but father-child interactions are also embedded in a broader relational web beyond the nuclear family as well as social norms and expectations. Fathers often receive support from grandparents, extended kin, community elders, and religious leaders in raising children, but this childrearing community may also punish the entire family through isolation if the child misbehaves. Therefore, the father as a principal moral guide is dutiful in teaching his children "proper" social and religious values and ensuring that they abide by relevant norms, such as those around masculine sex roles (Hossain & Madon, 2022). For example, Muslim fathers are responsible for teaching their children to believe in one God, to pray, and to fast (i.e., Ramadan), as well as life skills so that the children maintain a healthy diet, do well in school, and assist with household and other family tasks (Al-Husaini, 2015). Similarly, Hindu fathers have the sacred duty of preventing their children from socializing with the opposite sex and ensuring their daughters' virginity before marriage. In Malaysia, parents' subscription to the value of *Adat* and filial piety lowered children's psychopathology such as negative emotions (Ismail et al., 2009), and improved female children's academic success (Baharudin et al., 2014).

Father involvement in childrearing

Available literature reports varying levels of fathers' engagement in childcare tasks in Malaysian, Bangladeshi, and Indian families. Urban Indian fathers spent 2.7 hours per week with their older children, which appeared minimal compared to mothers' involvement (Saraff & Srivastava, 2010). However, Indian (as well as Bangladeshi and Malaysian) fathers take strong interests and invest in their children's education by assisting children with homework, arranging tutors, paying school fees and tuition, buying school supplies, and supporting their overall learning in school (Roopnarine & Gol-Guven, 2015).

In Bangladesh, middle-class fathers spent about 35 minutes per day on childcare tasks such as playing, reading, or talking to children (Jesmin & Seward, 2011). Although both rural and urban Bangladeshi fathers showed significant interest in children's education, mothers spent more time in childcare and academic needs than fathers (Hossain, 2013). Whereas urban fathers spent 51 percent as much time as mothers did (13.83 vs. 27.12 hours per week), rural fathers spent 30 percent as much time as mothers spent in routine childcare (3.61 vs. 12.06 hours per week), possibly because of rural fathers' access to multiple caregiving systems (Hossain & Atencio, 2017). This later study also reported rural fathers spent more time with boys than girls, whereas urban fathers spent a similar amount of time with sons and daughters. Younger, better-educated fathers and those married for a longer are more involved with their children. These findings vouch that residential locations, parental education, and marital union act as protective factors for fathers' involvement in childcare in Bangladeshi families.

In multi-ethnic Malaysia where the population is made up of Malay, Chinese, Indian, and indigenous groups, research on fathers' role is scattered. Rural and urban Malaysian fathers spent 4.16 and 2.56 hours each day on basic childcare activities, respectively (Hossain et al, 2005). Malay and Chinese-ethnic fathers spent far less time cleaning, feeding, holding, and playing with young children and infants than mothers did in both rural and urban families (Hossain et al., 2005; Noor, 1999), whereas indigenous Batek fathers and mothers showed egalitarian involvement in childcare (Endicott & Endicott, 2008). Because of Islamic beliefs, many Malay fathers practice inclusive parenting strategies depicting their own awareness and consciousness development as parents, and they convince themselves to equally invest in sons' and daughters' education, well-being, and health (Hossain & Madon, 2022), although fathers tend to allow more freedom for outdoor activities for boys than for girls following *Adat*.

Apart from participation in tasks directly related to the child, fathers' participation in household labor supposedly shapes the development of children's gender ideology by role modeling egalitarianism in children's future conjugal lives (Boo, 2020). The complex intersectionality of patriarchy, *Adat,* and religious codes craft an idiosyncratic scenario regarding the spousal distribution of household labor in South Asian and Malaysian families. Despite egalitarian Quranic teaching, Bangladeshi, Indian, and Malaysian fathers participate little in household labor. Contemporary Bangladeshi fathers, like their predecessors (Cain et al., 1979), spend less time in household labor than mothers in both rural and urban families. Surprisingly, whereas rural fathers spent about 56 percent as much time as mothers did in household labor (30.85 vs. 55 hours/week) each week, urban fathers spent only about 35 percenet as much time as mothers did (22.10 vs. 63.17/week) (Hossain, 2018). Similarly, fathers in both Malay and Chinese-ethnic urban professional Malaysian families spent 71 percent (3.32 vs. 4.67 hours per day) as much time as mothers did in household labor (Noor, 1999) despite their subscription to egalitarian sex roles. Rural and urban Malaysian fathers were recently found to spend 66 percent and 62 percent as much time as mothers did in major domains of household labor (Hossain & Madon, 2022). Interestingly, Malaysian fathers reportedly spent 3.9 times more time than non-fathers in meal preparation, implying that parental responsibilities may reduce the sex division of household labor in Malaysia (Khazanah Research Institute, 2019).

In sum, whereas Islamic values usher a tone of complementary sex roles in Muslim families, *Adat* and the *Laws of Manu* support patriarchal, sex-linked household labor division. Fathers in South Asia and Malaysia take part in household labor, but mothers perform most work regardless of their residential or employment status. As South and Southeast Asian societies undergo socioeconomic changes, the consequent redefinition and renegotiation of family roles and hierarchy might have implications for fathers' active involvement as parents and spouses. More research is needed to explore how fathers' caregiving in contemporary Malaysia is shaped by complex joint forces of *Adat*, Islamic dictum, filial piety, and evolving economic and technological development (Hossain & Juhari, 2015; Karim, 1992).

General Discussion and Conclusion

This chapter provides one of the first overviews of fathering and fatherhood across multiple Asian sub-regions that have only been examined separately in the extant scholarship. By laying out similarities and divergences in fathering contexts, values, and practices in China, Korea, Bangladesh, India, and Malaysia, this chapter offers theoretical and methodological insights for future fatherhood research in Asia and beyond.

The ecologies of fathering in Asia vary considerably alongside socioeconomic development, welfare schemes, and social values not only across sub-regions but also within national borders. Whereas fathers in today's East Asia (e.g., China, Korea) tend to have co-breadwinning spouses, fathers in South and Southeast Asia (e.g., Bangladesh, India) play a prominent role in financial provision. Different religions and ideologies, sometimes co-existing in the same region (Adat, patriarchy, Hinduism, and Islam), may jointly influence fatherhood ideals and practices in intersectional ways. Within China, the rural-urban inequality not only leaves some fathers in poverty but also makes long-term labor migration a conundrum for fathering; within Korea, the divide between regular and non-regular employment prevents a significant proportion of fathers from paternity leave entitlement. In addition, contemporary Asian families often face the changes and challenges of rapid globalization and modernization (Hossain, 2022). There is no single, static profile of "Asian" fathers, but a plethora of complex, nuanced, and dynamic situations. Future research can explore how Asian fathers and their families respond to their unique contextual footprints.

Meanwhile, seemingly divergent Asian societies shared characteristics in fathering ecology. Many Asian traditions (e.g., *Laws of Manu*, *Adat*,

Confucian ideals of *filial piety*) emphasize sex and age hierarchy where fathers are powerful figures with important responsibilities but are not necessarily expected to be involved in daily care work. These hierarchies have persisted (at least partially), reflected in fathers' limited involvement in early childcare across Asian societies despite profound social transformations. Another lasting role shared by Asian fathers from different belief systems is their identity as their children's educators instead of playmates, whereas the latter is often observed in Western families (Lamb, 2010). These patterns suggest that the assumption of a linear progression from "tradition" to "modernity" in fathers' roles and behaviors may be simplistic and need to be enriched by nuanced investigations of factors related to changes in fathers' roles and involvement.

Another major characteristic of Asian fatherhood is its embeddedness in the tapestry of a collectivistic lifestyle that sustains interdependent family relationships and multigenerational households. Whereas the accessibility of grandparents and other extended family members often creates a supportive environment for fathers (Hossain, 2014; Oshio et al., 2013), the readily available familial and societal support sometimes works insidiously letting fathers "off the hook" from childcare and household tasks and minimizing their active role as parents. As much of the fatherhood research is modeled after the nuclear family set-up prevalent in white, western middle-class families, we know little so far about whether and how Asian fathers "co-parent" with grandparents or other major caregivers. The inclusion of extended family members (or key extrafamilial figures) in fathering research not only resonates with Asian fathers' family and social contexts (Hossain, 2011) but may also conceptually and methodologically enrich or modify the nuclear-family assumption.

Finally, although much of the existing fathering research focused on infancy and early childhood where care work is most intense, Asian fathers are expected to be present in the later stages of their children's lives, if not more so than the early years, as authority figures that arrange their children's work and marriage or as recipients of filial care. The lifespan transition of paternal roles and father-child relationship as well as the association between parental and filial practices across different stages would be a fruitful avenue for future research.

References

Abdullah, R., Martinez, P., & Radzi, W. (2010). Islam and adat: Considering the wife's moral contribution in the division of harta sepencharian in Malaysia. *Indonesia and the Malay World*, *38*, 161–180.

Al-Husaini, H., M., H. (2015). *Untold Story, Ali bin Abi Thalib r.a.: Khalifah Gerbangnya Ilmu*. Pustaka Cordova.

Baharudin, R., Zulkefly, N. S., Yee, H. C., Yeng, C. W., & Jun, L. H. (2014). Parenting behavior of mothers and school adjustments of adolescents in Malaysia. In *Proceedings of the International Conference on Science, Technology and Social Sciences (ICSTSS) 2012* (pp. 29–42). Springer.

Boo, H. S. (2020). Familial influences on the division of household labour in Malaysian families. *Geografia-Malaysian Journal of Society and Space, 16*(3), 1–13.

Bronfenbrenner, U. (1977). Towards an experimental ecology of human development. *American Psychologist, 32*(7), 515–531.

Cain, M., Khanam, S. R., & Nahar, S. (1979). Class, patriarchy, and women's work in Bangladesh. *Population and Development Review*, 405–438.

Cao, S. & Lin, X. (2019). Masculinizing fatherhood: Negotiation of Yang and Jiao among young fathers in China. *Journal of Gender Studies, 28*(8), 937–947. https://doi.org/10.1080/09589236.2019.1625312.

Chang, K.-S. (2001). Accidental pluralism in family ideology: Compressed modernity and Korean families. *Korean Studies Quarterly, 24*(2), 161–202.

Chaudhury, N. (2013). The fathers' role in the Indian family: A story must be told. In D. Shwalb, B. Shwalb, & M. Lamb (Eds), *Fathers in cultural contexts* (pp. 68–94) Routledge.

Chen, X., Li, D., Liu, J., Fu, R., & Liu, S. (2019). Father migration and mother migration: Different implications for social, school, and psychological adjustment of left-behind Children in rural China. *Journal of Contemporary China, 28*(120), 849–863. https://doi.org/10.1080/10670564.2019.1594100.

China National Center for Children. (2017). 中国家庭教养中的父母角色：基于0–6岁儿童家庭现状的调查. [Parenting roles of Chinese families: Based on the investigation of 0–6 years children's families]. Social Sciences Academic Press (China).

Cho, Y.-K. (2011). 조선중기 재지사족 가문 아버지들의 자녀양육에 대한 검토. [Interests and characteristics for fathers nurturing children in the middle of the Joseon Dynasty]. *The Journal of Humanities Studies*, 38(1), 191–213.

Choi, S., Joung, E. H., & Choi, S. (2019). Mandatory parental leave for fathers and the emergence of a working dad. *Family and Culture, 31*(4), 1–29.

Choi, S. Y.-P. & Peng, Y. (2016). *Masculine Compromise: Migration, family, and gender in China.* University of California Press.

Choi, Y., Lee, T, Hwang, J., Ma, K., Joo, J., Kim, E., Lee, H., & Moon, H. (2016). *2016 년 양성평등 실태조사 분석 연구* [2016 Study on the status analysis of gender equality survey]. The Korean Ministry of Gender Equality and Family.

Cole, E. R. (2009). Intersectionality and research in psychology. *American Psychologist, 64*(3), 170–180. https://doi.org/10.1037/a0014564.

Dommaraju, P. & Wong, S. (2022). Grandparenthood and grandparenting in Asia. In S. I. Rajan (Ed.). *Handbook of Aging, Health and Public Policy: Perspectives from Asia* (pp. 1–13). Springer. https://doi.org/10.1007/978-981-16-1914-4_40-1.

Dou, D., Shek, D. T. L., & Kwok, K. H. R. (2020). Perceived paternal and maternal parenting attributes among Chinese adolescents: A meta-analysis. *International Journal of Environmental Research and Public Health, 17*(23), Article 23. https://doi.org/10.3390/ijerph17238741.

Endicott, K. M. & Endicott, K. L. (2008). *The headman was a woman: The gender egalitarian Batek of Malaysia*. Waveland Press.

Greenhalgh, S. (2014). 'Bare sticks' and other dangers to the social body: Assembling fatherhood in China. In M. C. Inhorn, W. Chavkin, & J.-A. Navarro (Eds), Globalized fatherhood (pp. 359–381). Berghahn Books.

Hertog, E., Kan, M-Y., Shirakawa, K., & Chiba, R. (2021). Do better-educated couples share domestic work more equitably in Japan? It depends on the day of the week. *Journal of Comparative Family Studies, 52*(2), 271–310.

Hong, S.A. (2018). Men's use of parental leave and the workplace culture, *Gender and Culture, 11*(1), 145–183.

Hossain, Z. (2013). Fathers in Muslim families in Bangladesh and Malaysia. In D. W. Shwalb, B. Shwalb, & M. E. Lamb (Eds), *Fathers in cultural context* (pp. 95–121). Routledge.

Hossain, Z. (2014). Parental beliefs and fathers' and mothers' roles in Malaysian families. In H. Selin (Ed.), *Parenting across cultures: Childrearing, motherhood and fatherhood in non-Western cultures* (pp. 77–90). Springer.

Hossain, Z. (2018). Division of domestic labor between mothers and fathers in rural and urban families in Bangladesh. *Journal of Behavioral and Social Sciences, 5*, 1–14.

Hossain, Z. & Atencio, D. J. (2017). Mothers' and fathers' perceived engagement in children's care and schooling in Bangladesh: A rural-urban comparison. *Journal of Comparative Family Studies*, 48, 289–311.

Hossain, Z. & Madon, Z. (2021). Distribution of household labor between mothers and fathers in rural and urban Malaysia. *Journal of Comparative Family Studies, 52*(4), 569–595.

Hossain, Z. & Madon, Z. (2022). Sociocultural and religious context of Malay parenting in Malaysia. In H. Selin (ed.) *Parenting across cultures* (pp. 175–192). Springer.

Hossain, Z., Roopnarine, J. L., Masud, J., Muhamed, A.A., Baharudin, R., Abdullah, R., & Juhari, R. (2005). Mothers' and fathers' childcare involvement with young children in rural families in Malaysia. *International Journal of Psychology, 40*(6), 385–394.

Hossain, Z. & Juhari, R. (2015). Fathers across Arab and non-Arab Islamic societies. In J. L. Roopnarine (Ed.). *Fathers across cultures: The importance, roles, and diverse practices of dads* (pp. 368–390). Praeger.

Hsu, H.-Y., Zhang, D., Kwok, O.-M., Li, Y., & Ju, S. (2011). Distinguishing the influences of father's and mother's involvement on adolescent academic achievement: Analyses of Taiwan Education Panel Survey Data. *Journal of Early Adolescence, 31*(5), 694–713. https://doi.org/10.1177/0272431610373101.

Huang, C.-Y., Shen, A. C.-T., Li, X., & Feng, J. Y. (2024). Happy parents, happy kids: Marital happiness, parenting styles, and children's behavioral outcomes in Chinese societies. *Family Relations*. Advanced online publication. https://doi.org/10.1111/fare.12997.

Hwang, W. & Lee, S. (2021). Guest editors' comments: Special issue: Understanding contemporary family issues in South Korea. *Journal of Comparative Family Studies, 52*(3), 311–316.

Ismail, N., Jo-Pei, T., & Ibrahim, R. (2009). The relationship between parental belief on filial piety and child psychosocial adjustment among Malay families. *Pertanika Journal of Social Science & Humanities, 17*, 215–224.

Jeoung, S. & Bae, E. (2022). Does fathers' use of parental leave promote degenderization of care? Focusing on fathers' experience of parental leave since the mid-2010s. *Journal of Korean Women's Studies, 38*(1), 111–146.

Jesmin, S. & Seward, R. (2011). Parental leave and fathers' involvement with children in Bangladesh: A comparison with Unit. *Journal of Comparative Family Studies, 42*(1), 95–112. https://doi.org/10.3138/jcfs.42.1.95.

Karim, J. W. (1992) *Women and culture between Malay Adat and Islam*. Westview Press.

Khazanah Research Institute (2019). *Time to care: Gender equality, unpaid care work and time use survey*. Khazana Research Institute. www.krinstitute.org/assets/contentMS/img/template/editor/Publications_Time%20to%20Care_Full%20report.pdf.

Kim, J. H. & Lee, S. (2014). The ideals and practices of fatherhood among highly educated and married males in their 30's. *Family and Culture, 26*(3), 71–104.

Kim, J. W. & Kwon, J. (2015). A qualitative study on the experience of fathers using parental leave. *Korea Social Policy Review, 22*, 265–302.

Kim, H. K. (2013). Failure of the patrilineal stem family system?: Familialism and individualization among the generation of the Economic Crisis of Korea in 1998. *Korean Journal of Sociology, 47*(2), 101–141.

Kim, H. H., Sun, J.-M., Kim, B.-Y., & Dong-Ki, K. (2008). 남성의 부성경험과 갈등에 관한 연구[*Research on men's paternal experiences and their work-father role conflict*]. Korean Women's Development Institute.

Kim, Y.-J. (2022). *Korean Fatherhood in Policy and Practice*. [Doctoral Thesis (compilation), School of Social Work]. Lund University. School of Social Work.

Kim, Y. & Kim, S. (2015). The effect of fathers' parental leave on gender role attitudes. *Korean Journal of Social Welfare Studies, 46*(4), 285–320.

Kim, Y.-J. & Kim, S. (2020). Relational ethics as a cultural constraint on fathers' parental leave in a Confucian welfare state, South Korea. *Social Policy & Administration, 54*(5), 684–698.

Korean Ministry of Health and Welfare (2017) *도와주는 아빠 NO! 함께하는 아빠 YES! 빅데이터로 본 아빠 육아* [Helping Father, No! Coparenting Father, Yes! Looking at paternal child care through big data]. Press release.

Kwon, Y. I. & Roy, K. M. (2007). Changing social expectations for work and family involvement among Korean fathers. *Journal of Comparative Family Studies, 38*(2), 285–305.

Lamb, M. E. (2000). The history of research on father involvement: An overview. *Marriage & Family Review, 29*(2–3), 23–42. https://doi.org/10.1300/J002v29n02_03

Lamb, M. E. (2010). *The role of father in child development* (5th ed.). Wiley.

Lau, E. Y. H. (2016). A mixed-methods study of paternal involvement in Hong Kong. *British Educational Research Journal, 42*(6), 1023–1040. https://doi.org/10.1002/berj.3248.

Lee, J. K. (2022). *한국가족: 신가족주의에서 포스트가부장제로* [Korean families: From neo-familism to post-patriarchy]. Ewha Womans University Press.

Lee, S. S. & Lim, M. J. (2023). Domestic research trends related to images of fathers: Focusing on perception of father's image [아버지상 관련 국내 연구동향 분석: 아버지에 대한 인식을 중심으로]. *Journal of Korean Council for Children & Rights, 27*(1), 115–134.

Lee, Y. (2022). Norms about childcare, working hours, and fathers' uptake of parental leave in South Korea. *Community, Work and Family,* 1–26.

Lee, Y. (2023). Online media experiences of caregiving fathers: A study of leave-taking fathers in South Korea. *Family Relations, 72*(2), 426–442.

Li, Q. & Zang, W. (2010). 父母外出对留守儿童健康的影响 [The health of left-behind children in rural China]. *Chinese Economic Quarterly, 10*(1), 341–360.

Li, X. (2020a). Fathers' involvement in Chinese societies: Increasing presence, uneven progress. *Child Development Perspectives, 14*(3), 150–156. https://doi.org/10.1111/cdep.12375.

Li, X. (2020b). How do Chinese fathers express love? Viewing paternal warmth through the eyes of Chinese fathers, mothers, and their children. *Psychology of Men & Masculinities, 22*(3), 500–511. https://doi.org/10.1037/men0000312.

Liu, J. (1995). 上海父亲育儿态度和观念的代际比较 [An intergenerational comparison of paternal child-rearing attitudes and ideas in Shanghai]. 心理科学 *[Journal of Psychological Science], 4,* 211–215, 255. https://doi.org/10.16719/j.cnki.1671-6981.1995.04.005.

Liu, Y., Dittman, C. K., Guo, M., Morawska, A., & Haslam, D. (2021). Influence of father involvement, fathering practices and father-child relationships on children in Mainland China. *Journal of Child and Family Studies, 30*(8), 1858–1870. https://doi.org/10.1007/s10826-021-01986-4.

Lu, W. (2010). "A pearl in the palm": A forgotten symbol of the father-daughter bond. *Late Imperial China, 31*(1), 62–97. https://doi.org/10.1353/late.0.0031

Masciadrelli, B. P., Pleck, J. H., & Stueve, J. L. (2006). Fathers' role model perceptions: Themes and linkages with involvement. *Men and Masculinities, 9*(1), 23–34.

Ministry of Gender Equality and Family (2022). *2021년 양성평등 실태조사 분석 연구* [2021 Study on the status analysis of gender equality survey].

Moon, M., Cho, S., & Kim, J. (2016). *한국인의 부모됨 인식과 자녀양육관 연구* [Perspectives and values of Koreans on becoming a parent and raising children]. Korea Institute of Child Care and Education.

Noor, N. (1999). Roles and women's well-being: Some preliminary findings from Malaysia. *Sex Roles, 41,* 123–145.

Ni, P., Hong, P., Pan, L., Han, X., Zhai, S., & He, J. (2024). Work arrangements and father involvement during COVID-19 lockdown: A mixed methods study. *Family Relations, 73*(1), 54–73. https://doi.org/10.1111/fare.12915.

Nuyen, A. T. (2009). Moral obligation and moral motivation in confucian role-based ethics. *Dao, 8*(1), 1–11.

Oshio, T., Nozaki, K., Kobayashi, M. (2013). Division of household labor and marital satisfaction in China, Japan, and Korea. *Journal of Family Economic Issues, 34,* 211–223.

Petts, R. J. & Knoester, C. (2020). Are parental relationships improved if fathers take time off of work after the birth of a child? *Social Forces, 98*(3), 1223–1256.

Petts, R. J., Knoester, C., & Waldfogel, J. (2020). Fathers' paternity leave-taking and children's perceptions of father-child relationships in the United States. *Sex Roles*, *82*(3–4), 173–188.

Park, H. & Walton-Moss, B. (2012). Parenting style, parenting stress, and children's health-related behaviors. *Journal of Developmental and Behavioral Pediatrics*, *33*, 495–503.

Riphenburg, C. J. (1998). Changing gender relations and the development process in Oman. In Y. Y. Haddad & J. L. Esposito (Eds), *Islam, gender and social change* (pp. 144–168). Oxford University Press.

Roopnarine, J. L. & Gol-Guven, M. (2015). Indian fathers: Traditional with changes on the horizon. In J. Roopnarine (Ed.), *Fathers across cultures: The importance, roles, and diverse practices of dads* (pp. 251–272). Praeger.

Roopnarine, J. L. & Hossain, Z. (1992). Parent–child interactions in urban Indian families in New Delhi: Are they changing? In J. L. Roopnarine and D. B. Carter (Eds), *Parent–child socialization in diverse cultures* (pp. 1–16). Ablex.

Saraff, A. & Srivastava, H. (2010). Patterns and determinants of paternal involvement in childcare: An empirical investigation in a metropolis of India. *Population Research and Policy Review*, *29*(2), 249–273.

Shin, Y.-J., Ki, J.-R., Woo, S., & Yoon, J. (2014). *Analysis on childcare behaviors after the expansion of family policies* [저출산 정책 확대에 따른 자녀 양육 행태 변화 분석]. Korea Institute for Health and Social Affairs.

Sriram, R. & Navalkar, P. G. (2012). Who is an 'ideal' father? Father, mother and childrens' views. *Psychology and Developing Societies*, *24*(2), 205–237.

Statistics Korea (2020, July 30). 2019 년 생활시간조사 결과 [2019 Result of time use survey]. Press release.

Statistics Korea (2022a). *육아휴직 통계 결과 (잠정)* [(Preliminary) Result of statistics on parental leave].

Statistics Korea (2022b). 2022 *년 8 월 경제활동인구조사 근로형태별 부가조사 결과* [August, 2022 Results of supplementary survey on economically active population by employment type].

Su, L. P., Kubricht, B., & Miller, R. (2017). The influence of father involvement in adolescents' overall development in Taiwan. *Journal of Adolescence, 59*, 35–44. https://doi.org/10.1016/j.adolescence.2017.05.010.

Tan, T. (2023). Changing fatherhood: A comparative study of Sweden, Germany and Japan. *Journal of Family Studies,* 1–16. https://doi.org/10.1080/13229400.2023.2179528.

Wang, L. & Keizer, R. (2024). 'I am a traditional but caring father': Narratives of paternal masculinity in urban Chinese families. *Journal of Gender Studies*. Advanced online publication. https://doi.org/10.1080/09589236.2023.2300426.

Xie, S. & Li, H. (2019). 'Tiger mom, panda dad': A study of contemporary Chinese parenting profiles. *Early Child Development and Care, 189*(2), 284–300. https://doi.org/10.1080/03004430.2017.1318870.

Xu, Y., Xu, D., Simpkins, S., & Warschauer, M. (2019). Does it matter which parent is absent? Labor migration, parenting, and adolescent development in China. *Journal of Child and Family Studies, 28*(6), 1635–1649. https://doi.org/10.1007/s10826-019-01382-z.

Yang, H., Hwang, J., Kwon, H., Jeon, Y., & Kim, J. (2021). What has happened after the parental leave? Analysis of interview research focusing on gender effects and continuing employment after the leave. *The Women's Studies, 109*(2), 69–99.

Zhang, J., Liu, Y., & Hu, T. (2021). A meta-analysis of the relationship between father involvement and problem behaviour among preschool children. *Early Child Development and Care, 191*(11), 1802–1824. https://doi.org/10.1080/03004430.2019.1679127.

Zhang, L., & Xu, A. (2008). 父亲参与研究：态度、贡献与效用. [Research on father involvement: Attitude, contribution and influences]. Shanghai Academy of Social Sciences Press.

Zhao, Q., Yu, X., Wang, X., & Glauben, T. (2014). The impact of parental migration on children's school performance in rural China. *China Economic Review, 31*, 43–54. https://doi.org/10.1016/j.chieco.2014.07.013.

Zhao, S. (2018). Changes in women's and men's child care time in China, 2004–2011: The contributions of cohort replacement and intra-cohort change. *Quality & Quantity, 52*(3), 1275–1289. https://doi.org/10.1007/s11135-017-0519-2.

10

EAST ASIAN PARENTING AND CHILDREN'S LEARNING AND EDUCATION

Yoko Yamamoto

Introduction

In societies where the importance of schooling and educational achievement is significant in the development and future of children, education becomes a key influence in shaping parenting practices and beliefs. Parents often adapt their parenting approaches to changing educational contexts and strategically invest their time and resources in their children's learning to increase their children's prospects (Doepke & Zilibotti, 2019; LeVine, 1988; Li & Yamamoto, 2020; Raymo & Dong, 2020). Education stands out as one of the central concepts in the studies of Asian parenting.

Since the 1970s, scholars in the field of child development and education have delved into understanding how East Asian parents support their children's learning and education. East Asian students have consistently exhibited remarkable academic performance in international tests, such as Trends in International Mathematics and Science Study (TIMSS) and Programme for International Student Assessment (PISA) (Raymo & Dong, 2020; Stevenson & Stigler, 1992; Stigler & Hiebert, 1999; Tucker, 2015). Educational researchers have endeavored to identify key elements explaining East Asian students' achievement by examining school curricula and teaching practices in addition to home environments (Rohlen & LeTendre, 1996; Stevenson & Stigler, 1992; Stigler & Hiebert, 1999; Tucker, 2015). However, East Asian students have also demonstrated high academic performance, irrespective of the school systems they encounter. For example, among students attending schools in the U.S., East Asian American students typically show higher academic achievement than students from other racial backgrounds (Byun &

DOI: 10.4324/9781003383949-10

Park, 2012; Kao & Thomson, 2003; Pearce & Lin, 2007: Zhou & Lee, 2017). If differences in educational systems, schools, and teacher practices across countries are not the primary factor explaining East Asian students' academic achievement, other factors beyond school environments could be responsible. This underscores the critical role played by East Asian families, especially their cultural practices, in children's education.

This chapter focuses on East Asian parents' practices and beliefs centered around children's learning and education by reviewing and highlighting the wealth of research on Chinese, Japanese, and Korean families. Various East Asian countries have exchanged frequent communications, which began as early as the 5th century CE, and political and economic interactions as neighboring nations (Thomas & Postlethwaite, 1983). Confucian philosophy originated in China has shaped cultural beliefs and practices in families and education across many East Asian countries, including Korea and Japan (Dittrich & Neuhaus, 2023; Ho & Lam, 2019; Li, 2012). However, there are substantial variations and differences in parenting and children's educational experiences across East Asian countries, owing to their distinct historical, political, and economic development, as well as the diverse trajectories of their educational systems (Ho & Lam, 2019; Raymo & Dong, 2020; Thomas & Postlethwaite, 1983).

In understanding parenting and children's education, it is also imperative to pay attention to variations within culture, particularly those related to family backgrounds. As in many other countries, there has been a significant gap in students' achievement depending on families' socioeconomic status (SES) within each East Asian country (Byun & Kim, 2010; Gao, 2001; Hannum et al., 2019; Kariya, 2009; Matsuoka, 2019; Raymo & Dong, 2020). Achievement gaps are powerfully associated with family SES, and some argue that the SES-related gap has increased over the last two decades in Japan and South Korea (Byun & Kim, 2010; Kariya, 2009). This is noteworthy because both Japan and South Korea exhibit relatively equitable public funding allocations to schools and standardized curricula, owing to the nationally administered educational systems (Kariya, 2009; Matsuoka, 2019; Raymo & Dong, 2020). These patterns compel scholars to scrutinize how parents of diverse socioeconomic statuses support their children's learning and education within and beyond the East Asian cultural contexts.

This chapter begins with East Asian parents' engagement in their children's learning and education at home and school, followed by their investment in supplementary education. Then the chapter delves into parental beliefs related to education, including parental aspirations and expectations, beliefs about learning, and parental roles related to education. Throughout the chapter, careful consideration is given to East Asia's sociocultural contexts, especially educational systems and school practices. The chapter concludes with implications and suggestions for future directions in studies of East Asian parenting and children's learning and education.

East Asian Parents' Engagement in Their Children's Learning and Education

Parental engagement in their children's education, or parental involvement, encompasses actions undertaken by parents both at home and school to support their children's learning, school experiences, and academic development (Hill et al., 2004; Hoover-Dempsey et al., 2005; Pomerantz et al., 2007). Substantial evidence demonstrates that parental engagement in children's education plays a pivotal role in their children's educational experiences and academic development. In general, parental involvement in their children's education is positively associated with children's valuation of learning, academic motivation, and educational aspiration and performance (Choi et al., 1994; Fan & Chen, 2001; Hill et al., 2004; Hoover-Dempsey et al., 2005; Kim, 2020; Pomerantz et al., 2007). This section focuses on East Asian parents' involvement in their children's learning and education at home and school and investment in supplemental educational opportunities.

Parental Engagement in Children's Learning and Education at Home

Scholars often attribute the generally high academic performance of East Asian and East Asian American students to their parent's involvement in their children's education (Chao, 2000; Chen & Stevenson, 1989; Choi et al., 1994; Huntsinger et al., 2000; Park & Kwon, 2009; Schneider & Lee, 1990). For example, cross-cultural studies demonstrate that parents in China are more involved in their children's education at home than parents in the U.S. (Chen & Stevenson, 1989; Cheung & Pomerantz, 2011). Whether they live in East Asia or other countries, providing direct and indirect support, such as teaching numbers, letters, and basic arithmetic skills to young children, is a relatively common practice among East Asian parents (Chao, 1994, 2000; Gao, 2011; Huntsinger et al., 2000; Park & Kwon, 2009; Sy, 2006; Yamamoto, 2015; Yamamoto et al., 2016a, 2016b). These practices are found to increase East Asian children's familiarity with academic and school-related tasks and facilitate their adjustment to a formal learning environment (Huntsinger et al., 2000; Sy, 2006; Yamamoto, 2015).

During the early years of schooling, East Asian parents may oversee their children's homework and provide additional opportunities to enhance their academic skills by assigning workbooks or enrolling them in after-school academic classes (Chao, 2000; Chen & Stevenson, 1989; Holloway et al., 2008; Huntsinger & Jose, 2009; Schneider & Lee, 1990; Yamamoto et al., 2016a). A study by Chen & Stevenson (1989) demonstrates that mothers and fathers with first and fifth graders in China and Taiwan spend more time providing homework assistance than parents in the U.S. and Japan. However, studies, including a meta-analysis, demonstrate that parents' homework help is not significantly associated with their children's achievement in East Asia, like the patterns found in the U.S. (Chen & Stevenson, 1989; Fan & Chen, 2001; Kim, 2020). Such results suggest the importance of assessing the quality of homework assistance beyond the quantity (Kim, 2020; Pomerantz et al., 2007). East Asian parents' involvement, especially when they have higher SES, may also encompass monitoring and managing children's learning, such as setting rules about television watching, restricting screen time or play time to increase learning- and academic-related time, and designating a study area within the household (Chao, 2000; Choi et al., 1994; Kim, 2020; Matsuoka, 2019; Schneider & Lee, 1990). Higher-SES parents are also likely to provide cognitively stimulating home environments by reading to their children and bringing them to museums and cultural activities (Holloway et al., 2008, 2016; Park & Kwon, 2009; Kariya, 2009; Matsuoka, 2019; Nakamura, 2019; Yamamoto et al., 2006, 2016a).

One unique aspect of East Asian parents' educational and learning-related support is their improvement-orientated approach. East Asian parents tend to highlight areas for improvement rather than focusing on positive performance or success when assisting their children's learning (Fung, 1999; Holloway, 1988; Ng & Wei, 2019; Yamamoto & Satoh, 2019). A study shows that Chinese parents are more likely to emphasize academic failure and less likely to praise 4th- and 5th-grade children's academic success than American parents (Ng et al., 2007). Ethnographic and fieldwork research also reveals that Japanese adults encourage children to reflect on areas to improve and rarely praise them for their accomplishments (Ben-Ari, 1997; Izumi-Taylor, 2009; Tsuneyoshi, 2008). East Asian parents and teachers tend to criticize work that does not reflect a child's commitment or effort but may praise them when tasks are completed with reflected effort (Tobin et al., 2009; Tsuneyoshi, 2008; Yamamoto et al., 2022b; Yamamoto & Satoh, 2019). The focus lies in cultivating children's motivation to learn and positive learning attitudes, especially developing abilities to work hard and persevere. This improvement-oriented approach may help foster East Asian children's master-oriented learning and motivation to persist (Duckworth,

2016; Dweck, 2006; Ng & Wei, 2019). For example, cross-cultural research shows that Japanese students demonstrate a prolonged attention span and greater task persistence, even with setbacks, compared to students in the U.S. (Blinco, 1992; Heine et al., 2001).

As children enter adolescence, East Asian parents' involvement in their children's education usually decreases (Matsuoka, 2019; Qu & Pomerantz, 2015). Parental involvement also shifts to focus on managing children's academic experiences and investment in supplemental education, such as cram schools, as children grow older (Raymo & Dong, 2020). Nevertheless, studies demonstrate that middle schoolers in China are likely to report greater parental involvement in their education, such as providing homework help, school-based involvement, conversations related to schooling, and purchasing extra workbooks, than students in the U.S. (Cheung & Pomerantz, 2011; Qu & Pomerantz, 2015).

Parents' Engagement at School

Beyond home, parents also engage in their children's education at school. School-based involvement encompasses parental actions that involve direct interactions and communications with schools or teachers, such as attending school events and parent–teacher meetings, communicating with teachers, volunteering at school, and engaging in parent–teacher organizations or associations (Hill et al., 2004; Hoover-Dempsey et al., 2005; Pomerantz et al., 2007). Parents' school-based involvement has received relatively little attention compared to home-based involvement in research on East Asian parenting (see Yamamoto et al., 2022a).

Although schools and educational policies in the U.S. consider school-based involvement a pillar of family engagement, this is not a prevalent practice among East Asian parents, including East Asian parents living in the U.S. or Canada (Kim et al., 2018; Lim, 2012; Turney & Kao, 2009; Yamamoto et al, 2016a; Yamamoto et al., 2022a; Zhou & Zhong, 2018). Analyses of national data in the U.S. demonstrate that Asian American parents, particularly Asian immigrant parents, generally report lower levels of school-based involvement for school-aged children when compared to Black or White parents (Pearce & Lin, 2007; Turney & Kao, 2009). In a Japan-U.S. cross-cultural study on mothers with second graders, more pronounced differences appeared in school-based involvement than home-based involvement (Yamamoto et al., 2016a). Mothers in the U.S. reported greater school-based involvement, such as communicating with teachers and visiting classrooms, than Japanese mothers, even after controlling for mothers' self-efficacy and sense of responsibility in supporting children's development and learning.

In many East Asian countries, there are parent–teacher meetings and school events, especially those showcasing students' performances, for which parents are invited to attend. However, schools usually discourage parents from making requests or volunteering in classrooms (Ho & Staub, 2018; Kim, 2019; Lee, 2005; Pang, 2004; Yamamoto, 2015; Yamamoto et al., 2016a, 2022a). Moreover, the centrally administered educational system with rigid and relatively standardized school curricula limits parents' ability to influence teachers' practices and children's academic experience at school (see Yamamoto et al., 2022a). Thus, parents may feel less motivated to make direct contact with teachers. Nevertheless, parents may contact teachers to seek advice and suggestions and consult about their children's academic and socioemotional experiences (Chen & Agbenyega, 2012; Ho & Staub, 2018; Holloway, 2010; Lee, 2005; Lim, 2012; Yamamoto, 2015; Yamamoto et al., 2022a). As the number of educated parents rises, parents with higher SES have spent time monitoring teacher practices and children's academic experiences at school (Hirota, 1999; Matsuoka, 2019; Yamamoto, 2015). When necessary, they may communicate directly with teachers or supplement their children's education by arranging tutoring or supplemental classes without interfering with school (Gao, 2011; Guo & Kiderry, 2018; Yamamoto, 2015).

Parental Investment in Supplemental Education

For a deeper understanding of how parents in different cultures support their children's education, it is crucial to consider the educational contexts of each country. For instance, standardized exams have been the predominant means to assess students' academic performance at schools and for high school and college admissions in many East Asian countries (Gao, 2011; Hannum et al., 2019; Kariya, 2009; Raymo & Dong, 2020). In response to such educational practices, arranging and providing supplementary educational opportunities, such as tutoring or private cram schools outside formal schooling, has become a common parental practice in East Asia (Bray, 2022; Byun & Kim, 2010; Hannum et al., 2019; Holloway et al., 2008, 2016; Kariya, 2009; Raymo & Dong, 2020). Participation in private supplemental schools is strongly associated with students' academic achievement and enrollment in competitive schools, such as 'key point' public high schools in China (Hannum et al., 2019; Kariya, 2009; Matsuoka, 2019; Raymo & Dong, 2020; Rohlen & LeTendre, 1996; Tucker, 2015). Parental investment in supplemental education often begins early, during elementary school. An OECD report indicates that more than 72 percent of primary school students in urban China, Hong Kong, and South Korea, and about half of primary school students in Japan have received private supplementary education (OECD, 2014). Supplemental education classes and schools, that aim to enhance children's academic skills, are also available in Asian ethnic enclaves in urban cities in the U.S. to cater to Asian American students (Byun & Park, 2012; Zhou & Lee, 2017). The widespread practice of using supplemental education might decrease parents' school-based involvement as parents perceive investing their resources in supplemental education rather than communicating with teachers as a critical form of parental involvement (Byun & Kim, 2010; Kariya, 2009; Yamamoto, 2015; Yamamoto et al., 2016a). Parents' increasing investment in supplemental education is problematized for contributing to educational inequality tied to family SES in East Asia (Bray, 2022; Byun & Kim, 2010; Hannum et al., 2019; Kariya, 2009; Matsuoka, 2019; Raymo & Dong, 2020).

Parental Beliefs Related to Learning and Education

Parents' beliefs serve as the driving force behind parenting practices, such as the decisions and choices they make to structure and organize children's learning and education-related activities, environments, and customs (Harkness et al., 2009; LeVine, 1988). Parents usually hold a sociocultural model, shared assumptions and perspectives in their community, that provides frameworks for understanding children's learning. A sociocultural model related to learning shapes parental beliefs about how children learn, how they should learn, what involves learning, and how parents should support children's learning (Harkness & Super, 2002; LeVine, 1988; Li & Yamamoto, 2020). Within the same society, diversities exist because individual characteristics, adaptation to environments, and various experiences and interactions influence parents' assessment and reconstruction of their beliefs. Nevertheless, sociocultural models help us understand implicit or taken-for-granted beliefs that play a pivotal role in steering East Asian parents' learning and education-related practices. In this section, we describe East Asian parents' educational aspirations and expectations, beliefs about learning and education, and parental roles.

Parental Aspirations and Expectations

When parents have high expectations of their children's education, they are more likely to be involved in their children's education (Doepke & Zilibotti, 2019; Yamamoto & Holloway, 2010). Parents' expectations of children's educational achievement or attainment emerge as among the most powerful and robust predictors of children's academic achievement (Fan & Chen, 2001; Kim, 2020; Yamamoto & Holloway, 2010). This pattern holds in the

East Asian context, as demonstrated in a meta-analysis by Kim (2020). It is important to clarify the distinction between parental aspirations and expectations, which are often used interchangeably by researchers. Parental aspirations usually refer to desires for their children's academic performance (e.g., grades; test scores) and educational attainment (e.g., desired final level of education). Parents' expectations incorporate a more realistic assessment and prediction based on factors, such as available resources and their children's abilities. Thus, parental expectations for their children's education tend to be lower than parental aspirations (see a detailed review by Yamamoto & Holloway, 2010).

There has been consistent evidence demonstrating that East Asian parents generally hold high aspirations and expectations of their children's education. East Asian parents in the U.S. typically expect higher academic achievement for their children, including better or satisfactory grades, and greater levels of education than parents in other racial groups (Okagaki & Frensch, 1998; Pearce & Lin, 2007; Schneider & Lee, 1990; Yamamoto & Holloway, 2010; Zhou & Lee, 2017). Studies also demonstrate that parents in East Asia, especially middle-SES parents, generally hold high educational expectations of their children's education (Dittrich & Neuhaus, 2023; Holloway, 2010; Ng & Wei, 2019; Yamamoto, 2015). The terms, such as Chinese "tiger mothers," "education fever" in South Korea, or "education mom (*kyōiku mama*)" in Japan, highlight East Asian parents' high parental expectations and intensive involvement in their children's education and ironically contributed to stereotyping East Asian parenting (Dittrich & Neuhaus, 2023; Hirota, 1999; Kim & Bang, 2017; Qin & Han, 2014; Raymo & Dong, 2020; Yamamoto et al., 2022a). Notably, studies on parental expectations and involvement have predominantly focused on middle-SES families in urban cities (Kim & Bang, 2017; Stevenson & Stigler, 1992; Yamamoto, 2016a).

The cultural emphasis on education is a key explanation scholars have employed to explain East Asian parents' high expectations of their children's education (Ho, 1996; Li, 2012; Schneider & Lee, 1990). Academic attainment often brings social respect in East Asian countries. Children's academic achievement and attainment are perceived to bring honor and pride to their families, especially their parents (Dittrich & Neuhaus, 2023; Hirota, 1999; Li, 2012; Ng & Wei, 2019; Qu & Pomerantz, 2015). Further, given the strong linkage between educational achievement, employment opportunities, and economic status along with economic development in contemporary East Asia, a crucial parenting goal has become to ensure children's optimal school experiences and academic development (Hirota, 1999; Kariya, 2009; Neuhaus, 2023; Raymo & Dong, 2020). Fundamentally, the belief in meritocracy within educational systems where parents perceive individual effort rather than family background determines educational achievement has heightened parents' expectations for their children's academic success (Hirota, 1999; Gao, 2001; Kariya, 2009).

Nevertheless, diversities in parental aspirations and expectations exist across and within East Asian countries. For example, a finding from an international survey demonstrates that Japanese mothers have comparatively modest aspirations regarding their children's college attainment compared to parents in other Asian nations, such as South Korea and Thailand, and the United States (National Women's Education Center, 2007). Other studies have demonstrated diverse aspirations for their children's educational attainment among Japanese mothers (Benesse Educational Research and Developmental Institute, 2015; Nakamura, 2019; Yamamoto & Hosokawa, 2017). Lower educational aspirations observed among Japanese parents reflect a gap linked to family SES and children's gender in addition to diversifying educational trajectories in Japan (Brinton, 1993; Holloway, 2010; Matsuoka, 2019; Yamamoto & Hosokawa, 2017). Indeed, in East Asian countries, parents' expectations for their children's education are significantly and positively associated with families' SES, like in other countries (Kim, 2019; Matsuoka, 2019; Nakamura, 2019; Yamamoto & Hosokawa, 2017; Zhang et al., 2007). Parents are likely to adjust their expectations based on available resources and perceived values of college education for their children's future (Doepke & Zilibotti, 2019; Yamamoto, 2015). Increasing educational costs for families, such as supplementary school expenses, contribute to lowered parental expectations for their children's educational trajectories, especially when parents have limited resources (Hannum et al., 2019; Matsuoka, 2019; Yamamoto, 2015). In Japan, parental aspirations for children's educational attainment decreased during the economic recession around 2000, especially among lower-SES parents (Benesse Educational Research and Developmental Institute, 2015; Yamamoto, 2015). Prologued economic stagnation and reduced employment opportunities during that period may have lessened Japanese parents' optimistic views about the value of college education and their capabilities to support their children's academic attainment (Yamamoto, 2015; Yamamoto & Hosokawa, 2017).

On the other hand, studies show that East Asian immigrant and East Asian American parents in the U.S. demonstrate consistently high academic expectations, regardless of SES (Mun & Hertzog, 2019; Naumann et al., 2012; Okagaki & Frensch, 1998; Pearce & Lin, 2007; Schneider & Lee, 1990; Yamamoto & Holloway, 2010; Zhou & Lee, 2017). Immigrant parents often view the U.S. as a land filled with opportunities as some families migrate to the U.S. in pursuit of a better education for their children (Zhou & Lee, 2017). Their optimistic views of children's educational experiences may elevate their educational expectations (Zhou & Lee, 2017). Further, concerns about future discrimination, especially in the labor market, owing to their racial and ethnic minority status are likely to elevate parents' educational expectations to compensate for such disadvantages (Fernández-Reino, 2016; Ng et al., 2017; Xie & Goyette, 2003). These findings suggest that East Asian parents' educational expectations shift in response to changing social and economic contexts, perceived educational opportunities, and perspectives on the utility of educational credentials.

High parental expectations are frequently addressed as a negative aspect of East Asian parenting, especially concerning their children's psychological and socioemotional development (Mun & Hertzog, 2019; Naumann et al., 2012; Qin, 2008; Zhou & Lee, 2017). When parental expectations do not align with children's expectations or academic performance, parent–child conflicts tend to increase and negatively impact children's psychological well-being (Mun & Hertzog, 2019; Naumann et al., 2012; Qin, 2008). Although inconsistent findings exist, several studies have found that, generally, educational expectations between East Asian parents and their children are congruent (Hao & Bonstead-Bruns, 1998; Kim & Bang, 2017). For example, based on their analysis of national data, Hao & Bonstead-Bruns (1998) demonstrated that Chinese and Korean immigrant parents and their children in the U.S. displayed higher educational expectations and a greater agreement in those expectations than White, Black, or Mexican immigrant families. Studies demonstrate that East Asian parents, especially mothers, often prioritize fostering affectionate, emotional bonds and reciprocal relationships with their children (Cheah et al., 2015; DeVos, 1996; Holloway, 2010; Kim & Choi, 1994; Raymo & Dong, 2020; Tsuneyoshi, 2008). Thus, children may become attuned to parents' expectations and become willing to internalize them, reciprocating the favor (DeVos, 1996; Tsuneyoshi, 2008). Further, filial piety emphasizes respect and care in familial relationships, involving children reciprocating the family's efforts in raising them by bringing honor to them (Ho, 1996; Li, 2012). Thus, children's recognition of parental expectations and involvement may increase their academic motivation (DeVos, 1996; Ho, 1996; Li, 2012; Yamamoto et al., 2022b). In a study conducted by Qu & Pomerantz (2015), Chinese students' sense of responsibility to parents did not decline from 7th to 8th grade, unlike American students. Moreover, students' continued sense of responsibility to parents was associated with maintaining their values on academic achievement and engagement in school, measured as self-regulated learning, during this adolescence period. In many cases, this sense of responsibility, or obligation, is not imposed. Instead, it reflects a voluntary commitment by children through nurturing affective familial relations (DeVos, 1996; Tsuneyoshi, 2008; Qu & Pomerantz, 2015; Yamamoto et al., 2022b).

Cultural Beliefs About Learning

Cultural models of learning enhance our more profound understanding of East Asian parents' beliefs about learning. The East Asian cultural model rooted in Confucianism views education as a process to cultivate children's social and moral development (Li, 2012). Learning and education are considered instrumental processes of acquiring and building knowledge, developing virtue, promoting personal effort, and encouraging contributions to others and society. This virtue-oriented cultural model contrasts with the Western model of mind-oriented learning, predominantly found in the U.S. and some European countries (Li, 2012; Li et al., 2010; Yamamoto, 2020). In this model, learning is generally considered a process of inquiry focusing on the mind and mental processes, involving positive feelings such as enjoyment, confidence, and pride. Examinations of parents' perceptions of intelligent children demonstrate that Asian immigrant parents tend to value noncognitive abilities, such as respecting adults and contributing to their families, whereas White parents tend to value cognitive abilities, such as verbal, reasoning, and mathematical skills in the U.S. (Li, 2012; Okagaki & Frensch, 1998; Yamamoto, 2016).

East Asian parents commonly perceive fostering effort as a central virtue that needs to be cultivated in and through children's learning (Holloway, 1988; Li, 2012; Tobin et al., 2009; Yamamoto & Satoh, 2019). The previously described improvement-oriented approach and East Asian parents' high expectations of their children's education connect with how they attribute the causes of children's academic success and failure. In East Asian cultures, adults commonly attribute academic outcomes to the exertion of effort rather than innate abilities, a more predominant perspective in the U.S. (Ben-Ari, 1997; Holloway, 1988; Li, 2012; Ng & Wei, 2019; Schneider & Lee, 1990; Stevenson & Stigler, 1992; Yamamoto & Satoh, 2019). There is a fundamental belief among East Asian adults that children can improve their performance by identifying weaknesses and putting in greater effort. Providing constructive criticism for young children is considered a means to encourage reflection, self-evaluation, and learning from mistakes (Fung, 1999; Izumi-Taylor, 2009; Tobin et al., 2009; Yamamoto & Satoh, 2019). Struggles are understood as a natural process and fundamental for children's growth, helping them learn to manage frustrations and develop self-reliance skills, fostering a sense of accomplishment and pride (Ben-Ari, 1997; Izumi-Taylor, 2009; Holloway, 2010; Li, 2012; Stigler & Hiebert, 1999; Tsuneyoshi, 2008; Yamamoto & Satoh, 2019). East Asian parents' attributing children's academic outcomes to effort is likely to increase their educational expectations, as they believe that dedicating more effort to schoolwork can improve children's academic performance (Yamamoto &

Holloway, 2010). However, as a result of globalization and exposure to Western norms, East Asian parents have increasingly valued cultivating self-esteem and providing positive feedback, such as praise (Yamamoto & Satoh, 2019).

The vigilance of one's shortcomings and limitations and a focus on self-improvement are closely tied to the concept of humility—a moderate view of self, awareness of one's limits, and openness to new ideas (DeVos, 1996; Li, 2012, 2016; Tsuneyoshi, 2008; Yamamoto & Li, 2012; Yamamoto et al., 2022b). East Asian parents often consider humility a crucial virtue and character to cultivate in children and for their learning (DeVos, 1996; Fung, 1999; Yamamoto et al., 2022b). Humility, which encourages self-control by regulating one's inflated sense of self and self-enhancement, is believed to enable children to acknowledge their novice status and guide them in taking necessary steps to exert efforts in learning (Fung, 1999; Li, 2016; Yamamoto et al., 2022b). A case study on a low-income Chinese immigrant family demonstrates that cultivating humility in young children may help them become humble yet resilient learners by enhancing their appreciation for learning and hard work, especially when families' resources are limited (Yamamoto et al., 2022b). However, the cultivation of humility involving encouraging sympathetic listening, indirect communication, and deference toward authority may not align with U.S. classroom learning and practices that highly value honing students' persuasive verbal skills and active verbal engagement (Lareau, 2003; Tateishi, 2007; Yamamoto & Li, 2012). East Asian American students are generally observed to be quiet and less expressive in U.S. classrooms (Tateishi, 2007; Yamamoto & Li, 2012). Such evaluations potentially negatively impact East Asian American children's school experiences. A study conducted by Yamamoto and Li (2012) demonstrates that teachers at White-dominant preschools tend to assess quieter Chinese American children less positively in terms of their engagement in learning and peer relations. On the other hand, teachers in Asian-dominant preschools tend to assess quieter Chinese American children more favorably in terms of engagement in learning and adaptation to school. These studies present strengths and challenges arising from East Asian families' cultural socialization when cultural contexts between home and school differ (Kim & Choi, 1994; Qin, 2008; Yamamoto & Li, 2012; Yamamoto et al., 2022b).

Parents' Beliefs About Their Roles in Children's Education

Parents' beliefs about their roles in supporting children's learning and education play a critical role in explaining East Asian parents' patterns of involvement, especially their greater involvement at home. Although there are variations across East Asian countries, mothers are generally perceived as primary caretakers of children and responsible for children's education, more than fathers (Holloway, 2010; Shwalb et al., 2010; Raymo & Dong, 2020; Yamamoto, 2015). The traditional East Asian family model supports distinctive gender-based parental roles and responsibilities with fathers providing a good role model as an educator and disciplinarians for their children, especially sons, and mothers giving warmth, daily care, and nurturance, including children's educational matters (Ho & Lam, 2019; Holloway, 2010; Li, 2012; Shwalb et al., 2010; Yamamoto, 2016). Economic development and work conditions (e.g., long work hours) in East Asia have further reinforced fathers' roles as breadwinners and mothers' responsibilities as teachers and supporters of children's learning and development, although Chinese fathers tend to be more involved than Japanese fathers (Holloway, 2010; Li, 2020; Shwalb et al., 2010).

Research consistently demonstrates a strong sense of responsibility for teaching, disciplining, and assisting their children's learning and education among East Asian and East Asian immigrant mothers, regardless of SES (Kim & Bang, 2017; Kim et al., 2018; Ng & Wei, 2019; Yamamoto, 2015; Yamamoto et al., 2016a). East Asian parents tend to perceive guiding their children's learning and cultivating their education as a parental duty and responsibility, although there are variations associated with SES (Chao, 1994, 2000; Holloway, 2010; Li, 2012; Lim, 2012; Ng & Wei, 2019; Yamamoto et al., 2016a). A prevailing view is that children are born naturally good yet need adult guidance and instruction for optimal development and learning (Chao, 1994, 2000; Cheah et al., 2015; Yamamoto et al., 2022a). These beliefs encourage parents, especially mothers, to actively engage in their children's education, sometimes necessitating sacrifices for their own needs (Holloway, 2010; Ng & Wei, 2019; Yamamoto, 2016).

In East Asian culture, the quality of an affectionate bond with their children is highly valued. Still, parents may be less likely to directly express parental warmth through verbal or physical affection (e.g., hugs and kisses) (Cheah et al., 2015). Instead, they tend to focus on functional and instrumental care (e.g., caretaking) to express their love and warmth to their children. Supporting children's learning and engaging in education-related activities is considered a parental duty and a way to express parental care and love in East Asia (Cheah et al., 2015; Ng & Wei, 2019). Parents may engage in various learning- or education-related activities for their children. This involvement includes daily reminders to foster students' positive learning attitudes, gathering information about schools and extra-curricular lessons, financial support, driving to lessons and classes, managing children's schedules, and preparing favorite foods and snacks to bolster their children's studies (Chao, 1994, 2000; Cheah et al., 2015; Holloway, 2010; Li, 2012; Ng & Wei, 2019; Yamamoto, 2015; Yamamoto et al., 2022a).

Nevertheless, as described before, parents in East Asia tend to focus on their roles in supporting their children's education at home rather than at school. This tendency is related to parental perceptions of teachers' roles. Traditionally, East Asian parents perceive teachers as masters and authorities possessing professional knowledge, wisdom, and accumulated experience (Chen & Agbenyega, 2012; Guo & Kilderry, 2018; Holloway & Yamamoto, 2003; Li, 2012; Stevenson & Stigler, 1992; Stigler & Hiebert, 1999; Rohlen & LeTendre, 1996), although teachers' authority and occupational prestige have declined in Japan and South Korea (Akiba et al., 2023; Holloway & Yamamoto, 2003; Yamamoto, 2015). Parents and teachers are believed to have distinct roles, maintaining a clear boundary between the two. Parents often entrust school-related decisions to teachers and schools, believing that teachers have a better knowledge of children's school lives and that schools are responsible for their educational experiences at school (Kim, 2019; Stevenson & Stigler, 1992; Yamamoto et al., 2022a, 2005). One study demonstrates that Chinese parents with a kindergartner perceive teachers as leaders, with parents' roles primarily being seen as learning from them and mainly supporting and following the decisions made by teachers (Chen & Agbenyega, 2012). The prevailing concept of 'parent education' in East Asia has traditionally centered on teachers' providing knowledge and practical parenting advice to parents, aiming to educate parents (Chen & Agbenyega, 2012; Holloway & Yamamoto, 2003; Tobin et al., 2009; Yamamoto et al., 2005).

School expectations of parental roles also contribute to reinforcing parental roles in supporting children's schooling and education at home. Several studies show that schools in East Asia typically anticipate parents to support their children's school attendance, oversee the completion of homework assignments for young children, and understand and offer support for children's academic progress (Chen & Agbenyega, 2012; Holloway, 2010; Holloway & Yamamoto, 2003; Kim, 2019; Pang, 2004; Tobin et al., 2009; Yamamoto et al., 2016a). Research in China, Japan, and South Korea reveals that kindergarten and elementary school teachers may offer explicit instructions on what parents should or could do to assist their children's homework assignments or activities and suggestions about daily routines, such as sleeping, eating, and other habits outside of school hours (Chen & Agbenyega, 2012; Holloway, 2010; Holloway & Yamamoto, 2003; Kim, 2019; Lee, 2005; Tobin et al., 2009). Although research on parental roles has paid limited attention to school and educational contexts, these studies suggest that family-school relations and school practices significantly shape East Asian parents' beliefs about their roles. Moreover, these elements influence the extent and quality of parental engagement in children's learning and education, both at home and school (Yamamoto et al., 2024).

Conclusion and Future Directions

This chapter delved into East Asian parents' practices and beliefs related to children's education and learning. The East Asian sociocultural model serves as a valuable framework for understanding parental beliefs and practices concerning education in East Asia (LeVine, 1988; Li & Yamamoto, 2020). The wealth of research demonstrates shared beliefs and practices related to children's learning and education among East Asian parents, despite variations across the countries. However, variations in parental beliefs and practices across and within each country, such as those associated with SES, underscore parents' adaptation to cultural beliefs through their interactions with their life contexts and environments.

In studies of parental practices and beliefs related to education, it is essential to pay attention to the educational contexts of each country, including educational systems, school practices, and school-family relations, that impact parents' beliefs and practices related to children's education. Educational institutions often reflect the mainstream cultural models and function to reward and enhance the reproduction of dominant cultural beliefs and practices (Bourdieu & Passeron, 1977; Lareau, 2003). As a major educational institution, school plays a central role in children's attainment of social norms and culturally valued skills and knowledge (Ben-Ari, 1997; Bourdieu & Passeron, 1977; Tobin et al., 2009). Educational systems and policies also shift depending on countries' economic and political standings and goals (Doepke, & Zilibotti, 2019; Tucker, 2015). In response to such changes, parents often negotiate and change their beliefs about learning and education and ways of supporting their children's education (Kariya, 2009; Tucker, 2015). As elaborated in this chapter, the East Asian sociocultural models emphasizing parental roles, values on learning, effort orientation, and East Asian educational practices emphasizing standardized exams and meritocracy through academic attainment, are intertwined and collectively contribute to elevating East Asian parents' expectations of their children's education and engagement in children's learning and education. There is a need for more research that examines parenting, especially parental beliefs and practices related to learning, that considers educational systems and school practices.

Owing to space constraints, this chapter did not cover various important factors impacting parents' beliefs and practices related to education in East Asia, such as gender, religion, and regions (e.g., urban vs. rural areas). For example, a rise in Christianity in South Korea might have changed traditional Confucian-based beliefs and practices (Baik, 2019). Children's gender has also been a powerful factor impacting parents' beliefs, including their expectations, practices, and investment in education in East Asia (Brinton, 1993; Hannum et al., 2019; Holloway, 2010; Ng &Wei, 2019; Raymo & Dong, 2020; Yamamoto, 2016; Yamamoto & Hosokawa, 2017; Zhang et al., 2007). China (107th), Japan (125th), and South Korea (105th) all demonstrated low standings among the 146 countries on the global gender gap index in 2023 (World Economic Forum, 2023). In particular, examining the intersection between SES and gender concerning parental beliefs and practices would help us understand how educational inequality associated with gender and SES persists and can be reduced, a critical theme in East Asian countries (Kariya, 2009; Yamamoto. 2016; Zhang et al., 2007).

Overall, most studies on East Asian parents' educational beliefs and practices focus on mothers, especially middle-SES mothers. Thus, empirical research focused on how East Asian fathers' involvement in their children's education influences children's educational processes or outcomes is still relatively limited. While strong associations between fathers' occupations or educational levels and children's educational outcomes are evident in East Asia, especially in studies examining social class reproduction, these studies have not specifically examined fathers' daily practices (Byun & Park, 2012; Kariya, 2009; Matsuoka, 2019; Raymo & Dong, 2020). Research has documented the importance of fathers' care and involvement in children's lives in their children's academic achievement, self-esteem, and internalizing and externalizing behaviors (Ho & Lam, 2019; Li, 2020; Shwalb et al., 2010; Su et al., 2017). Further investigations into the roles of fathers in children's education and learning would deepen our understanding of similarities and differences between fathers' and mothers' practices, and how their support impacts children's educational experiences and outcomes in East Asia and beyond.

References

Akiba, M., Byun, S., Jiang, X., Kim, K., & Moran, A. J. (2023). Do teachers feel valued in society? Occupational value of the teaching profession in OECD Countries. *AERA Open, 9*. https://doi.org/10.1177/23328584231179184.

Baik, C.-H. (2019). Some influences of Confucianism on Korean Christian family life: Confucian? Christian? or Confucian-Christian? *Theology Today, 76*(3), 242–251. https://doi.org/10.1177/0040573619859019.

Ben-Ari, E. (1997). *Body projects in Japanese childcare: Culture, organization and emotions in a preschool*. Curzon Press.

Benesse Educational Research and Developmental Institute. (2015). *Yōji no seikatsu ankēto* [A survey on the life of young children]. https://berd.benesse.jp/jisedai/research/detail1.php?id=4770.

Blinco, P. M. A. (1992). A cross-cultural study of task persistence of young children in Japan and the United States. *Journal of Cross-Cultural Psychology, 23*(3), 407–415. https://doi.org/10.1177/0022022192233010.

Bourdieu, P. & Passeron, J. (1977). *Reproduction in education, society and culture.* Sage Publications.

Bray, M. (2022). Shadow education in Asia and the Pacific: Features and implications of private supplementary tutoring. In W. O. Lee, P. Brown, A. L. Goodwin, & A. Green (Eds), *International handbook on education development in Asia-Pacific* (pp. 1–23). Springer. https://doi.org/10.1007/978-981-16-2327-1_10-1.

Brinton, M. (1993). *Women and the economic miracle: Gender and work in post-war Japan.* University of California Press.

Byun, S. Y. & Kim, K. K. (2010). Educational inequality in South Korea: The widening socioeconomic gap in student achievement. In E. Hannum, H. Park, & Y. G. Butler (Eds), *Globalization, changing demographics, and educational challenges in East Asia* (Vol. 17, pp. 155–182). Emerald Group Publishing Limited. doi: 10.1108/S1479–3539(2010)17.

Byun, S. Y. & Park, H. (2012). The academic success of East Asian American youth: The role of shadow education. *Sociology of Education*, *85*(1), 40–60. https://doi.org/10.1177/0038040711417009.

Chao, R. K. (1994). Beyond parental control and authoritarian parenting style: Understanding Chinese parenting through the cultural notion of training. *Child Development, 65*(4), 1111–1119. https://doi.org/10.1111/j.1467-8624.1994.tb00806.x.

Chao, R. K. (2000). The parenting of immigrant Chinese and European American mothers: Relations between parenting styles, socialization goals, and parental practices. *Journal of Applied Developmental Psychology, 21*(2), 233–248. https://doi.org/10.1016/S0193-3973(99)00037-4.

Cheah, C. S., Li, J., Zhou, N., Yamamoto, Y., & Leung, C. Y. (2015). Understanding Chinese immigrant and European American mothers' expressions of warmth. *Developmental psychology, 51*(12), 1802–1811. https://doi.org/10.1037/a0039855.

Chen, C. S. & Stevenson, H. W. (1989). Homework: a cross-cultural examination. *Child development, 60*(3), 551–561. https://doi.org/10.1111/j.1467-8624.1989.tb02736.x.

Chen, F. & Agbenyega, J. (2012). Chinese parents' perspectives on home-kindergarten partnership: A narrative research. *Australasian Journal of Early Childhood, 37*(2), 95–105. https://doi.org/10.1177/183693911203700213.

Cheung, C. S. & Pomerantz, E. M. (2011). Parents' involvement in children's learning in the United States and China: implications for children's academic and emotional adjustment. *Child development, 82*(3), 932–950. https://doi.org/10.1111/j.1467-8624.2011.01582.x.

Choi, Y. E., Bempechat, J., & Ginsburg, H. P. (1994). Educational socialization in Korean American children: A longitudinal study. *Journal of Applied Developmental Psychology, 15*(3), 313–318. https://doi.org/10.1016/0193-3973(94)90033-7.

DeVos, G. A. (1996). Psychological continuities in Japanese social motivation. In D. W. Shwalb & B. J. Shwalb (Eds), *Japanese childrearing: Two generations of scholarship* (pp. 44–84). Guilford Press.

Dittrich, K. & Neuhaus, D. (2023) Korea's 'education fever' from the late nineteenth to the early twenty-first century. *History of Education, 52*(4), 539–552. doi: 10.1080/0046760X.2022.2098391.

Doepke, M. & Zilibotti, F. (2019). *Love, money, and parenting: How economics explains the way we raise our kids*. Princeton University Press. https://doi.org/10.2307/j.ctvc77fr1.

Duckworth, A. L. (2016). *Grit: The power of passion and perseverance*. Scribner.

Dweck, C. S. (2006). *Mindset: The new psychology of success*. Random House.

Elman, B. A., Duncan, J. B., & Ooms, H. (2002). *Rethinking Confucianism: Past and present in China, Japan, Korea, and Vietnam*. UCLA Asian Pacific Monograph Series.

Fan, X. & Chen, M. (2001). Parental involvement and students' academic achievement: A meta-analysis. *Educational Psychology Review, 13*, 1–22. https://doi.org/10.1023/A:1009048817385.

Fernández-Reino, M. (2016). Immigrant optimism or anticipated discrimination? Explaining the first educational transition of ethnic minorities in England. *Research in Social Stratification and Mobility, 46*, 141–156. https://doi:10.1016/j.rssm.2016.08.007.

Fung, H. (1999). Becoming a moral child: The socialization of shame among young Chinese children. *Ethos, 27*, 180–209. https://doi.org/10.1525/eth.1999.27.2.180.

Gao, L. (2011). *Impacts of cultural capital on student college choice process in China*. Lexington Books.

Guo, K. & Kilderry, A. (2018). Teacher accounts of parent involvement in children's education in China. *Teaching and Teacher Education, 69*, 95–103. https://doi.org/10.1016/j.tate.2017.09.018.

Hannum, E., Ishida, H., Park, H., & Tam, T. (2019). Education in East Asian societies: Postwar expansion and the evolution of inequality. *Annual Review of Sociology, 45*, 625–647. https://doi.org/10.1146/annurev-soc-073018-022507.

Hao, L. & Bonstead-Bruns, M. (1998). Parent–child differences in educational expectations and the academic achievement of immigrant and native students. *Sociology of Education, 71*(3), 175–198. https://doi.org/10.2307/2673201.

Harkness, S. & Super, C. M. (2002). Culture and parenting. In M. H. Bornstein (Ed.), *Handbook of parenting* Volume 2: *Biology and ecology of parenting* (pp. 253–280). Lawrence Erlbaum Associates.

Harkness, S., Super, C. M., Bermúdez, M. R., Moscardino, U., Rha, J., Mavridis, C. J., Bonichini, S., Huitrón, B., Welles-Nyström, B., Palacios, J., Hyun, O., Soriano, G., & Zylicz, P. O. (2009). *Parental ethnotheories of children's learning*. www.celf.ucla.edu/2010_conference_articles/Harkness_et_al_2009.pdf.

Heine, S. J., Kitayama, S., Lehman, D. R., Takata, T., Ide, E., Leung, C., & Matsumoto, H. (2001). Divergent consequences of success and failure in Japan and North America: An investigation of self-improving motivations and malleable selves. *Journal of Personality and Social Psychology, 81*(4), 599–615. https://doi.org/10.1037/0022-3514.81.4.599.

Hill, N. E., Castellino, D. R., Lansford, J. E., Nowlin, P., Dodge, K. A., Bates, J. E., & Pettit, G. S. (2004). Parental academic involvement as related to school behavior, achievement, and aspirations: Demographic variation across adolescence. *Child Development, 75,* 1491–1509. https://doi.org/10.1111/j.1467-8624.2004.00753.x.

Hirota, T. (1999). *Nihonjin no shitsuke wa suitai shitaka: Kyōiku suru kazoku no yukue* [Has Japanese child-rearing declined? The direction of education-oriented families]. Kōdansha Gendai Shinsho.

Ho, D. Y. F. (1996). Filial piety and its psychological consequences. In M. H. Bond (Ed.), *Handbook of Chinese psychology* (pp. 155–165). Oxford University Press.

Ho, E. S. C. & Staub, K. V. (2018). Home and school relationships in Switzerland and Hong Kong. In S. B. Sheldon & T. A. Turner-Vorbeck (Eds), *The Wiley handbook of family, school, and community relationships in education* (pp. 289–314). John Wiley & Sons, Inc. https://doi.org/10.1002/9781119083054.ch14.

Ho, H. & Lam, Y. W. (2019). Father involvement in East Asia. In The Wiley Handbook of family, school, and community relationships in education (pp. 333–356). John Wiley & Sons, Inc. https://doi.org/10.1002/9781119083054.ch16.

Holloway, S. D. (1988). Concepts of ability and effort in Japan and the United States. *Review of Educational Research, 58*(3), 327–345. https://doi.org/10.2307/1170258.

Holloway, S. D. (2010). *Women and family in contemporary Japan*. Cambridge University Press. https://doi.org/10.1017/CBO9780511761317"https://doi.org/10.1017/CBO9780511761317.

Holloway S. D., Campbell E. J., Nagase A., Kim S., Suzuki S., Wang Q., Iwatate, K., & Baak S. Y. (2016). Parenting self-efficacy and parental involvement: Mediators or moderators between socioeconomic status and children's academic competence in Japan and Korea? *Research in Human Development, 13,* 258–272. https://doi.org/10.1080/15427609.2016.1194710.

Holloway, S. D. & Yamamoto, Y. (2003). Sensei! Early childhood education teachers in Japan. In O. Saracho & B. Spodek (Eds), *Contemporary perspectives in early childhood education: Studying teachers in early childhood setting* (pp. 181–207). Information Age Publishing.

Holloway, S. D., Yamamoto, Y., Suzuki, S., & Dalesandro, J. (2008). Determinants of parental involvement in early schooling: Evidence from Japan. *Early Childhood Research & Practice, 10*(1). https://ecrp.illinois.edu/v10n1/holloway.html.

Hoover-Dempsey, K. V., Walker, J. M. T., Sandler, H. M., Whetsel, D., Green, C. L., Wilkins, A. S., & Closson, K. (2005). Why do parents become involved? Research findings and implications. *The Elementary School Journal, 106*(2), 105–130. https://doi.org/10.1086/499194.

Huntsinger, C. S. & Jose, P. E. (2009). Parental involvement in children's schooling: Different meanings in different cultures. *Early Childhood Research Quarterly, 24,* 398–410. https://doi.org/10. 1016/j.ecresq.2009.07.006.

Huntsinger, C. S., Jose, P. E., Larson, S. L., Balsink Krieg, D., & Shaligram, C. (2000). Mathematics, vocabulary, and reading development in Chinese American and European American children over the primary school years. *Journal of Educational Psychology, 92*(4), 745–760. https://doi.org/10.1037/0022-0663.92.4.745.

Izumi-Taylor, S. (2009). Hansei: Japanese preschoolers learn introspection with teachers' help. *Young Children, 64*(4), 86–90.

Kao, G. & Thompson, J. S. (2003). Racial and ethnic stratification in educational achievement and attainment. *Annual Review of Sociology, 29*(1), 417–442. https://doi.org/10.1146/annurev.soc.29.010202.100019.

Kariya, T. (2009). *Kyōiku to byōdō* [Education and equality]. Chuō Kōron Shinsha.

Kim, J. & Bang, H. (2017) Education fever: Korean parents' aspirations for their children's schooling and future career. *Pedagogy, Culture & Society, 25*(2), 207–224. doi: 10.1080/14681366.2016.1252419.

Kim, S. W. (2019) Left-behind children: Teachers' perceptions of family-school relations in rural China. *Compare: A Journal of Comparative and International Education, 49*(4), 584–601. doi.org/10.1080/03057925.2018.1438885.

Kim, S. W. (2020). Meta-analysis of parental involvement and achievement in East Asian countries. *Education and Urban Society, 52*(2), 312–337. https://doi.org/10.1177/0013124519842654.

Kim, U. & Choi, S.H. (1994). Individualism, collectivism, and child development: A Korean perspective. In P. M. Greenfield, R. Rodney, & R. R. Cocking (Eds), *Cross-cultural roots of minority child development* (pp. 227–258). Psychology Press.

Kim, Y. A., An, S., Kim, H. C. L., & Kim, J. (2018). Meaning of parental involvement among Korean immigrant parents: A mixed-methods approach. *Journal of Educational Research, 111*(2), 127–138. https://doi.org/10.1080/00220671.2016.1220355.

Lareau, A. (2003). *Unequal childhoods: class, race and family life.* University of California Press.

Lee, S. (2005). Selective parent participation: Structural and cultural factors that influence school participation among Korean parents. *Equity & Excellence in Education, 38*(4), 299–308. https://doi.org/10.1080/10665680500299734.

LeVine, R. (1988). Human parental care. In R. LeVine, P. M. Miller, & M. M. West. (Eds), *Parental behaviors in diverse societies: New Directions for Child Development.* (pp. 3– 12). Jossey Bass. https://doi.org/10.1002/cd.23219884003.

Li, J. (2012). *Cultural foundations of learning: East and West* Cambridge University Press. https://doi.org/10.1017/CBO9781139028400.

Li, J. (2016). Humility in learning: A Confucian perspective. *Journal of Moral Education, 45*(2), 1–19. https://doi-org/10.1080/03057240.2016.1168736.

Li, J., & Yamamoto, Y. (2020). Western and East Asian sociocultural learning models: Evidence from cross-cultural and immigrant research. *Asian Journal of Social Psychology, 23*, 174–186. https://doi.org/10.1111/ajsp.12384.

Li, J., Yamamoto, Y., Luo, L., Batchelor, A., & Bresnahan, R. (2010). Why attend school? Chinese immigrant and European American preschoolers' views and outcomes. *Developmental Psychology, 121*, 9–25. https://doi.org/10.1037/a0019926.

Li, X. (2020). Fathers' involvement in Chinese societies: Increasing presence, uneven progress. *Child Development Perspectives, 14*(3), 150–156. https://doi.org/10.1111/cdep.12375.

Lim, M. (2012). Unpacking parent involvement: Korean American parents' collective networking. *School Community Journal, 22*(1), 89–109. www.adi.org/journal/2012ss/LimSpring2012.pdf.

Matsuoka, R. (2019). *Kyōiku kakusa: kaisō chiiki gakureki [Educational gaps: social class, regions, and educational credentials].* Chikuma Shobō.

Mun, R. U., & Hertzog, N. B. (2019). The influence of parental and self-expectations on Asian American women who entered college early. *Gifted Child Quarterly, 63*(2), 120–140. https://doi.org/10.1177/0016986218823559.

Nakamura, E. (2019). Tōkei dēta karamiru kosodate to gakuryoku [Child-rearing and academic performance based on data]. In N. Isa (Ed.), *Gakuryoku wo sasaeru kazoku to kosodate senryaku: Shūgaku zengo ni okeru daitoshiken deno tsuiseki chōsa* (pp. 69–87). Akashi Shoten.

National Women's Educational Center (2007). *Heisei 16 nendo 17 nendo kateikyōiku ni kansuru kokusaihikaku chōsa hōkokusho* [Report of international comparisons about family education from 2004 to 2005]. www.nwec.jp/about/publish/2005/ndpk5s0000000zft.html.

Naumann, L. P., Guillaume, E. M., & Funder, D. C. (2012). The correlates of high parental academic expectations: An Asian-Latino comparison. *Journal of Cross-Cultural Psychology, 43*(4), 515–520. https://doi.org/10.1177/0022022112438398.

Ng, F. F., Pomerantz, E. M., & Lam, S. F. (2007). European American and Chinese parents' responses to children's success and failure: Implications for children's responses. *Developmental Psychology, 43*(5), 1239–1255. https://doi.org/10.1037/0012-1649.43.5.1239.

Ng, F. F., Sze, I. N., Tamis-LeMonda, C. S., & Ruble, D. N. (2017). Immigrant Chinese mothers' socialization of achievement in children: A strategic adaptation to the host society. *Child Development, 88*(3), 979–995. https://doi.org/10.1111/cdev.12701.

Ng, F. F. & Wei, J. (2019). Delving into the minds of Chinese parents: What beliefs motivate their learning-related practices? *Child Development Perspectives, 14*(1), 61–67. https://doi.org/10.1111/cdep.12358.

OECD (2014). Supplementary education in East Asia. *Lessons from PISA for Korea*, OECD Publishing. https://doi.org/10.1787/9789264190672-5-en.

Okagaki, L. & Frensch, P. A. (1998). Parenting and children's school achievement: A multiethnic perspective. *American Educational Research Journal, 35*(1), 123–144. https://doi.org/10.2307/1163454.

Pang, I. (2004). School–family–community partnership in Hong Kong – Perspectives and challenges. *Educational Research for Policy and Practice, 3*, 109–125. https://doi.org/10.1007/s10671-004-5556-7.

Park, J.-H. & Kwon, Y. I. (2009). Parental goals and parenting practices of upper-middle-class Korean mothers with preschool children. *Journal of Early Childhood Research, 7*(1), 58–75. https://doi.org/10.1177/1476718X08098354.

Pearce, R. R. & Lin, Z. (2007). Chinese American post-secondary achievement and attainment: A cultural and structural analysis. *Educational Review, 59*(1), 19–36. https://doi.org/10.1080/00131910600796827.

Pomerantz, E. M., Moorman, E. A., & Litwack, S. D. (2007). The how, whom, and why of parents' involvement in children's academic lives: More is not always better. *Review of Educational Research, 77*(3), 373–410. https://doi.org/10.3102/003465430305567.

Qin, D. B. (2008). Doing well vs. feeling well: Understanding family dynamics and the psychological adjustment of Chinese immigrant adolescents. *Journal of Youth and Adolescence, 37*(1), 22–35. https://doi.org/10.1007/s10964-007-9220-4.

Qin, D. B. & Han, E-J. (2014). Tiger parents or sheep parents? Struggles of parental involvement in working-class Chinese immigrant families. *Teachers College Record, 116*(8), 1–32. https://doi.org/10.1177/016146811411 6008.

Qu, Y. & Pomerantz, E. M. (2015). Divergent school trajectories in early adolescence in the United States and China: An examination of underlying mechanisms. *Journal of Youth and Adolescence,* 44, 2095–2109. https://doi.org/10.1007/s10964-014-0201-0.

Raymo, J. M. & Dong, H. (2020). Parental resources and child well-being in East Asia: An overview. *Chinese Journal of Sociology,* 6(2), 197–218. https://doi.org/10.1177/2057150X20908093.

Rohlen, T. & LeTendre, G. (Eds) (1996). *Teaching and learning in Japan*. Cambridge University Press. https://doi.org/10.1017/CBO9781139174480.

Schneider, B. & Lee, Y. (1990). A model for academic success: The school and home environment of East Asian students. *Anthropology and Education Quarterly, 21*(4), 358–377. https://doi.org/10.1525/aeq.1990.21.4.04x0596x.

Shwalb, D.W., Nakazawa, J., Yamamoto, T., & Hyun, J-H. (2010). Fathering in Japan, China, and Korea: Changing contexts, images, and roles. In M. Lamb (Ed.), The role of the father in child development (pp. 341–387). John Wiley & Sons, Inc.

Stevenson, H. W. & Stigler, J. W. (1992). *The learning gap: Why our schools are failing and what we can learn from Japanese and Chinese education*. Summit Books.

Stigler, J. W. & Hiebert, J. (1999). *The teaching gap: Best ideas from the world's teachers for improving in the classroom.* The Free Press.

Su, L. P., Kubricht, B., & Miller, R. (2017). The influence of father involvement in adolescents' overall development in Taiwan. *Journal of Adolescence, 59,* 35–44. https://doi.org/10.1016/j.adolescence.2017.05.010.

Sy, S. R. (2006). Rethinking parent involvement during the transition to first grade: A focus on Asian American families. *The School Community Journal, 16*(1), 107–125. www.adi.org/journal/ss06/SySpring2006.pdf.

Tateishi, C. A. (2007). Why are the Asian-American kids silent in class? Taking a chance with words. *Rethinking Schools, 22*(2), 20–23.

Thomas, R. M. & Postlethwaite, T. N. (1983). Describing change and estimating its causes. In R. M. Thomas & T. N. Postlethwaite (Eds), *Schooling in East Asia* (pp. 1–36). Pergamon.

Tobin, J. J., Hsueh, Y., & Karasawa, M. (2009). *Preschool in three cultures revisited: China, Japan, and the United States*. University of Chicago Press.

Tsuneyoshi, R. (2008). *Kodomotachi no mittsu no kiki: Kokusaihikaku kara miru nihon no mosaku* [Three risks facing Japanese children]. Keisō Shobō.

Tucker, M. S. (2015). *Surpassing Shanghai: An agenda for American education built on the world's leading systems*. Harvard Education Press.

Turney, K. & Kao, G. (2009). Barriers to school involvement: Are immigrant parents disadvantaged? *The Journal of Educational Research, 102*(4), 257–271. https://doi.org/10.3200/JOER.102.4.257-271.

World Economic Forum (2023). *Global gender gap report*. www3.weforum.org/docs/WEF_GGGR_2023.pdf.

Xie, Y. & Goyette, K. (2003). Social mobility and the educational choices of Asian Americans. *Social Science Research, 32*, 467–498. https://doi.org/10.1016/S0049-089X(03)00018-8.

Yamamoto, Y. (2015). Social class and Japanese mothers' support for young children's education: A qualitative study. *Journal of Early Childhood Research, 13*(2), 165–180. https://doi.org/10.1177/1476718X13482303.

Yamamoto, Y. (2016). Gender and social class differences in Japanese mothers' beliefs about children's education and socialisation. *Gender and Education, 28*(1), 72–88. https://doi-org/10.1080/09540253.2015.1091917.

Yamamoto, Y. (2020). Young children's beliefs about school learning in Japan and the United States: Cultural and socioeconomic comparisons. *Early Childhood Research Quarterly, 50*(2), 28–37. https://doi.org/10.1016/j.ecresq.2019.06.013.

Yamamoto, Y. & Holloway, S. D. (2010). Parental expectations and academic performance in sociocultural contexts. *Educational Psychology Review, 22*(3), 189–214. https://doi.org/10.1007/s10648-010-9121-z.

Yamamoto, Y., Holloway, S. D., & Suzuki, S. (2006). Maternal involvement in preschool children's education in Japan: Parenting beliefs and socioeconomic status. *Early Childhood Research Quarterly, 21*, 332–346. https://doi.org/10.1016/j.ecresq.2006.07.008.

Yamamoto, Y., Holloway, S. D., & Suzuki, S. (2016a). Parental engagement in children's education: Motivating factors in Japan and the U.S. *School Community Journal, 26*(1), 45–66. www.adi.org/journal/2016ss/YamamotoEtAlSpring2016.pdf.

Yamamoto, Y. & Hosokawa, S. (2017). Maternal aspirations and expectations for their children's educational attainment in Japan: Relations to gender and mothers' educational levels. *International Psychology Bulletin, 21*(3), 25–33.

Yamamoto, Y. & Li, J. (2012). Quiet in the eye of the beholder: Teacher perceptions of Asian immigrant children. In C. Garcia Coll (Ed.), *The impact of immigration on children's development. Contributions to Human Development* (Vol. 24, pp. 1–17). Karger. https://doi.org/10.1159/000331021.

Yamamoto, Y., Li, J., & Bempechat, J. (2022a). Reconceptualizing parental involvement: A sociocultural model explaining Chinese immigrant parents' school-based and home-based involvement. *Educational Psychologist, 57*(4), 267–280. https://doi.org/10.1080/00461520.2022.2094383"https://doi.org/10.1080/00461520.2022.2094383.

Yamamoto, Y., Li, J., & Bempechat, J. (2024). A cultural model of family-school relations: East Asian immigrant parents' involvement in children's education. In M. Williams-Johnson & N. P. Rickert (Eds.), *Critical analysis of parental involvement in school: Working with families across sociocultural contexts*. Routledge.

Yamamoto, Y., Li, J., Li, A., LaFave, R., & Reichling, C. J. (2022b). Raising humble children: Asian immigrant families' socialization and children's school experiences. In M. J. Strickland (Ed.), *Composing storylines of possibilities: Immigrant and refugee families navigating school* (pp. 37–54). Information Age Publishing.

Yamamoto, Y., Li, J., & Liu, JL. (2016b). Does socioeconomic status matter for Chinese immigrants' academic socialization? Family environment, parental engagement, and preschoolers' outcomes. *Research in Human Development, 13*(3), 191–206. https://doi.org/10.1080/15427609.2016.1194706.

Yamamoto, Y. & Satoh, E. (2019). Ganbari: Cultivating perseverance and motivation in early childhood education in Japan. In O. Saracho (Ed.), *Contemporary research on motivation in early childhood education* (pp. 227–246). Information Age Publishing.

Zhang, Y., Kao, G., & Hannum, E. (2007). Do mothers in rural China practice gender equality in educational aspirations for their children? *Comparative Education Review, 51*(2), 131–157. https://doi.org/10.1086/512023.

Zhou, G. & Zhong, L. (2018). Chinese immigrant parents' involvement in their children's school-based education: Behaviours and perceptions. In Y. Guo (Ed.), *Home-school relations: International perspectives* (pp. 89–111). Springer. https://doi.org/10.1007/978-981-13-0324-1_6.

Zhou, M. & Lee, J. (2017). Hyper-selectivity and the remaking of culture: Understanding the Asian American achievement paradox. *Asian American Journal of Psychology, 8*(1), 7–15. https://doi.org/10.1037/aap0000069.

11

PARENTING AND BEHAVIOR PROBLEMS OF CHILDREN AND ADOLESCENTS IN ASIAN FAMILIES

Jennifer E. Lansford, Liane P. Alampay, Lei Chang, and Saengduean Yotanyamaneewong

Introduction

One of the most important roles for parents globally is to socialize their children to be well-functioning members of their respective societies. The specific strategies parents use to socialize desired behaviors and prevent maladaptive behaviors vary across cultural groups. In addition, parents in different cultural groups differ to some extent in which behaviors are deemed problematic and which desirable, although there are many cultural similarities as well. This chapter begins with a consideration of ethnotheories regarding parents' understandings of children's adaptive and problematic behaviors as well as how to manage those behaviors before considering Asian cultural values in relation to parenting. The chapter then focuses on parenting styles, parental discipline, and parental monitoring as central ways that parents influence their children's adaptive behaviors and behavior problems. The chapter next considers implications for practice and policy, suggests directions for future research, and concludes.

We acknowledge at the outset that Asia comprises many diverse cultures, which are often lumped together and considered homogeneous relative to Western contexts. Cultural contexts apart from China are typically underrepresented, even within studies of Asian parents. Asian countries represent the full range from low-income to high-income, differences in predominant religion (Buddhist, Hindu, Muslim), and differences in socio-political contexts, all of which can affect parenting and child behaviors. Although we make some generalizations about Asian parenting in relation to behavior

DOI: 10.4324/9781003383949-11

problems of children and adolescents, it is important to recognized variability within Asian countries, cultural contexts, and families.

History and Theory

Understanding parents' ethnotheories regarding children's desirable and undesirable behaviors is important when conceptualizing parenting and the behavior problems of children and adolescents (Olson et al., 2019). Parents in some cultural contexts may regard particular behaviors as especially problematic, whereas parents in other contexts may not regard these same behaviors as problematic at all. For example, parents in Thailand were found to regard children's externalizing behaviors (such as aggression) as more problematic than internalizing behaviors (such as depression and anxiety) because externalizing behaviors are more disruptive to other people than internalizing behaviors are (Weisz et al., 1993). Because externalizing problems can interfere with group harmony, these problems may carry more stigma in cultural contexts characterized as collectivistic (e.g., focused on group harmony) than individualistic (e.g., focused on individual goals; Lau et al., 2016).

When mothers in Japan and the United States were asked to describe desirable and undesirable behaviors of preschoolers, they generated similar descriptions of desirable behaviors, including cooperativeness and good manners (Olson et al., 2001). Mothers' descriptions of undesirable behaviors differed, however. Mothers in Japan focused on the undesirability of socially insensitive and uncooperative behaviors such as disrespect and rudeness; they did not mention concerns with emotional problems such as anxiety or low self-esteem. By contrast, mothers in the United States focused on aggressive and disruptive behaviors as well as on emotional problems. Similarly, when European American and Taiwanese mothers were asked how to foster their preschoolers' positive adjustment, almost all European American mothers described promoting children's high self-esteem; however, almost no Taiwanese mothers mentioned promoting self-esteem, and when they did, self-esteem was more often described as a liability that could contribute to poor self-control or other problem behaviors such as rudeness or stubbornness (Miller et al., 2012). In studies of school-aged children, inhibited social behaviors, such as shyness, that can foster social harmony are valued more and are considered indicators of social competence more in China, Indonesia, and Korea than in Canada and the United States, where more assertive behaviors are valued more and are associated with better adjustment (Chen, 2018).

Parents in different countries also have different views regarding the appropriateness of expressing different emotions. For instance, Tamang

Nepalese parents believe that anger should be suppressed, perhaps because of the high importance they place on respect for authority and group harmony (Cole et al., 2002). Likewise, children in India report not expressing anger and sadness in social settings because of their parents' disapproval of such displays (Raval et al., 2007). Parents' emphasis on their children's emotional restraint and impulse control has been described as being more common in several Asian countries than in Canada and the United States (Chen, 2018; Lee et al., 2013).

Not only do parents in different countries hold different beliefs about which child behaviors are problematic, parents also attribute problem behaviors to different causes, which affects how parents manage these behaviors (Bayram Özdemir & Cheah, 2015). For example, Japanese mothers are likely to perceive their preschoolers' disruptive behaviors as a reflection of developmental immaturity normative at that age and therefore respond tolerantly with sensitivity and redirection rather than punishment (Tobin et al., 2009). With respect to academic achievement, Chinese and Japanese parents are more likely than parents from Canada and the United States to believe that achievement is a function of hard work and effort rather than innate abilities, which is related to Chinese and Japanese parents' efforts to encourage their children to work harder (Rothbaum & Wang, 2010).

Despite these generalizations about between-country differences in parents' views regarding children's misbehavior and how to manage misbehavior, it is also important to recognize that cultures are not static over time and also that within-country variability can be common in parents' beliefs and behaviors. With respect to historical time, globalization, technology uptake, and migration from rural to urban areas can all affect parents' beliefs about children's behaviors. For example, in China, parents' positive regard for children's shyness was higher in the past and in rural settings than it is in contemporary urban settings (Chen, 2018). Regional (urban versus rural), socioeconomic, racial/ethnic, and other demographic factors can contribute to within-country variability (Cole et al., 2006; Keller, 2018). For example, in Nepal, elders hold different beliefs about children's displays of anger and shame depending on whether they are Tamang or Brahmin, reflecting the discrepancy in social status of these groups (Cole et al., 2006).

Asian Cultural Values and Parenting

In general, Asian parenting research indicates that, first, parenting frameworks, which encompass aspects of acceptance-rejection, warmth-control, and authoritative-authoritarian parenting dimensions, explain variations in Asian parenting similarly to results widely reported in Western research. Therefore, these frameworks are considered universal rather than specific to the Western context (Guo et al., 2005; Lu & Chang, 2013; Wang & Chang, 2009). Second, within the universal parenting frameworks, variations in Asian parenting may also be elucidated by identifying additional parenting practice patterns that are culturally meaningful but that have not been the primary focus of Western research (Lu & Chang, 2013; Wang & Chang, 2008).

Although the cross-cultural literature has reported more Chinese parenting work compared with other Asian cultural groups, Chao and Tseng (2002) conducted a comprehensive review of Asian parenting and concluded that various communities share cultural similarities, owing to the significant influence of Confucian and Buddhist philosophies in these contexts, particularly in China and other countries in East Asia (Kelley & Tseng, 1992). These shared cultural features underscore the family as a collective entity, prioritize family and community harmony, and most notably, highlight the importance of parental involvement in their children's education and academic performance. Against these two backdrops, we delve into one of the most distinctive aspects of Chinese parenting—the concept of "guan."

Deeply rooted in Confucian philosophy, particularly in the concept of filial piety, "guan," which translates to "to care for" and "to govern" offspring (Chao, 1994), encompasses a multifaceted set of behaviors in which Chinese parents engage to ensure the educational success of their children. In Chinese culture, parents are regarded as a child's first and eternal teachers, responsible for modeling exemplary behavior to establish a lifelong foundation for their child's development. They are expected to offer guidance and advice even as their child matures into adulthood. Contrary to the more open, permissive, and child-centered educational concepts in Western cultures, "guan" underscores behavioral training aimed at aligning the child with adult expectations (Hays, 1996). In contrast to the Western approach, which values communication and the expression of affection while promoting democratic control and discipline, "guan" emphasizes one-sided governance by parents and the child's obedience and understanding (Lin, 2003). Parental governance under the concept of "guan" encompasses the regulation and restriction of a child's activities to prevent negative outcomes. Examples may include monitoring and limiting the child's use of phones or the internet, structuring the child's daily routines, and imposing strict rules and behavioral expectations. However, "guan" also implies parental accommodation (Chao, 1994), which involves parents sacrificing their own interests for the well-being of their children (Lin, 2003). Parental accommodation may extend to providing nutritious meals, sacrificing leisure time, and offering financial support for the child's education. Last but not least, "guan" also entails the parent–child relationship, characterized by a hierarchical structure, enduring bonds, and the core principle of filial piety (Chao, 1996).

Guan parenting is distinct from both authoritative and authoritarian parenting styles (Stewart & Bond, 2002). Authoritative parenting aims for a balance between parental control and emotional support. In contrast, guan places a higher emphasis on parental control over emotional support. However, guan parenting advocates parental sacrifice to promote provisioning and other benefits for the children. Therefore, in comparison to authoritative parenting, guan differs more markedly from authoritarian parenting. Authoritarian parenting emphasizes strict obedience to parental authority without much explanation or emotional support. Guan parents may set strict rules and expectations for their children, but they also provide explanations and observe the rules of reward and punishment without anger or resentment (Wang & Chang, 2008). Guan may, on the surface, resemble an authoritarian parenting style, owing to its foundation in the cultural principle of filial piety and the related hierarchical and non-democratic parent–child relationship. Guan parenting can have both positive and negative effects on children's development. On the positive side, guan parents often provide their children with the resources and support required for academic success. On the other hand, this style of parenting may exert excessive pressure on children to achieve, leading to heightened stress and anxiety (Chao, 1996).

Other culturally meaningful and indigenous parenting practices also are important in Asian contexts. For example, the concept of *utang na loob* (immeasurable debt of being) in the Philippines has been described as being central to family interdependence and the obligations that children perceive themselves as having to their parents (Alampay, 2014). Similarly, the *Ashrama* theory of family life in India captures how *kal, des,* and *patra* (time, place, and person) are central to understanding parent–child relationships (Chaudhary & Sriram, 2020). These and other cultural values are socialized by parents and reflected in children's adaptive and maladaptive behaviors.

Parenting Styles and Behavior Problems of Children and Adolescents

Warmth and control are the cornerstones of parenting styles defined by high levels of both warmth and control (authoritative), high levels of warmth but low levels of control (permissive), low levels of warmth but high levels of control (authoritarian), and low levels of warmth and control (neglecting) parenting (Baumrind, 1967; Maccoby & Martin, 1983). A large body of research has examined how these four parenting styles are related to children's and adolescents' behavior problems. Early research concluded that authoritarian parenting was related to fewer behavior problems in Asian children than in European American children, who were the original participants in studies that yielded the framework for these parenting styles; however, more recent research has suggested that compared with authoritative parenting, authoritarian parenting is also related to more behavior problems for Asian children (see Sorkhabi, 2005, for a narrative review). A randomized controlled trial of a parenting intervention in Pakistan demonstrated that as authoritative parenting increased, adolescents' challenging behaviors decreased (Kauser & Pinquart, 2019).

Recent meta-analyses have shown that an increasing proportion of Asian parents tend to adopt authoritative parenting styles. East Asian countries such as China, Japan, Korea, Singapore, and Taiwan show the most adoption of authoritative styles (Kim, 2019; Yim, 2022). Research in southeast Asian countries such as the Philippines and Thailand also found similar results (Benito, 2022; Hosiri et al., 2018; Rhucharoenpornpanich et al., 2010). Although authoritative parenting is the most widely accepted style across the Asian continent, studies conducted in Malaysia and Vietnam indicate a bigger mix between authoritarian and authoritative parenting styles (Ghani et al., 2014; Keshavrz & Baharudin, 2009; Nguyen et al., 2020).

It is important to note that definitions of authoritative parenting may not align completely with those in Western countries. For instance, although many Thai parents accept the concept of an authoritative style, in cultural practice, their parenting style may not neatly fit into the distinct categories used to describe Western parenting. Thai children may not be encouraged to express themselves as much as their Western counterparts. Simultaneously, Thais tend to avoid conflict and seek compromise with their children. Consequently, Thai parents may not strictly adhere to being entirely authoritative or authoritarian (Yotanyamaneewong et al., 2021). Therefore, the meaning of parenting styles is likely to be influenced by the cultural norms of each country.

As noted earlier, the trend in parenting styles across many Asian countries appears to be leaning toward the adoption of the authoritative style. This inclination may be indicative of the positive outcomes associated with authoritative parenting. In a meta-analysis, authoritative parenting was linked with lower levels of internalizing and externalizing problems in various regions, including Asia (Pinquart & Kauser, 2018). Parenting practices consistent with an authoritative style, such as parental warmth and understanding, also are associated with children's academic achievement, well-being, and mental health (Kim, 2019; Nguyen, 2020). Authoritative parenting has also been linked to positive moral behavior (Ghani et al.,

2014) and moral reasoning (Pinquart & Fisher, 2022). Asian parenting practices are often characterized by strictness and high demands, which may result in negative consequences for children. However, it is important to acknowledge that this strictness and demanding nature can also be viewed as a means for parents to express their love and care toward their children. Starting from their love and concern for their children, combined with the swift advancement of technology, significant urbanization, and improved education, Asian parents are gradually adjusting their parenting practices to address the needs and well-being of their children (Chang et al., 2011).

Longitudinal research including families from China, the Philippines, and Thailand revealed bidirectional relations between parental warmth and control on the one hand and children's externalizing and internalizing behaviors from age eight to 13 on the other (Lansford et al., 2018). That is, children who exhibited more externalizing and internalizing problems elicited less subsequent warmth and more subsequent control from parents. Parent effects were less consistent than child effects, but earlier in childhood, parents who exhibited less warmth and more control had children with more subsequent externalizing and internalizing problems (Lansford et al., 2018). As the cornerstones of parenting styles, warmth and control are important both in terms of setting an overall emotional climate for parent–child relationships and in terms of specific parenting practices that are related to adaptive or problematic behavior of children and adolescents.

Parental Discipline

One of the main ways that parents attempt to manage their children's behaviors is through discipline. Parents' discipline strategies range from proactive (e.g., explaining behavioral expectations for a new situation to prevent children's misbehaviors) to reactive (e.g., punishing a child for misbehaviour after it occurs). Across cultural groups, including in Asian families, inductive forms of discipline, such as offering explanations and teaching children to make amends if they have hurt someone, are preferred to punitive forms of discipline, such as spanking or yelling (e.g., Helwig et al., 2014). In a study of mother–child dyads in six countries, including China, India, the Philippines, and Thailand, more frequent corporal punishment was related to more child aggression and anxiety (Lansford et al., 2005). Children in these countries whose mothers used more corporal punishment and harsh verbal discipline reported feeling that their mothers regarded them with more hostility, which in turn predicted more child aggression and anxiety (Lansford et al., 2010).

Despite the association between corporal punishment and more child behavior problems, corporal punishment remains common in many countries.

For example, in nationally representative samples, 14 percent of caregivers in Mongolia and 35 percent of caregivers in Vietnam reported believing it is necessary to use corporal punishment to rear a child properly, and 40 percent of caregivers in Mongolia and 5 percent of caregivers in Vietnam reported that they or another caregiver in their household had severely physically punished (hit on the head or beat with an implement) their two- to four-year-old child in the last 30 days (Lansford & Deater-Deckard, 2012).

In addition to forms of discipline that are common in Asian and non-Asian contexts alike, parents in some Asian countries have been found to use "shaming" as a form of discipline. Shaming was originally documented in qualitative research with Taiwanese families that showed how parents attempted to teach their preschoolers right from wrong and to motivate their children to make amends by instilling shame after misbehavior (Fung, 1999). In comparative research with seven- to 14-year-olds in China and Canada, children in Canada reported that shaming is less common than did children in China; children in both countries thought that shaming is detrimental to children's psychological well-being and sense of self-worth and that inductive reasoning is more effective than shaming (Helwig et al., 2014).

Research with mothers in Hong Kong and Taiwan also demonstrates that the discipline responses parents use depend on how children misbehave and the circumstances surrounding the misbehavior (Fung et al., 2017). For example, in response to open-ended questions following the presentation of hypothetical vignettes, mothers reported that their discipline responses would differ at home versus in public, as a function of who was present (just family members or also friends or acquaintances), and whether children's misbehaviors entailed violations of social conventions, morals, or rules about safety. Mothers also indicated that they would try particular responses first but have contingency plans for additional disciplinary responses if their initial response was unsuccessful (Fung et al., 2017).

In addition to factors related to children's misbehaviors and the circumstances surrounding them, intergenerational continuity is often found in parents' use of different discipline strategies. For example, parents whose own parents used corporal punishment are more likely to use corporal punishment with their children than parents who did not experience corporal punishment (Wang et al., 2014). Cultural norms regarding the desirability of particular parenting practices can be passed from one generation to the next, for better or worse. Intergenerational transmission of maladaptive parenting is related to more child internalizing and externalizing problems, but intergenerational transmission, including in Asia, can be disrupted by factors such as increases in income and participation in parenting programs (Rothenberg et al., 2023).

Parental Monitoring

Parental monitoring has long been considered as a protective factor in development, as it is consistently associated with decreased risk of behavior problems in children across different cultural contexts. Monitoring, also referred to in the literature as behavioral control, entails knowing about children's activities, whereabouts, and peer groups, as well as providing supervision and structure, as when setting rules and limits for children to follow (Fosco et al., 2012). Current conceptualizations of monitoring unpack parental knowledge according to how parents obtain information about their children, namely, via parents' solicitation of information, and via their children's disclosure of information to their parents (Kerr et al., 2010). Particularly in the adolescent period, parental knowledge more likely comes from adolescents' disclosures, as parents encounter increasing bids for privacy (Ranganathan & Montemayor, 2014). However, studies on parental monitoring in families in Asia do not always specify parental monitoring or knowledge with respect to parent solicitation or adolescent disclosure of information; in other reports, parental control and rule-setting are also included under the rubric of monitoring.

Substantial research has shown that monitoring children and adolescents, when measured as extent of parental knowledge (e.g., "how much do you know about what your child does after school"), is related to lower levels of aggressive behaviors, delinquency, and substance use (Fosco et al., 2012) and buffers the impacts of neighborhood and peer risks (Chao & Otsuki-Clutter, 2011). Studies in Asian contexts likewise report these benefits of parental knowledge. For instance, parental knowledge (labeled as behavioral control) was persistently and negatively linked with antisocial behavior across time for large samples of adolescents in Bangladesh, China, and India (Barber et al., 2005). In addition to decreased antisocial behaviors and risk involvement, positive academic outcomes such as school engagement, adjustment, and performance, have also been associated with higher parental monitoring among elementary and high school children in China, Korea, and Malaysia (Bae et al., 2015; Li et al., 2003; see review of Ng & Wang, 2019). In Vietnam, parental knowledge was also negatively related to the likelihood of school bullying and mental health problems among adolescents (Nguyen et al., 2019).

Mechanisms of Effects and the Role of Adolescent Disclosure

Parental knowledge is thought to function as a deterrent to child and adolescent misbehaviors and to disrupt the influence of deviant peers in the critical transition from childhood to early adolescence (Fosco et al.,

2012). In the Philippines, for instance, Filipino mothers in risky environments not only directly ask children about their plans; they also solicit information from neighbors, children's friends, and teachers about their children's whereabouts (Jocson & Garcia, 2017). This work highlights the role that community members can play in parents' attempts to monitor their children.

Given that parental knowledge may be derived from adolescent disclosures of information, the protective effect may also reflect a family environment where children are open with their parents about their activities or where they reveal information in response to parental involvement and interest (Hawk, 2016). Among adolescents in Beijing, China, parental knowledge and solicitation of information was indirectly associated with adolescents' trust in their parents via enhanced positive and open parent–child communication (Ying et al., 2015). Adolescent disclosure has also been consistently linked with positive adjustment among Chinese youth (Qin & Pomerantz, 2013).

Certain conditions can influence adolescent disclosure, however. For adolescents in rural China, as with North American and European youth, disclosure to parents is less likely when adolescents perceive that their privacy is being invaded via covert parental monitoring (e.g., eavesdropping in adolescents' conversations) (Hawk, 2016) or overly restrictive control (Ying et al., 2015). This reluctance to disclose when their privacy is invaded reflects a developmentally normative resistance to parent behaviors that impinge on the personal domain of adolescents, even in a cultural context that emphasizes parental authority over the child (Hawk, 2016). Altogether, the positive effect of parental knowledge in deterring antisocial behaviors may reflect all these mechanisms, whereby parents solicit information, and adolescents disclose.

Problem behaviors likewise decrease with higher levels of monitoring that is defined in terms of supervision and setting rules. The structure and guidance provided by parents is thought to increase self-regulation abilities that curb impulsive behaviors (Barber et al., 2005). In Korea, for instance, enhanced self-regulation with respect to time use (towards academic activities) mediated the association of parental knowledge and limit-setting with school achievement (Lee et al., 2012).

Nuancing Monitoring and Behavioral Control in Asian Contexts

In studies of families in Asia, higher levels of control are considered a hallmark of Asian parenting, alongside strictness, respect for parental authority, and expectations of filial piety or familial obligations (Ng & Wang, 2019).

Supervising and regulating children's behaviors is seen as a primary responsibility of parents in order to foster much valued academic success and harmonious relationships, and indeed can be considered as expressions of love and support for the child (Ng & Wang, 2019). The relatively culturally unique concept of *guan* (Chao, 1994) similarly emphasizes "governing" or directive control and behavioral regulation of the child, as well as "caring for" the child and close parent–child relationships.

Given the foregoing, rule-setting may be expected to be higher in Asian contexts. In a cross-sectional study that compared parents' rules among Filipino, U.S. American, and Chilean teenagers, Filipino adolescents reported that their parents set rules and expectations over significantly more areas in their lives, including issues that are considered in the personal domain (i.e., perceived as affecting only the self) (Darling et al., 2005). Conflict between parents and adolescents can arise when adolescents believe that parents are setting too many rules or setting rules in domains in which they have no authority.

Legitimacy Beliefs

Key to whether adolescents comply with their parents' rules are adolescents' beliefs about the legitimacy of parental authority over domains where rules are set (Smetana, 2011). Filipino teens reported being less obliged to comply with rules on which they disagreed with their parents and were not within the domain of legitimate parental jurisdiction. Not only do legitimacy beliefs potentially qualify or moderate the impact of rule-setting on problem behaviors; they may also predict internalizing symptoms for youth who perceive parental control over issues they deem to be in their personal purview, as was found among Japanese adolescents (Hasebe et al., 2004). Similarly, adolescents in rural and urban China whose parents made decisions across all domains (including personal) had higher levels of depressive symptoms and higher school misconduct (Wang & Faldowski, 2014).

These findings suggest that despite the norm of parental supervision and governance in Asian contexts, across adolescence there is a normative shift toward decreasing legitimacy of parental authority and decreasing rules in the personal domain. More contemporary studies of urban Chinese families also surmise that culture change and socioeconomic development have shifted norms and values toward greater support for children's independence versus rule enforcement and unquestioning obedience (Long et al., 2021). Supporting the aforementioned studies, contemporary longitudinal studies show a general decrease in monitoring and rule-setting across the ages of 10 to 17 years old in China, the Philippines, and Thailand (Lansford et al., 2021).

Implications for Practice and Policy

Parenting styles, discipline, and monitoring have all been the focus of parenting interventions. In any attempt to alter parenting and, thereby, child behavior, it is important to take into account the cultural contexts in which families are situated. A poignant example that illustrates the harm that can be done by trying to intervene from a Western perspective in Asian contexts occurred following the 2004 tsunami in the Indian Ocean (Christopher et al., 2014). Well-intentioned Western psychologists came to Sri Lanka following the tsunami, which killed over 36,000 people and destroyed over 300,000 homes, to offer support, assuming that a mental health crisis and suicidality would spike. However, these beliefs were not shared by the local community (and ultimately did not come to pass; Rodrigo et al., 2009), which was more focused on obtaining food, shelter, and clothing; reuniting with missing family members; conducting funeral rites; and getting children back to school. In addition to not offering services that were directly connected with local needs, the psychological services offered were in conflict with local norms regarding appropriate social interactions, privacy, emotional displays, and more. In addition, the psychologists actually detracted from the community's own response by using limited resources (food, clean water, shelter) and by not drawing on local wisdom regarding how best to alleviate grief and suffering and instead increasing anxiety by making culturally inappropriate demands (Christopher et al., 2014).

A more promising approach to intervention is to have local experts adapt any programs that were developed elsewhere to make them culturally appropriate for their new setting. For example, Parenting for Lifelong Health is a program designed to prevent child maltreatment that was originally developed in South Africa but has been carefully adapted for use in the Philippines and Thailand (Alampay et al., 2018; McCoy et al., 2021). By balancing the perspectives of cultural insiders who could provide insights into local childrearing goals and values with scientific evidence on components of effective parenting programs from cultural outsiders, the program ultimately could be implemented more effectively and at larger scale than would have been possible without this adaptation (Mamauag et al., 2021).

Sets of international standards exist to help countries considering creating or adapting parenting programs that ultimately aim to improve child outcomes by improving parenting (UNICEF, 2017). For example, UNICEF (2017) provides guidance regarding attending to the developmental stage of the child, involving all key caregivers, and continuously improving through monitoring and evaluation. Adopting an implementation science perspective has also been informative in understanding a range of factors, such as securing buy-in from key stakeholders, integrating programs into existing infrastructure, training the workforce, and making sure that the program addresses needs identified by local communities, that contribute to the success of parenting programs in a range of contexts (Lansford et al., 2022). A review and meta-analysis of parenting programs implemented in East and Southeast Asia demonstrated the potential for these programs to reduce harsh discipline and violence against children and to improve parent–child interactions (McCoy et al., 2020).

One of the most pressing policy issues related to parenting and children's behavior problems is the push to outlaw corporal punishment that was originally instigated by the United Nations (1989) Convention on the Rights of the Child and is currently instantiated in the Sustainable Development Goals guiding the international development agenda through 2030 (United Nations, 2017). As of December 2024 a total of 67 countries have outlawed all forms of corporal punishment, including by parents in the home, but Japan and Nepal are the only two Asian countries that have outlawed all forms of corporal punishment (Global Initiative to End Corporal Punishment, 2024). The Association of Southeast Asian Nations adopted a Regional Plan of Action on the Elimination of Violence Against Children to address the obligations of countries in the region to advance this issue (ASEAN Secretariat, 2017). Going forward, protection of children from violence in all forms will continue to be an important policy issue in parent–child relationships, as well as an issue addressed in programs that try to reduce child behavior problems by enhancing parenting.

Future Directions

Compared with many Western countries, countries in Asia have been historically under-represented in the study of psychology, including developmental psychology (Thalmayer et al., 2021). Even within Asia, some countries are more under-represented in the parenting and child development literature than others; for example, research in China has burgeoned in recent years, whereas research in Cambodia, Laos, and Myanmar is still nascent. Differences within Asia are important to understand for many of the same reasons that it is important to understand differences (and similarities) between Asian countries and countries in other regions. Science is advanced by greater attention to the full range of contexts in which parenting and child development occur, and future research should continue to prioritize the inclusion of Asian samples that have been historically under-represented.

Another important direction for future research on parenting and behavior problems of children and adolescents in Asian families will be to understand how cultural values that are important in Asian contexts but are unknown in Western contexts in which many theories of parenting originated may be central to understanding Asian parenting. Finally, future research will benefit from careful work on measurement both conceptually and empirically. Even a component of parenting that is universally beneficial for children, such as parental warmth and acceptance (Khaleque & Ali, 2017), may be expressed differently in different cultural contexts. For example, Chinese immigrant parents in the United States are more likely to express warmth by supporting their children's education and providing for basic physical needs like nutritious food than to use physical affection and direct praise, which are more common among European American parents (Cheah et al., 2015). Conceptualizing constructs in ways that are culturally appropriate and measuring these constructs in ways that validly capture how they are expressed in particular cultural groups is important to avoiding a deficit perspective on parenting and child behavior that may otherwise result from the misapplication of constructs and measures in contexts for which they were not originally designed.

Conclusion

Because parents' ethnotheories regarding desirable and undesirable child behaviors as well as how to manage these behaviors differ across cultures, an effort to understand parenting and behavior problems of children and adolescents in Asian families should be grounded in an understanding of these ethnotheories and Asian cultural values. Relations between parenting styles and child behaviors are largely similar in Asian countries and Western countries, although the concept of "guan" parenting has been documented specifically in Asian families. Harsh verbal discipline and corporal punishment are associated with more child behavior problems in Asian countries, whereas inductive forms of discipline, such as reasoning, are related to fewer child behavior problems. Parental monitoring is generally a protective factor that decreases children's behavior problems and is nuanced in Asian families by cultural values that endorse the legitimacy of parental authority. Programs to improve parent–child relationships and, in turn, child outcomes, are more effective if they are culturally adapted for local contexts; such programs have been found to have desired effects in Asian countries. Current policy efforts in several Asian countries involve moving toward child protection targets in the Sustainable Development Goals operationalized as outlawing corporal punishment. Examining variability within and across Asian countries, attending to indigenous cultural concepts as they relate to parenting and child behaviors, and conceptualizing and measuring constructs in culturally meaningful ways are all important future directions.

References

Alampay, L. P. (2014). Parenting in the Philippines. In H. Selin & P. Schvaneveldt (Eds), *Parenting across cultures: Childrearing, motherhood and fatherhood in non-Western cultures* (pp. 105–121). Springer.

Alampay, L. P., Lachman, J. M., Landov, B. V., Madrid, B. J., Ward, C. L., Hutchings, J., Alinea, C. D., & Gardner, F. (2018). Preventing child maltreatment in low- and middle-income countries: Parenting for Lifelong Health in the Philippines. In S. Verma & A. Petersen (Eds), *Developmental science and Sustainable Development Goals for children and youth* (pp. 277–293). Springer.

ASEAN Secretariat (2017). ASEAN regional plan of action on elimination of violence against children. Available https://asean.org/wp-content/uploads/2021/01/ASEAN-Regional-Plan-of-Action-on-the-Elimination-of-Violence-against-Children-RPA-on-EVAC-2016-in-collaboration-with-SOMSWD-ENG.pdf.

Bae, D. & Wickrama, K. A. S. (2015). Family socioeconomic status and academic achievement among Korean adolescents: Linking mechanisms of family processes and adolescents' time use. *Journal of Early Adolescence, 35*(7), 1014–1038.

Barber, B. K., Stolz, H. E., & Olsen, J. A. (2005). Parental support, psychological control, and behavioral control: Assessing relevance across time, method, and culture. *Monographs of the Society for Research in Child Development, 70*.

Baumrind, D. (1967). Child care practices anteceding three patterns of preschool behavior. *Genetic Psychology Monographs, 75*, 43–88.

Bayram Özdemir, S. & Cheah, C. S. L. (2015). Turkish mothers' parenting beliefs in response to aggressive and socially withdrawn behaviors. *Journal of Child and Family Studies, 24*, 687–702.

Benito, L. D. (2022). Parenting styles of teen mothers in a selected city in Mindanao, Philippines. *Randwick International of Social Sciences Journal, 3*(3), 472–476.

Chang, L., Chen, B-B., & Ji, L. (2011). Attributions and attitudes of mothers and fathers in China. *Parenting: Science and Practice, 11*, 102–115.

Chao, R. K. (1994). Beyond parental control and authoritarian parenting style: Understanding Chinese parenting through the cultural notion of training. *Child Development, 65*, 1111–1119.

Chao, R. K. (1995). Chinese and European American cultural models of the self reflected in mothers' childrearing beliefs. *Ethos, 23*, 328–354.

Chao, R. & Otsuki-Clutter, M. (2011). Racial and ethnic differences: Sociocultural and contextual explanations. *Journal of Research on Adolescence, 21*(1), 47–60.

Chao, R. K. & Tseng, V. (2002). Parenting of Asians. In M. H. Bornstein (Series Ed.), *Handbook of parenting: Vol. 4. Social conditions and applied parenting* (2nd ed., pp. 59–93). Lawrence Erlbaum Associates.

Chaudhary, N. & Sriram, S. (2020). Psychology in the "Backyards of the World": Experiences From India. *Journal of Cross-Cultural Psychology, 51*(2), 113–133.

Cheah, C. S., Li, J., Zhou, N., Yamamoto, Y., & Leung, C. Y. (2015). Understanding Chinese immigrant and European American mothers' expressions of warmth. *Developmental Psychology, 51*, 1802–1811.

Chen, X. (2018). Culture, temperament, and social and psychological adjustment. *Developmental Review, 50*, 42–53.

Christopher, J. C., Wendt, D. C., Maracek, J., & Goodman, D. M. (2014). Critical cultural awareness: Contributions to a globalizing psychology. *American Psychologist, 69*, 645–655.

Cole, P. M., Bruschi, C. J., & Tamang, B. L. (2002). Cultural differences in children's reactions to difficult situations. *Child Development, 73*, 983–996.

Cole, P. M., Tamang, B. L., & Shrestha, S. (2006). Cultural variations in the socialization of young children's anger and shame. *Child Development, 77*, 1237–1251.

Darling, N., Cumsille, P., & Alampay, L. (2005). Rules, legitimacy of parental authority, and obligation to obey in Chile, the Philippines, and the United States. In J. Smetana (Ed.), *Changing boundaries of parental authority during adolescence* (pp. 47–60). Jossey-Bass.

Fosco, G., Stormshak, E., Dishion, T., & Winter, C. (2012). Family relationships and parental monitoring during middle school as predictors of early adolescent problem behavior. *Journal of Clinical Child and Adolescent Psychology, 41*(2), 202–213.

Fung, H. (1999). Becoming a moral child: The socialization of shame among young Chinese children. *Ethos, 27*, 180–209.

Fung, H., Li, J., & Lam, C. K. (2017). Multi-faceted discipline strategies of Chinese parenting. *International Journal of Behavioral Development, 41*, 472–481.

Ghani, F. B. A., Kamal, S. L. A., & Aziz, A. A. (2014). The implication of parenting styles on the akhlak of Muslim teenagers in the south of Malaysia. *Procedia: Social and Behavioral Sciences, 114*, 761–765.

Global Initiative to End Corporal Punishment (2024). Retrieved from www.endcorporalpunishment.org.

Guo, B., Wang, Y., & Chang, L. (2005). Classroom effects on the relations between children's social behaviors and school adjustment. *Acta Psychologica Sinica, 37*, 239–244.

Hasebe, Y., Nucci, L., & Nucci, M. S. (2004). Parental control of the personal domain and adolescent symptoms of psychopathology: A cross-national study in the United States and Japan. *Child Development, 75*(3), 815–828.

Hawk, S. (2016). Chinese adolescents' reports of covert parental monitoring: Comparisons with overt monitoring and links with information management. *Journal of Adolescence, 55*, 24–35.

Hays, S. (1996). *The cultural contradictions of motherhood*. Yale University Press.

Helwig, C. C., To, S., Wang, Q., Liu, C., & Yang, S. (2014). Judgments and reasoning about parental discipline involving induction and psychological control in China and Canada. *Child Development, 85*, 1150–1167.

Hosiri, T., Wannasewok, K., Chaiharn, P., Phattharayuttawat, S., Manussirivithaya, V., & Ngamthipwatthana, T. (2018). Parenting style and hardiness of students in a Thai military academy. *Journal of the Medical Association of Thailand, 101*, 19–23.

Jocson, R. & Garcia, A. (2017). Low-income urban Filipino mothers' experiences with community violence. *International Perspectives in Psychology: Research, Practice, Consultation, 6*, 133–151.

Kauser, R. & Pinquart, M. (2019). Effectiveness of an indigenous parent training program on change in parenting styles and delinquent tendencies (challenging behaviors) in Pakistan: A randomized controlled trial. *Journal of Experimental Child Psychology, 188*, 104677.

Keller, H. (2018). Parenting and socioemotional development in infancy and early childhood. *Developmental Review, 50*, 31–41.

Kelley, M. L. & Tseng, H. M. (1992). Cultural differences in child rearing: A comparison of immigrant Chinese and Caucasian American mothers. *Journal of Cross-Cultural Psychology, 23*, 444–455.

Kerr, M., Stattin, H., & Burk, W.J. (2010). A reinterpretation of parental monitoring in longitudinal perspective. *Journal of Research on Adolescence, 20*(1), 39–64.

Keshavarz, S. & Baharudin, R. (2009). Parenting style in a collectivist culture of Malaysia. *European Journal of Social Science, 10*(1), 66–73.

Khaleque, A. & Ali, S. (2017). A systematic review of meta-analyses of research on interpersonal acceptance–rejection theory: Constructs and measures. *Journal of Family Theory & Review, 9*, 441–458.

Kim, S. W. (2019). Meta-analysis of parental involvement and achievement in East Asian countries. *Education and Urban Society, 52*, 312–337.

Lansford, J. E., Betancourt, T. S., Boller, K., Popp, J., Altafim, E. R. P., Attanasio, O., & Raghavan, C. (2022). The future of parenting programs: II Implementation. *Parenting: Science and Practice, 22*, 235–257.

Lansford, J. E., Chang, L., Dodge, K. A., Malone, P. S., Oburu, P., Palmérus, K., . . . Quinn, N. (2005). Physical discipline and children's adjustment: Cultural normativeness as a moderator. *Child Development, 76*, 1234–1246.

Lansford, J. E. & Deater-Deckard, K. (2012). Childrearing discipline and violence in developing countries. *Child Development, 83*, 62–75.

Lansford, J. E., Malone, P. S., Dodge, K. A., Chang, L., Chaudhary, N., Tapanya, S., . . . Deater-Deckard, K. (2010). Children's perceptions of maternal hostility as a mediator of the link between discipline and children's adjustment in four countries. *International Journal of Behavioral Development, 34*, 452–461.

Lansford, J. E., Rothenberg, W. A., & Bornstein, M. H. (2021). *Parenting across cultures from childhood to adolescence*. Routledge.

Lansford, J. E., Rothenberg, W. A., Jensen, T. M., Lippold, M. A., Bacchini, D., Bornstein, M. H., Chang, L., Deater-Deckard, K., Di Giunta, L., Dodge, K. A., Malone, P. S., Oburu, P., Pastorelli, C., Skinner, A. T., Sorbring, E., Steinberg, L., Tapanya, S., Uribe Tirado, L. M., Alampay, L. P., & Al-Hassan, S. M. (2018). Bidirectional relations between parenting and behavior problems from age 8 to 13 in nine countries. *Journal of Research on Adolescence, 28*, 571–590.

Lau, A. S., Guo, S., Tsai, W., Nguyen, D. J., Nguyen, H. T., Ngo, V., & Weiss, B. (2016). Adolescents' stigma attitudes toward internalizing and externalizing disorders: Cultural influences and implications for distress manifestations. *Clinical Psychological Science, 4*(4), 704–717.

Lee, E. H., Zhou, Q., Eisenberg, N., & Wang, Y. (2013). Bidirectional relations between temperament and parenting styles in Chinese children. *International Journal of Behavioral Development, 37*, 57–67.

Lee, J., Yu, H., & Choi, S. (2012). The influences of parental acceptance and parental control on school adjustment and academic achievement for South Korean children: The mediation role of self-regulation. *Asia Pacific Education Review, 13*, 227–237.

Li, X., Fang, X., Stanton, B., Lizeng, S., & Wu, Y. (2003). Parental monitoring among adolescents in Beijing, China. *Journal of Adolescent Health, 33*, 130–132.

Lin, W. Y. (2003). The influence of parents' theories of human nature on parenting belief: The case of theories of intelligence. *Indigenous Psychological Research in Chinese Societies, 20*, 253–293.

Long, Q., Rothenberg, W. A., Liu, Q., & Chang, L. (2021). Four domains of parenting in China. In J. E. Lansford, W. A. Rothenberg, & M. H. Bornstein (Eds), *Parenting across cultures from childhood to adolescence: Development in nine countries* (pp. 22–40). Routledge.

Lu, H. J. & Chang, L. (2013). Parenting and child socialization of only children in urban China: An example of authoritative parenting. *Journal of Genetic Psychology, 174*, 335–343.

Maccoby, E. E. & Martin, J. A. (1983). Socialization in the context of the family: Parent–child interaction. In P. H. Mussen (Series Ed.) & E. M. Hetherington (Vol. Ed.), *Handbook of child psychology: Vol. 4, Socialization, personality, and social development* (4th ed., pp. 1–101). Wiley.

McCoy, A., Lachman, J. M., Ward, C. L., Tapanya, S., Poomchaichote, T., Kelly, J., Mukaka, M., Cheah, P. Y., & Gardner, F. (2021). Feasibility pilot of an adapted parenting program embedded within the Thai public health system. *BMC Public Health, 21*, 1009.

McCoy, A., Melendez-Torres, G. J., & Gardner, F. (2020). Parenting interventions to prevent violence against children in low- and middle-income countries in East and Southeast Asia: A systematic review and multi-level meta-analysis. *Child Abuse & Neglect, 103*, 104444.

Miller, P. J., Fung, H., Lin, S., Chen, E. C.-H., & Boldt, B. R. (2012). How socialization happens on the ground: Narrative practices as alternate socializing pathways in Taiwanese and European-American families. *Monographs of the Society for Research in Child Development, 77*(Serial No. 302), 1–140.

Ng, F. F. & Wang, Q. (2019). Asian and Asian American parenting. In M. H. Bornstein (Ed.), *Handbook of parenting. Vol. 4. Special conditions and applied parenting* (3rd ed., pp. 108–169). Routledge.

Nguyen, H., Nakamura, K., Seino, K., & Al-Sobaihi, S. (2019). Impact of parent–adolescent bonding on school bullying and mental health in Vietnamese cultural setting: Evidence from the global school-based health survey. *BMC Psychology, 7*, 16.

Nguyen, Q-A. N., Tran, T. D., Tran, T-A., Nguyen, T. A., & Fisher, J. (2020). Perceived parenting styles and emotional intelligence among adolescents in Vietnam. *The Family Journal: Counseling and Therapy for Couples and Families, 28*, 441–454.

Olson, S. L., Kashiwagi, K., & Crystal, D. (2001). Concepts of adaptive and maladaptive child behavior: A comparison of U.S. and Japanese mothers of preschool-age children. *Journal of Cross-Cultural Psychology, 32*, 43–57.

Olson, S., Lansford, J. E., Evans, E. M., Blumstein, K. P., & Ip, K. I. (2019). Parents' ethnotheories of maladaptive behavior in young children. *Child Development Perspectives, 13*, 153–158.

Pinquart, M. & Fischer, A. (2022). Associations of parenting styles with moral reasoning in children and adolescents: A meta-analysis. *Journal of Moral Education, 51*(4), 463–476.

Pinquart, M. & Kauser, R. (2018). Do the associations of parenting styles with behavior problems and academic achievement vary by culture? Results from a meta-analysis. *Cultural Diversity & Ethnic Minority Psychology, 24*(1), 75–100.

Qin, L. & Pomerantz, E. (2013). Reciprocal pathways between American and Chinese early adolescents' sense of responsibility and disclosure to parents. *Child Development, 84*(6), 1887–1895.

Ranganathan, C. & Montemayor, R. (2014). Parental efficacy, parental monitoring efficacy, and monitoring among Asian-Indian parents of adolescents living in Chennai, India. *Journal of Adolescence, 37*(8), 1363–1372.

Raval, V. V., Martini, T. S., & Raval, P. H. (2007). "Would others think it is okay to express my feelings?" Regulation of anger, sadness, and physical pain in Gujarati children in India. *Social Development, 16*, 79–105.

Rhucharoenpornpanich, O., Chamratrithirong, A., Fongkaew, W., Rosati M. J., Miller, B. M., & Cupp, P. K. (2010). Parenting and adolescent problem behaviors: A comparative study of sons and daughters in Thailand. *Journal of the Medical Association of Thailand, 93*(3), 293–300.

Rodrigo, A., McQillin, A., & Pimm, J. (2009). Effect of the 2004 Tsunami on suicide rates in Sri Lanka. *Psychiatric Bulletin, 33*, 179–180.

Rothbaum, F. & Wang, Y. Z. (2010). Fostering children's malleable views of the self and the world: Caregiving practices in East Asian and European American communities. In B. Mayer & H. J. Kornadt (Eds), *Soziokultureller context und mensschliche Entwicklung [Sociocultural context and human development]* (pp. 101–120). VS Verlag.

Rothenberg, W. A., Lansford, J. E., Uribe Tirado, L. M., Yotanyamaneewong, S., Alampay, L. P., Al-Hassan, S. M., Bacchini, D., Chang, L., Deater-Deckard, K., Di Giunta, L., Dodge, K. A., Gurdal, S., Liu, Q., Long, Q., Oburu, P., Pastorelli, C., Skinner, A. T., Sorbring, E., Tapanya, S., Steinberg, L., & Bornstein, M. H. (2023). The intergenerational transmission of maladaptive parenting and its impact on child mental health: Examining cross-cultural mediating pathways and moderating protective factors. *Child Psychiatry and Human Development, 54*, 870–890.

Smetana, J. (2011). *Adolescents, families, and social development: How teens construct their worlds*. Wiley-Blackwell.

Sorkhabi, N. (2005). Applicability of Baumrind's parent typology to collective cultures: Analysis of cultural explanation of parent socialization effects. *International Journal of Behavioral Development, 29*, 552–563.

Stewart, S. M. & Bond, M. H. (2002). A critical look at parenting research from the mainstream: Problems uncovered while adapting western research to non-western cultures. *British Journal of Developmental Psychology, 20*, 379–392.

Thalmayer, A. G., Toscanelli, C., & Arnett, J. J. (2021). The neglected 95% revisited: Is American psychology becoming less American? *American Psychologist, 76*, 116–129.

Tobin, J., Hsueh, Y., & Karasawa, M. (2009). *Preschool in three cultures revisited: China, Japan, and the United States*. University of Chicago Press.

UNICEF (2017). *Standards for ECD parenting programs in low and middle income countries*. UNICEF.

United Nations (1989). Convention on the Rights of the Child. https://www.ohchr.org/en/professionalinterest/pages/crc.aspx.

United Nations. (2017). Sustainable Development Goals: 17 goals to transform our world. Retrieved from www.un.org/sustainabledevelopment/sustainable-development-goals.

Wang, M., Xing, X., & Zhao, J. (2014). Intergenerational transmission of corporal punishment in China: The moderating role of marital satisfaction and gender. *Journal of Abnormal Child Psychology, 42*, 1263–1274.

Wang, Q. & Chang, L. (2009). Parenting and child socialization in contemporary China. In M. H. Bond (Ed.), *Handbook of Chinese psychology* (2nd ed.). Oxford University Press.

Wang, Y. & Chang, L. (2008). *Urban parenting in China: Research and reflections*. Fudan University Press.

Wang, Y. & Faldowski, R. (2014). Beliefs in the legitimacy of decision authority among Chinese adolescents and parents: A person-centered approach. *Journal of Adolescence, 37*(7), 1121–1132.

Weisz, J. R., Sigman, M., Weiss, B., & Mosk, J. (1993). Parent reports of behavioral and emotional problems among children in Kenya, Thailand, and the United States. *Child Development, 64*(1), 98–109.

Yim, E. P-Y. (2022). Effects of Asian cultural values on parenting style and young children's perceived competence: A cross-sectional study. *Frontiers in Psychology, 13*, 905093.

Ying, L., Ma, F., Huang, H., Guo, X., Chen, C., & Xu, F. (2015) Parental monitoring, parent–adolescent communication, and adolescents' trust in their parents in China. *PLoS ONE, 10*(8), e0134730.

Yotanyamaneewong, S., Rothenberg, W. A., & Tapanya, S. (2021). Four domains of parenting in Thailand. In J. E. Lansford, W. A. Rothenberg, & M. H. Bornstein (Eds), *Parenting across cultures from childhood to adolescence* (pp. 172–192). Routledge.

12

CHILDREARING IN NEPAL

Pamela M. Cole and Yeunjoo Kim

Nepal, a nation of almost 31 million people (World Population Review, December 17, 2023), is among the least developed nations in the world (United Nations Conference on Trade and Development, 2023). Nearly 80 percent of the population lives in villages, most as subsistence farmers with little disposable income (National Statistics Office, 2022). Yet, despite what it lacks in economic resources, Nepal is rich in its cultural diversity. Historically, its slow rate of development has contributed to many people living in remote villages where their culturally distinct practices are preserved; they have experienced few outside influences that could dilute their cultural practices. For example, it can take days to walk to a larger town and interact with other ethnic groups. If there is no electricity, there is no access to international influences broadcast on television.

Nepal's most recent census identified 142 castes and ethnicities in its population (National Statistics Office, 2022). The castes stem from Nepal's historical identity as a Hindu nation; although the caste system is no longer legal, Nepal society is still influenced by the ancient hereditary stratification of society by caste and over 80 percent of its population identified as Hindu in the most recent census (National Statistics Office, 2022). Other Nepali citizens identify as minorities and practice other religions, particularly Buddhism and Islam, and increasingly, Christianity. Those practicing Buddhism are mainly indigenous peoples, e.g., Sherpa, Tamang, most of whom resided in the Himalayan region before Nepal became a nation and whose cultures predate the arrival of Hindus from the Indian subcontinent. Nepal strives to cultivate a unified national identity that is distinct from its neighbors, India and China, while it also strives to appreciate and preserve its cultural diversity;

DOI: 10.4324/9781003383949-12

modern Nepal acknowledges the need to recognize the rights of all groups, despite persistent inequities among them (Bhandari, 2016; Breen, 2018).

We introduce our chapter with this snapshot of Nepali's cultural diversity to underscore the challenge of characterizing childrearing in Nepal—in such a poor nation there is very little research conducted to describe childrearing values and practices—and its cultural diversity contributes to variations that preclude any singular description of them. In this chapter, we offer an initial portrait of commonalities and variations among Nepali peoples in how they raise their children. We first address some traditional childrearing characteristics that appear common among Nepal's peoples, highlighting ways that they differ from many Western styles of childrearing. We next draw upon a sparse and varied collection of published studies, using them to shed light on major issues involving the context and style of childrearing in Nepal. We then discuss insights we gained in studying emotion socialization among two Nepali groups—Brahman and Tamang families in the rural middle hills of Nepal. We emphasize the challenges of conducting culturally meaningful research on childrearing, how we attempted to address them, and how our learning reinforces for us the value of understanding childrearing through different cultural lenses.

Childrearing versus Parenting

In a book on parenting, you may wonder why we chose the term "childrearing." It reflects the first point of departure between Western scientific models of parenting and how most Nepali families enact the important function of raising children. To our knowledge, there are no words in Nepal's many languages that translate directly to the terms parent or parenting. But mothers and fathers, and the family members with whom they live, try to raise healthy children who become competent adults in their cultural setting, goals that appear universal across cultures (LeVine et al., 1996; Whiting, 1963; Whiting & Whiting, 1979). We first present two cultural threads that influence how children are raised and appear common to many Nepali groups and explain why we use the term childrearing.

First, among both conjoint families that typify many subsistence agricultural communities in the hilly and mountainous regions and the nuclear families that have become more common in the capital, Kathmandu, and other major towns, every person is referred to by a kinship term (not their given name). Even biologically unrelated individuals are referred to by kinship terms. That means that the self is defined by one's relationships with the person with whom they are interacting, a self-construal often described as relational-interdependent (Cross et al., 2000). Whereas in many Western nations, persons are identified by their given names, and each seen as a unique individual, Nepali persons are identified by their relation to the person with whom they are interacting. For example, a Nepali woman is called sister, mother, sister-in-law, paternal aunt, maternal aunt, etc., depending upon whom she is with. And she shares those terms of address with all other Nepali woman.

Second, all family members, thus broadly defined, participate in caring for children. Most Nepali terms used to refer to childrearing include the word that translates to care. The raising of children is a communal activity and not the strict purview of the parents. Indeed, when a person visits a household, the visit typically begins by identifying the proper kinship terms (if not already established) and teaching the children to use the proper term with the visitor. e.g., uncle on the mother's side. This is so central to Nepali society that time is spent coaxing even the youngest children to use the proper term. This family member then is expected to engage in behaviors that Western models call parenting. Here is an example of an interaction witnessed by the first author:

> Saria, a British woman who came to Nepal to trek the famous Annapurna Circuit, visits her guide's family upon their return to Kathmandu. The visit begins with an animated discussion as to the proper kinship term to use with Saria. Because she is older than Rajan, the guide, he refers to her as older sister (*didi* in Nepali). Because this term identifies Saria as his sister (not sister-in-law), it indicates she is a family member on the paternal side. Therefore, Rajan's wife Sita calls Saria sister-in-law (*bhauju*) and the children are told to refer to Saria as paternal aunt (*phupu*). With the proper kinship terms identified, tea and biscuits are served. Rajan's children, ages 2, 4, and 6 years, sit quietly on the rug and eye the biscuits intensely. The four-year-old suddenly rises and snatches a biscuit. The Nepali adults in the room all begin to scold the child. Then they tell the new *phupu* to scold the child. Taken aback, Saria is reluctant to do so. Rajan explains that by scolding him, the child and everyone will see that she is invested in the family and is loving the child. Saria makes a weak attempt, sternly telling the child to wait for a biscuit. Everyone laughs heartily but the four-year-old, who drops his head and whimpers quietly. "*Laj laagyo, lobhi*?" an aunt taunts; "*hamro nayan phupule hamro chhoralai lobhi chhani cinnubhayo*" (trans: Are you ashamed, greedy? Our new auntie knows our son is greedy."). "*Au, mero lobhi chhora, ahile biscuit khau*," Rajan says (trans: Come, my greedy son, eat a biscuit now). He puts his son on his lap; he hugs him and cajoles the humbled child into taking a biscuit. Saria is again taken aback by this shaming, followed by Rajan's lovingly coaxing the child to eat the biscuit.

Although this anecdote depicts an uncommon situation, an encounter with a new aunt who is not Nepali, it is an interaction familiar to Nepalis, who can relate it to times when a new person visits their home. Everyone is related, those relationships are important to know. They reflect the family's hierarchy as well as its cohesion, and all family members, closely related or otherwise, are expected to be actively involved in childrearing. Of course, a one-time visit does not capture the daily lives of caregivers; the anecdote highlights the salience of how interrelated Nepali people are and how that cultural value influences interactions with children.

More typically, children are raised by all the family members living in the home. In a conjoint family, this includes the child's living paternal grandparents, the parents, the father's brothers, and their wives if married, the father's unmarried sisters, and older siblings. The patrilocal conjoint family is common in South Asia, representing 64.5 percent of families in Nepal (Khalil & Mookerjee, 2019). The number of nuclear families is increasing slowly, due in part to social trends, such as migration to cities (i.e., leaving ancestral villages), a gradual increase in females receiving more education (Acharya, 2021), and economic trends, especially notable increases in migration outside of Nepal, largely among men, to earn income and send remittances to Nepal to provide for their families (Adhikari et al., 2023).

In sum, despite its diversity, the traditional constitution of the Nepali family and the roles of all family members in childrearing distinguishes the Nepali family from the families depicted in most of the child development literature on parenting. There is not a specific word for parents; to convey that idea, Nepalis refer to *amaaba* (mother/father). The terms referring to raising children usually include the word for care as in caregiving. Despite this difference from the way parenting is conceptualized in most of the child development literature, Nepali caregivers appear to focus on a few basic aspects of child-rearing that are universal: supporting the life and health of children and guiding them to become competent adults in their setting (LeVine et al., 1996; Whiting, 1963). How they socialize their children varies not only in comparison to families in North America or Europe (which have notable diversity within their nations), but among the different ethnic groups within Nepal, as we will discuss later in this chapter. Now, we turn to the small body of research that has been done in Nepal that may help us begin to understand childrearing in the Nepali context.

Studies of Childrearing in Nepal

We searched studies of childrearing in Nepal through PsycINFO and Google Scholar with the following keywords: "Nepal*" "parent*" "famil*" and "child*" or "childrearing" or "caregiv*." We used both search engines to locate articles from psychology and other disciplines, e.g., sociology, economics, anthropology, education, that might shed light on the context of childrearing in Nepal. We identified a limited and diverse set of studies. Most were limited in their methods. Many samples were small and participant characteristics were either not described or described in limited fashion. Most used qualitative methods, typically interviews. Those using quantitative methods mainly relied on self-report questionnaires developed in the United States and translated into Nepali (e.g., Alabama Parenting Scale; Kunwor et al., 2021; Khadka et al., 2021). Details of translation methods, and in some cases adaptations to increase cultural relevance, were not provided. Cultural variations within Nepal were rarely considered. Observational studies were uncommon.

Raval (2023) underscored how little is known of child socialization in Asian marginalized communities and emphasized the limitations of conceptualizing socialization with frameworks developed in North America or Europe. Unique, nuanced, and complex variations in childrearing may be obscured when investigated through the lens of Western models. Despite these concerns, our search revealed clear scientific interest in Nepali childrearing, even if resources for conducting research were limited. To summarize what we learned, we begin with two contextual factors—economic need and societal values—that must be considered to understand childrearing in Nepal. Considering them is consistent with the ecological model of human development (Bronfenbrenner, 1979). That is, to understand childrearing, it is important to understand factors that impinge on the family microsystem and may influence how children are raised.

Economic need

Economic challenges are significant concerns for most Nepali families, many of whom live in poverty (An et al., 2018). Qualitative interviews reveal that economic need is one of the most common concerns of Nepali adults (e.g., Burkey et al., 2016). The need for income influences family life. For many decades, children had to leave school without acquiring a secondary school diploma. Although education is usually valued, children stop attending school to contribute to farming and caring for younger children. In village life, farming is the priority as that is how families have enough food throughout the year. This set of priorities is reminiscent of Maslow's (1943) hierarchy of needs; the family's physical survival takes precedence over education.

Another way to meet basic needs is for one or more members to leave the home in search of income. Rural children, typically the heartiest, are sent to Kathmandu to earn income on the city streets (Panter-Brick, 2002).

Adults and older school age children leave villages to seek manual labor jobs in other regions (e.g., construction projects; KC, 2004). Others, particularly those from indigenous groups, seek jobs in tourism (e.g., porters for treks or mountaineering; Law & Rodway, 2008). About one third of Nepali households have had at least one household member migrate, either internationally or internally, who sent remittances to support their families (Thapa et al., 2019). Since, the late 1990s, internal migration has yielded to employment outside Nepal; adults, primarily men, pay workforce companies to secure jobs in other nations (e.g., Southeast Asia, Middle East). This form of migration is so substantial that it has, more than any intervention, not only increased household income but increased Nepal's GDP (International Labour Organization, 2023).

The trend of a family member leaving the household disrupts family functioning (e.g., Kaimal & Paul, 2021; Rai & Dangal, 2021; Rai et al., 2023). Evidence suggests that caregiver migration places children at risk for behavior problems, such as substance use, aggression, disobedience, and stealing, as well as increasing child labor and even child migration (Rai et al., 2023). Yet not all forms of parental migration appear detrimental. Large-scale studies using Nepali versions of the Strengths and Difficulties Questionnaire or the Child Behavior Checklist reported that international migration by one parent, versus both or neither parent, was associated with *better* child outcomes; this was the case if the departed caregiver was not the mother or if the remittances provided income for mother and children to relocate to urban areas for better schooling (Kharel et al., 2021; Ma et al., 2022; Speck & Müller-Böker, 2020; Rai & Dangal, 2021). Possibly, particularly for rural families who are disproportionately represented by international migration (Thapa et al., 2019), the perceived sacrifice by the absent caregiver and the resulting advantages are beneficial, despite the disruption of family structure.

Societal values

There are societal values in Nepal that provide context for how Nepali caregivers raise their children. Historically, Nepal is regarded as a collectivistic, hierarchical society. Each person's priority is the good of the group rather than of the self; one depends on the group for well-being. Each person accepts unequal distribution of power, and respects and complies with authority figures to foster social cohesion (Hofstede, 1980). Outside family life, hierarchy is instantiated in the Hindu caste system and its influence on intergroup relations. Although social harmony is highly valued, social hierarchy is also important. Harmony is not always reflected in social interactions; higher caste members can be angry and aggressive toward members of the *dalit* class, who perform essential work for the castes, work that is deemed impure and a threat to the spiritual purity of higher caste members (Cameron, 1998). Although caste was once legally codified and every ethnic group, even those who were not Hindu, were placed in an elaborate hierarchical system, it is no longer legally sanctioned. Nonetheless, caste continues to influence intergroup relations and allocation of resources (Pathak & Schündeln, 2022; Subedi, 2016).

A strict hierarchy also characterizes family life. In most homes, father (or grandfather if present) is head of the household and not to be questioned or disobeyed. The mother is the authority for the women in the family but subservient to the will of the father. In vignette-based interviews, primary school children understand that you should not feel angry, or if you feel so, you should not display anger (Cole et al., 2002). Mother and father must be respected because they gave one life; friends must cooperate. Even children reinforce hierarchy; they always know who is elder, use the proper kinship term (e.g., *dai* for older brother), and respect the older child even if there is a conflict (Cole, Walker, et al., 2006).

The degree to which these values influence childrearing are barely understood. Moral knowledge, which explicitly conveys these values, is taught in school at every grade level (Shrestha & Parajuli, 2019). Qualitative interviews with caregivers, teachers, and community leaders describe childrearing practices refer to respect for authority, obedience, interpersonal harmony, and cooperation, all as a result of self-control (An et al., 2018; Burkey et al., 2016; Langer et al., 2019). When compared with German and Korean mothers, Nepali mothers of primary school children more often refer to using punitive reactions (reprimands, discouragement) in response to self-focused emotions (e.g., pride about individual accomplishments; Cho et al., 2022).

Interviews and questionnaires may be prone to espousing societal values and may or may not reflect actual childrearing behavior. Our research team's observations, both empirical and anecdotal, indicate that most families convey love and support of children; they engage in teaching, scolding, and corporal punishment, although when and how much depends upon the culture group observed (Cole, Tamang et al., 2006).

Childrearing practices and beliefs

Viewed through the lens of Western models of parenting (e.g., Baumrind, 1967), childrearing in Nepal is generally seen as authoritarian, more harsh than warm, more controlling than democratic. As we know, applying a model developed in another nation risks mischaracterization (Raval et al., 2018). Generally, childrearing in Nepal is marked by strictness, consistent with both economic realities and hierarchical societal values. Caregivers expect children not to ask for things that the family cannot afford or acquire, and to be willing to sacrifice their own needs and desires in deference to the good of the family (An et al., 2018). Recall that childrearing is a shared responsibility within most Nepali families. Older children care for younger children and contribute to household work; girls also cook and clean, assist in farming and childcare, and in some cases contribute to decisions that affect family life (Langer et al., 2019). Again, the available data comes from interviews and questionnaires, not observations.

Several qualitative interview studies address caregivers' ethnotheories about desirable child behavior (Harkness et al., 2015). Ethnotheories are one aspect of the developmental niche, a framework for conceptualizing cultural variations in childrearing (Super & Harkness, 1986). In-depth interviews with adults from different Nepali castes and ethnic groups reveal a common ethnotheory, that the caregiver's role is to foster children's *ujjala bhavishya*, i.e., bright future (Burkey et al., 2016). A bright future involves good family relationships and educational, social, and economic success; a dark future is defined by division from family and community and failure, shame, and/or poverty. Education is valued as the means to secure a better life, such that adults emphasize school attendance, academic competence, and earning income that can change the family's status (An et al., 2018). Yet, despite these values, children may not complete education because of a higher priority of providing for their families' immediate needs.

It is unclear from these studies whether and to what degree different Nepali caste and ethnic groups share these values equally. Hindus, who represent 81 percent of the population, emphasize the importance of *sanskar*, defined as the purification and enhancement of inner consciousness that emerges from the development of conscience (Novianti et al., 2023). Hindu caregivers are expected to mentor and nurture children's moral development as well as academic and social development. As the learned caste, Brahmans emphasize excelling in school (Cole et al., 2006). The beliefs of other groups, e.g., Buddhists and Muslims, may influence childrearing in ways that emphasize other priorities. For example, Tamang elders, who ascribe to Tibetan Buddhism, describe competent children as having social grace and not being angry (Cole et al., 2006). Caregiver interviews also reveal that raising children is difficult during planting and harvesting seasons, especially in families in which a caregiver has migrated for income (Pant, 2021). In rural villages, adults may work in the fields and household up to 14 hours a day (Panter-Brick, 1989). Notably, caregiver engagement with children appeared to increase during and immediately after the COVID-19 global pandemic (Miller et al., 2022), but then dropped lower than it had been before the pandemic, perhaps owing to pandemic-related stressors affecting agriculture and food insecurity especially in low-resource regions (Adhikari et al., 2021).

When asked, Nepali caregivers believe certain childrearing practices are critical to children's *ujjala bhavishya*—caregiver engagement, warm and positive interactions, supervision, meeting basic needs and supporting schooling (Hossain et al., 2015; Miller et al., 2022). In general, and especially in less resourced nations, these childrearing values are linked to the psychological and physical well-being of youth (Jeong et al., 2018; Vijayalakshmi et al., 2007). Western models have traditionally characterized Nepali caregiving as authoritarian (high control, low warmth), although recent questionnaire evidence suggests respondents may be endorsing authoritative values—openness to children's perspectives, providing structure, and being involved and warm toward children (Khadka et al., 2021; Kunwor et al., 2021). Nonetheless, the extent to which Nepali caregivers behave in ways that Western models define as authoritative or generally positive may depend on household wealth and caregiver availability (Miller et al., 2022).

Nepali parents rarely endorse the use of physical punishment for children's rule violations (Burkey et al., 2016). Rather, interviewees state it is better to verbally admonish misbehaving children. They use the term *samjhaune* (to be reminded) as the way to influence children's *dimaag* (brain-mind) development (An et al., 2018; Burkey et al., 2016; Langer et al., 2019). Nepali scholars suggest the move away from physical punishment may be due to some families having increased awareness of information regarding childrearing and child development, awareness that is linked to economic improvements in household income, especially in urban locales (Kunwor et al., 2021; Langer et al., 2019; Shrestha et al., 2019). Scolding, admonishing, and reminding, however, do not always change children's behavior and can lead to caregivers using threats without consequences; this has been described as inconsistent caregiving from the perspective of Western models of parenting (Khadka et al., 2021).

The evidence thus far has several acknowledged limitations. For example, women sometimes refuse to participate (e.g., Speck & Müller-Böker, 2020). Women can be concerned about sharing their personal opinions, about not knowing the answer researchers want, or about repercussions in the home or community for participation. Time is also an issue; villagers spend considerable time working, especially during the many months ranging from planting to harvesting, which limits their availability (Panter-Brick, 1989). Further, there are questions about the construct and cultural validity of questionnaires, including those administered orally to parents who are illiterate (Ma et al., 2022). Interviews and questionnaires reflect societal beliefs about childrearing. Whether they reflect a caregiver's actual beliefs, or their actual practices, is unknown.

Culturally sensitive observational research is rare. Time usage studies provide valuable observations that shed light on childrearing in Nepali households. Among many ethnic groups throughout Nepal, conjoint households share the responsibilities of childcare (Levine, 1988). However, not all families are conjoint. Tamang families in one rural village preferred nuclear family life. This preference placed multiple, conflicting demands on caregivers, including pregnant/lactating mothers (Panter-Brick, 1986). Throughout much of Nepal, the year is absorbed by subsistence farming. In nuclear families, which have many fewer household members, mothers and fathers must spend considerable time in fieldwork, growing the food that the family needs to survive throughout the year. They often bring young children to the fields. Thus, models and methods that assume the importance of high levels of interaction between mothers and their children do not capture the realities of many rural Nepalis.

As part of a larger study (Cole, Tamang et al., 2006), we observed how Brahman and Tamang caregivers interacted with three- through five-year-olds with a particular interest in how they responded when children appeared angry or ashamed. We conducted home observations after harvesting and harvest festivals when adults had more time at home. We worked with villages where more than 90 percent of households were from the one of these two groups. We compared Brahman and Tamang families because Nepalis perceive these two groups as very different (Jacobson, 2000). Brahmans are high caste Hindus, the learned caste, and despite our participants being poor subsistence farmers, they nonetheless conveyed their status as high caste. In contrast, Tamang are an indigenous minority, whose language is no longer written, and whose village life appears to have a more egalitarian social structure than in Brahman villages (Holmberg, 1992). Higher castes regard Tamang as backward and unintelligent, in part because they consume alcohol.

Our observations revealed many similarities among the two groups but also some interesting differences. First, there was a higher rate of caregiver-child interaction in Tamang households. Second, Brahmans and Tamang were similar on all but four of the 16 Structural Analysis of Social Behavior (Benjamin, 1979) codes, a system for describing dyadic interactions in terms of warmth and control. The four differences described Tamang children as more trusting and their caregivers as more nurturing in their control relative to Brahmans. Brahman children had greater autonomy and caregivers expressed less overt warmth. Third, both groups were equally likely to ignore child anger but when they did respond, both engaged in scolding, physical punishments, or cajoling. However, Brahman caregivers were more likely to engage in teaching angry children (*samjhaune*) than the Tamang who were more likely to first tease angry children, and then when the children appeared ashamed, they provided physical affection and/or food. Teasing typically resulted in Tamang children's appearing ashamed, an emotion that is highly valued in Nepal and especially by Tamang. Brahman caregivers mainly ignored child shame, whereas Tamang caregivers sometimes ignored but also engaged in teaching (*samjhaune*) and nurturing the ashamed child more than Brahmans. These findings may explain why (a) Brahman children show more anger, and endorse angry responses to hypothetical situations; and (b) Tamang children show more shame, and endorse shame as a response to those same situations.

Future Directions

To understand childrearing across communities within and between nations, there is a critical need to strive for culturally meaningful approaches (Bornstein & Chen, Chapter 1 in this volume; Raval, 2023). We next discuss how we conducted research in Nepal, with cultural groups other than our own. We discuss how we tried to form mutual understanding of the research concepts, how we grappled with the fact that the culture of science conflicted at times with Nepali cultures, and how we attempted to ensure our interpretations of the data were consistent with Brahman and Tamang views on childrearing.

The research team

In conducting cross-cultural comparative research, which includes collaborations with Japanese colleagues (e.g., Mizuta et al.,1996), we quickly appreciated the value of having collaborators from the cultural group (insiders) and non-members (outsiders) (Liu & Burnett, 2022). Outsiders note differences with their own experience that insiders may take for granted, and insiders provide insight and detail on the behavior of members of their group. In Nepal, the team was a white U.S. female, five Tamang staff (three men, two women), and one Brahman woman. All had previously traveled throughout Nepal, except one Tamang and one Brahman woman who lived in or near participating villages.

In approaching potential participant villages, Nepali staff described us as "beggars," seeking support to conduct research on children's emotions. We spent days talking with the leaders in each village to reach a common understanding of the study goals and methods and to consider how our presence could be of value to the village. Because cultural pressures to conform might make it difficult for someone to refuse to participate, we did not compensate individuals (we did give children pencils) but developed projects with the help of village leaders, e.g., a girls' latrine at a school, a new school roof). In this way, the whole village benefited regardless of whether every villager participated (almost all did).

A critical issue at the time was our U.S. federal funding; we were perceived as representatives of the U.S. government at a time when there was a domestic war between Nepali security forces and Maoist rebels. The rebels who lived in the woods frequently took goods (jewelry, animals) from families and there was concern that they would think we had given money to villagers. Extensive discussions helped us address these issues to everyone's satisfaction, aided in large part by our Nepali staff.

We were also sensitive to the experience of each participant. We did not realize how uncomfortable mothers would be trying to respond to our open-ended interview about children. As we began to appreciate this discomfort, we switched to interviewing village elders (leaders, lamas and priests, grandparents) who were very interested in our work and easily offered ideas. Children were also anxious about providing the right answer to our questions. They were all school age children who had learned that the teacher knew the right answer and that they might be punished if they failed to provide that answer. Our Nepali research staff began to coax the children, supplying answers. Extensive discussions helped them understand that science requires that they not be the respondents and that with patience children would provide their own answers.

The methods

The task that took the most time was working out the cultural equivalence of concepts and the meaningfulness of the questions we asked. We spent more days working through these issues with village leaders than we did collecting the data. For example, there is no word in the participants' languages (Nepali and Tamang) for emotion. Anthropologists refer to *man* (Nepali; Kohrt & Harper, 2008) and *sem* (Tamang; Desjarlais, 2003) as referring to 'heartmind', which we came to understand as referring to internal states—both thinking and feeling. We then spent days making informal observations in villages, listening and then hearing the terms that appeared to be equivalents to our English language terms.

In our first foray into cross-cultural research in Nepal (Cole et al., 2002), our insider collaborators noted that Americans seemed preoccupied with the emotion anger. If we wished to understand negative emotion in Nepal, we should study *laj* (self-conscious negative emotions, like shame). We added shame to our procedures, which yielded interesting results and made more sense to the Nepali staff. We also spent time addressing whether there were meaningful equivalents to the emotion terms happy, angry, ashamed, and okay. To this end, we again spent time just observing in villages; when we perceived an event involving a child that appeared emotionally evocative to us, we asked villagers what happened, including asking about the child's internal state. We found terms that were used frequently and consistent with the English language terms. For example, when a child's desire or goal was blocked, they appeared angry to us; Brahmans explained that the child's *ris uthyo* (anger rose) and Tamang said *bhomo khaba* (anger came).

Home observations of three- through five-year-olds and caregivers were conducted by female research assistants (RAs) who were from the region and of the same ethnic group as the participants. Sara Harkness, our consultant, advised us to have RAs follow the child and record everything they observed, including emotional reactions. The observations were recorded in copies (notebooks) rather than video or audio, which would likely distract and interfere with the ongoings in the home. The notes were written in the native tongues of the participants and included verbatim interactions. The notes were later transcribed into English by staff members who were fluent in all three languages and the English transcriptions were coded by two teams. One team (Nepali and American) used the Structural Analysis of Social Behavior (SASB; Benjamin, 1979), a circumplex model of social interaction, to capture the degree of control and warmth reflected in caregiver responses to children's expressed anger and shame. The SASB, developed in the United States, has been used with European but not to our knowledge with Asian participants. Another team (Nepali and American) developed a system for coding antecedent and consequent events when children displayed anger or shame (see Cole et al., 2006 for further details).

Interpreting findings

We questioned whether the coding systems we used captured Tamang and Brahman interactions with children fairly. Each group has biases about the other group. To address this issue, we conducted slide presentations to mental health professionals in Kathmandu who identified with each of these groups. In both cases, the professionals remarked at the familiarity of the portraits. For example, a Brahman psychologist said the findings captured his own upbringing and noted that although there was not much open affection in his household, he always felt loved. A Tamang mental health worker commented that the importance of not being angry was very important in Tamang society. We felt reassured enough that we proceeded with conference presentations and publishing the findings.

The second concern was the question of why—why was anger acceptable to feel (although not to show) in the Brahman context but unacceptable to Tamang, who clearly valued a submissive stance in situations that

Brahman (and U.S.) children would feel angry (Cole et al., 2002). One possibility is that being high caste might support the experience of anger, as has been shown in research on interactions between high caste and lowest caste members (Cameron, 1996). As for the Tamang, the Tibetan Buddhism that guides their lives identifies emotions, and particularly anger, as destructive states (Goleman, 2000). However, we had not measured these values and were unclear that they were adequate explanations. There are other possibilities. For example, majority/minority status might explain the differences; being an indigenous minority group member in a majority Hindu culture in which Brahmans are the highest caste might influence when and where one can convey anger or shame. Expressing anger to persons who have relative power and regard themselves as having higher status may lead to undesirable outcomes in a society where civil rights are generally not prioritized. Therefore, minority persons may assume a humble posture, appear ashamed even if they do not feel such (Cameron, 1996). The open question is whether caregivers from different cultural groups have different expectations and practices that influence how they socialize children's anger and shame.

In sum, it is critical that we broaden and deepen our understanding of parenting throughout the world, with all the different ways that groups identify. Doing so requires openness, patience, and learning, including reading beyond the immediate literature that informs the constructs studied. We found that scholars from other fields informed our work considerably. We are grateful for what we learned from Brahman and Tamang villagers and staff members, which helped us not only conduct but understand our research. Nepal lacks the resources to conduct the type of research that would address parenting at the standards that are required by mainstream outlets. Thus, it is hard to both conduct high quality research and share the learned information widely. We hope that others will collaborate with scholars in Nepal, including across fields of expertise, and further our understanding of how children are raised in such a richly interesting nation.

References

Acharya, D. R. (2021). Status of girls' participation in higher education in Nepal. *International Journal of Multidisciplinary Perspectives in Higher Education, 6*(2), 68–85.

Adhikari, J., Rai, M. K., Baral, C., & Subedi, M. (2023). Labour migration from Nepal: Trends and explanations. In: Rajan, S.I. (eds) *Migration in South Asia*. IMISCOE Research Series. Cham: Springer. https://doi.org/10.1007/978-3-031-34194-6_5.

Adhikari, J., Timsina, J., Khadka, S. R., Ghale, Y., & Ojha, H. (2021). COVID-19 impacts on agriculture and food systems in Nepal: Implications for SDGs.

Agricultural Systems, 186(June 2020), 102990. https://doi.org/10.1016/j.agsy.2020.102990.

Adhikari, R. P., Upadhaya, N., Gurung, D., Luitel, N. P., Burkey, M. D., Kohrt, B. A., & Jordans, M. J. D. (2015). Perceived behavioral problems of school aged children in rural Nepal: A qualitative study. *Child and Adolescent Psychiatry and Mental Health, 9*(1), 1–9. https://doi.org/10.1186/s13034-015-0061-8.

An, D., Eggum-Wilkens, N. D., Chae, S., Hayford, S. R., Yabiku, S. T., Glick, J. E., & Zhang, L. (2018). Adults' conceptualisations of children's cocial competence in Nepal and Malawi. *Psychology and Developing Societies, 30*(1), 81–104.

Baumrind, D. (1967). Child care practices anteceding three patterns of preschool behavior. *Genetic Psychology Monographs, 75*(1), 43–88.

Benjamin, L. S. (1979). Use of structural analysis of social behavior (SASB) and Markov chains to study dyadic interactions. *Journal of Abnormal Psychology, 88*(3), 303–319. https://doi.org/10.1037/0021-843X.88.3.303.

Bhandari, K. (2016). Understanding Nepali nationalism. *Studies in Ethnicity and Nationalism, 16*(3), 416–436. https://doi.org/10.1111/sena.12208.

Breen, M. G. (2018). Nepal, federalism and participatory constitution-making: deliberative democracy and divided societies. *Asian Journal of Political Science, 26,* 33–39. https://doi.org/10.1080/02185377.2018.1515639.

Bronfenbrenner, U. (1979). *The ecology of human development: Experiments by nature and design*. Cambridge, MA: Harvard University Press.

Burkey, M. D., Ghimire, L., Adhikari, R. P., Wissow, L. S., Jordans, M. J. D., & Kohrt, B. A. (2016). The ecocultural context and child behavior problems: A qualitative analysis in rural Nepal. *Social Science and Medicine, 159*, 73–82. https://doi.org/10.1016/j.socscimed.2016.04.020.

Cameron, M. M. (1998). *On the edge of the auspicious: Gender and caste in Nepal.* Urbana-Champaign, IL: University of Illinois Press.

Cole, P. M., Bruschi, C. J., & Tamang, B. L. (2002). Cultural differences in children's emotional reactions to difficult situations. *Child Development, 73*(3), 983–996. https://doi.org/10.1111/1467-8624.00451.

Cole, P. M., Tamang, B. L., & Shrestha, S. (2006). Cultural variations in the socialization of young children's anger and shame. *Child Development, 77*(5), 1237–1251. https://doi.org/10.1111/j.1467-8624.2006.00931.

Cole, P. M., Walker, A. R., & Lama-Tamang, M. (2006). Emotional aspects of peer relations among children in rural Nepal. In X. Chen, D. C. French & B. H. Schneider (Eds), *Peer relationships in cultural context* (pp. 148–169). Cambridge University Press.

Cross, S. E., Bacon, P. L., & Morris, M. L. (2000). The relational-interdependent self-construal and relationships. *Journal of Personality and Social Psychology, 78*, 791–808. https://psycnet.apa.org/doi/10.1037/0022-3514.78.4.791.

Desjarlais, R. R. (2003). *Sensory biographies: Lives and deaths among Nepal's Yolmo Buddhists* (Vol. 2). University of California Press.

Goleman, D. (2003). *Destructive emotions: how can we overcome them? A scientific dialogue with the Dalai Lama.* New York: Bantam Books.

Harkness, S., Mavridis, C. J., Liu, J. J., & Super, C. M. (2015). Parental ethnotheories and the development of family relationships in early and middle childhood. In L. A. Jensen (Ed.), *The Oxford handbook of human development and culture: An interdisciplinary perspective* (pp. 271–291). Oxford University Press. https://doi.org/10.1093/oxfordhb/9780199948550.013.17.

Hofstede, G. (1980). *Culture's consequences: International differences in work-related values*. Beverly Hills, CA: Sage Publications.

Holmberg, D. (1992). *Order in paradox: Myth and ritual among Nepal's Tamang*. Ithaca, NY: Cornell University Press.

Hossain, S. M., Huq, S., Adhikari, B., Eusuf Zai, S. Z., & Haque, S. M. T. (2015). Parenting skills and child behavior: A cross-sectional study in some selected areas of Nepal. *South East Asia Journal of Public Health, 5*(1), 44–48.

International Labour Organization. (2023). *Labour migration in Nepal*. www.ilo.org/kathmandu/areasofwork/labour-migration/lang--en/index.htm.

Jacobson, C. (2000). Glimpses from the margin: Images of caste and ethnicity in Nepal's middle hills. *Himalaya: The Journal of the Association for Nepal and Himalayan Studies*, 1–2, 31–41. https://digitalcommons.macalester.edu/himalaya/vol20/iss1/9?utm_source=digitalcommons.macalester.edu%2Fhimalaya%2Fvol20%2Fiss1%2F9&utm_medium=PDF&utm_campaign=PDFCoverPages.

Jeong, J., Pitchik, H. O., & Yousafzai, A. K. (2018). Stimulation interventions and parenting in low- and middle-income countries: A meta-analysis. *Pediatrics, 141*(4), e20173510. https://doi.org/10.1542/peds. 2017–3510.

Kaimal, L. S. & Paul, A. M. (2020). A sociological preview on the effects of migration on families left behind in homeland. *Asian Review of Social Sciences, 9*(1), 9–13. https://doi.org/10.51983/arss-2020.9.1.1613.

KC, B. K. (2004). Internal migration in Nepal. In *Population Monograph of Nepal* (pp. 121–168). Kathmandu: Central Bureau of Statistics.

Keller H. (2007). *Cultures of infancy*. Mahwah, NJ: Lawrence Erbaum.

Khadka, J. (2021). Parental behavior across Nepali schools' parents and children demographic characteristics. *Journal of Community Psychology, 49*(7), 2704–2718. https://doi.org/10.1002/jcop.22509.

Khalil, U. & Mookerjee, S. (2019). Patrilocal residence and women's social status: Evidence from South Asia. *Economic Development and Cultural Change, 67*, 401–438. https://www.journals.uchicago.edu/doi/epdf/10.1086/697584.

Kharel, M., Akira, S., Kiriya, J., Ong, K. I. C., & Jimba, M. (2021). Parental migration and psychological wellbeing of left-behind adolescents in Western Nepal. *PLoS ONE, 16*(1 January), 1–13. https://doi.org/10.1371/journal.pone.0245873.

Kohrt, B. A. & Harper, I. (2008). Navigating diagnoses: Understanding mind–body relations, mental health, and stigma in Nepal. *Culture, Medicine, and Psychiatry, 32*, 462–491.

Kunwor, A., Khadka, B., Pariyar, M., Ghimire, N., Panta, P., & Baraili, S. (2021). Exploring parental involvement practices of child rearing in five major cities of Nepal. *SXC Journal of Management and Social Sciences, 1*(1), 33–43.

Langer, J. A., Ramos, J. V., Ghimire, L., Rai, S., Kohrt, B. A., & Burkey, M. D. (2019). Gender and Child Behavior Problems in Rural Nepal: Differential Expectations and Responses. *Scientific Reports, 9*(1), 1–10. https://doi.org/10.1038/s41598-019-43972-3.

Law, A. & Rodway, G. W. (2008). Trekking and climbing in the Solu Khumbu district of Nepal: impact on socioeconomic status and health of lowland porters. *Wilderness & Environmental Medicine, 19*, 210–217.

Levine, N. E. (1988). Women's work and infant feeding: A case from rural Nepal. *Ethnology*, 27, 231–251. https://doi.org/10.2307/3773519.

LeVine, R. A., Dixon, S., LeVine, S., Richman, A., Leiderman, P. H., Keefer, C. H., & Brazelton, T. B. (1996). *Child care and culture: Lessons from Africa. Cambridge University Press.* https://doi.org/10.1017/CBO9780511720321.

Liu, X. & Burnett, D. (2022). Insider-outsider: Methodological reflections on intercultural collaborative research. *Humanities and Social Science Communications*, 9, 314. https://doi.org/10.1057/s41599-022-01336-9.

Ma, J., Mahat, P., Brøndbo, P. H., Handegård, B. H., Kvernmo, S., & Javo, A. C. (2022). Family correlates of emotional and behavioral problems in Nepali school children. *PLoS ONE, 17*(1 January), 1–17. https://doi.org/10.1371/journal.pone.0262690

Maslow A. H. (1943). A theory of human motivation. *Psychological Review, 50,* 370–396.

Miller, L. C., Neupane, S., Joshi, N., Lohani, M., & Shrestha, B. (2023). Trajectories of child growth, child development, and home child-rearing quality during the Covid pandemic in rural Nepal. *Child: Care, Health and Development, 49*(5), 800–810. https://doi.org/10.1111/cch.13078.

Mizuta, I., Zahn-Waxler, C., Cole, P. M., & Hiruma, N. (1996). A cross-cultural study of preschoolers' attachment: Security and sensitivity in Japanese and US dyads. *International Journal of Behavioral Development, 19*, 141–159. https://doi.org/10.1080/016502596385992.

National Statistics Office (2022). *National population and housing census 2021: National report on caste/ethnicity, language, and religion*. Thapathali, Kathmandu, Nepal: National Statistics Office.

Novianti, R., Suarman, & Islami, N. (2023). Parenting in Cultural Perspective: A Systematic Review of Paternal Role Across Cultures. *Journal of Ethnic and Cultural Studies, 10*(1), 22–44. https://doi.org/10.29333/ejecs/1287.

Pant, R. (2021). Transnational parenting from the views of fathers: A study on Nepalese immigrants living in Portugal (master's thesis). University Institute of Lisbon, Portugal.

Panter-Brick, C. (1989). Motherhood and subsistence work: The Tamang of rural Nepal. *Human Ecology, 17*, 205–228. doi: 10.1007/BF00889713.

Panter-Brick, C. (2002). Street children, human rights, and public health: A critique and future directions. *Annual Review of Anthropology, 31*(1), 147–171.

Pathak, P. & Schündeln, M. (2022). Social hierarchies and the allocation of development aid: Evidence from the 2015 earthquake in Nepal. *Journal of Public Economics, 209*, 104607. https://doi.org/10.1016/j.jpubeco.2022.104607.

Rai, D. R. & Dangal, M. R. (2021). The Effect of Migration on Family in Nepal: A Review on the Family Structure, Livelihood, Education, Aging Parents, Reproductive Health and Marital Relationship. *Open Journal for Anthropological Studies, 5*(2), 49–60. https://doi.org/10.32591/coas.ojas.0502.02049r.

Rai, D. R., Dangal, M. R., & Sharma, S. (2023). Effect of Parental Seasonal Labor Migration on Children's Care and Educational Performance in Rural Nepal. *Open Journal for Sociological Studies, 7*(1), 1–10. https://doi.org/10.32591/coas.ojss.0701.01001r.

Raval, V. V. (2023). From the margins to the center: Advancing research on caregiver socialization of emotion in Asia. *Child Development Perspectives, 17*(3–4), 142–148. https://doi.org/10.1111/cdep.12487.

Raval, V. V., Li, X., Deo, N., & Hu, J. (2018). Reports of maternal socialization goals, emotion socialization behaviors, and child socio-emotional functioning in China and India. *Journal of Family Psychology, 32*(1), 81–91. https://doi.org/10.1037/fam00 00336.

Shrestha, B. K. & Parajuli, T. R. (2019). Teaching practices of moral education in public and private schools of Nepal. *World Wide Journal of Multidisciplinary Research and Development, 5*(1), 1–6.

Shrestha, M., Ulak, M., Strand, T. A., Kvestad, I., & Hysing, M. (2019). How much do Nepalese mothers know about child development? *Early Child Development and Care, 189*(1), 135–142. https://doi.org/10.1080/03004430.2017.1304391.

Speck, S. & Müller-Böker, U. (2020). Population ageing and family change: older people's perceptions of current changes in family composition in rural Nepal. *European Bulletin of Himalayan Research, 55*, 7–37. https://doi.org/10.4000/ebhr.234.

Subedi, M. (2016). Caste/ethnic dimensions of change and inequality: implications for inclusive and affirmative agendas in Nepal. *Nepali Journal of Contemporary Studies, 16*(1), 1–16.

Super, C. M., & Harkness, S. (1986). The developmental niche: A conceptualization at the interface of child and culture. *International Journal of Behavioral Development, 9*(4), 545–569. https://doi.org/10.1177/016502548600900409

Thapa, N., Paudel, M., Guragain, A. M., Thapa, P., Puri, R., Thapa, P., Aryal, K. K., Paudel, B. K., Thapa, R., & Stray-Pedersen, B. (2019). Status of migration and socio-reproductive impacts on migrants and their families left behind in Nepal. *Migration and Development, 8*(3), 394–417. https://doi.org/10.1080/21632324.2019.1567097.

United Nations Conference on Trade and Development (2023, November 7). *Least Developed Countries Report 2023*. UNCTAD. https://unctad.org/publication/least-developed-countries-report-2023.

Vijayalakshimi, K., Kumar, C. V., & Rajamanickm, H. (2007). Child rearing practice and psychological problems of children. *Nursing and Midwifery Research Journal, 2*, 49–56. https://doi.org/10.33698/nrf0065.

Whiting, B. B. (1963). *Six cultures: Studies of child-rearing*. New York: Wiley and Sons.

Whiting, B. B. & Whiting, J. W. (1979). *Children of six cultures: A psycho-cultural analysis*. Cambridge, MA: Harvard University Press.

World Population Review (2023, December 17). *Nepal Population 2023*. https://worldpopulationreview.com/countries/nepal-population.

13

FILIAL PIETY, PARENT–CHILD RELATIONSHIPS, AND PARENTING IN TAIWAN

Kuang-Hui Yeh

Parents are considered important contributors to their children's social behavior and adaptive development, and parenting style is regarded as the most important way to influence this process. However, what role should parents play in raising their children? The answer is likely multifaceted and may vary from person to person and culture to culture. Generally speaking, the basic functions of parenting include ensuring the survival and well-being of the child, as well as socializing the child according to the social norms, values, and acceptable behaviors of a particular culture or society at least.

Over the past three decades, concerning how to ensure the survival and well-being of children and socialize them, Taiwan's mainstream discourse has evolved with different arguments, making today's Taiwanese parents full of anxiety and uneasiness about parenting (Lan, 2019). When psychologists talk about parenting issues, they often look for factors from the characteristics of parents and children and family. But parenting is not only the interpersonal interaction between individuals within the family, it is also subject to the influence of the parenting rationality of social and cultural construction (Arendell, 1997). Suppose a society makes people feel that the gap between the rich and the poor is polarized, and competition for status and life is fierce. In that case, parents in society will put cultivating their children's "survival skills" ahead of "happy growth" (Doepke & Zilibotti, 2019). But if the gap between the rich and the poor is small and the return on investment in education is not high in society, parents will have little incentive and no need to worry about how to parent their children. Therefore, to explore the causes of Taiwanese parental anxieties and difficulties,

DOI: 10.4324/9781003383949-13

we also need to examine the root causes of the problem from the perspective of social structure and cultural changes in Taiwan, especially from the ideological change of the social trends on parenting. These arguments in Taiwan have been intertwined by the entanglement between Chinese traditional and Western parenting concepts, and the impact of the globalization trends (Lan, 2014; Wu, 2016).

In addition, parents from different social classes have different relationships to the projection of modernity and different levels of involvement in the globalization process (Lan, 2019; Wu, 2016), which also contributes to the divergence of the parenting arguments. Despite differences in parenting ideologies, most contemporary Taiwanese parents hope that the ways they raise their children should not be the same as those of their parents, such as beating and scolding, and demanding absolute obedience from their children, especially in the era of globalization. But in the face of an uncertain global future, how to be a competent parent makes today's Taiwanese parents collectively feel anxious and uneasy.

The purpose of this article is twofold. The first is to examine how people have made corresponding adjustments to the changes of filial piety concepts and family values during the evolvement in Taiwan's social, cultural, and economic structures under the impact of modernization and globalization from 1965 to the present, and how these adjustments have changed parent–child interactions and parenting styles. The second is to provide suggestions for parenting that Taiwanese parents can adopt in the future, as the trend of globalization continues impacting people's quality of life and challenging children's physical and psychological adaptation, for resolving their own increasing anxieties and uneasiness about raising their children.

Filial Piety, Parent–Child Relationships, and Children's Well-Being

Filial piety, consistently acknowledged as the cornerstone of all other Chinese family values, occupies a distinctive position in the field of parent–child relationships and parenting studies within Chinese societies (Ho, 1994; Yeh et al., 2013). Beyond its role in setting family norms, filial piety assumes a crucial role as the ethical bedrock for maintaining social order and fostering a stable society (Ho, 1996; Yeh, 1997). Over millennia, it has steadfastly provided the moral framework shaping Chinese patterns of parent–child relations and socialization (Bedford & Yeh, 2019). Despite the impact of Western cultures and modernization on the connotation and influence of Chinese filial piety in contemporary times, it continues to wield a significant influence on the dynamics of Chinese parent–child interactions. Since 1986, consistent findings in population-based studies have highlighted that family harmony and filial piety stand out as the most significant values in the daily lives of Taiwanese people, garnering widespread agreement (see Huang & Chu, 2012). One large-scale longitudinal study (Huang & Chen, 2024) in Taiwan even showed that after controlling for several demographic variables, greater adherence to filial piety in adolescence (aged 13–15) predicts higher independence and interdependence in emerging adulthood (aged 22). However, based on the Dual Filial Piety Model, which integrates Chinese historical, philosophical, and social trends to construct a comprehensive model of filial piety (Yeh, 2003; Yeh & Bedford, 2003; Bedford & Yeh, 2019), modern Chinese filial piety comprises at least two higher-order factors corresponding to two central filial attributes: reciprocity and authoritarianism. The former, operating following the Confucian principle of favoring the intimate, is termed *reciprocal filial piety* (RFP), while the latter, following the Confucian principle of respecting the superior, is referred to as *authoritarian filial piety* (AFP).

An individual's development of RFP hinges on the deep affection, mutual understanding, and trust fostered in interactions with loving parents throughout the growth process. This results in children harboring spontaneous feelings for their parents and cultivating a conscious sense of love and respect to parents. Conversely, the development of AFP is rooted in children gradually learning to regulate their behavior and needs, gaining acceptance and recognition from parents, and subsequently extending these principles to seek societal and cultural approval by adhering to parental expectations or embodying the role of "good children." Importantly, it's noteworthy that reciprocal and authoritarian filial piety are not mutually exclusive; they can coexist within an individual or a society simultaneously (Bedford & Yeh, 2019). The relative proportions of each that an individual possesses are shaped by their upbringing experiences in real interactions with parents, while the societal emphasis on either is contingent on the political, social, and economic milieu.

The filial piety most widely acknowledged by contemporary Taiwanese is RFP rather than AFP (Yeh, 1997; Yeh, 2003; Yeh & Olwen, 2003; Wu & Yeh, 2021). Prior research consistently demonstrates that higher levels of RFP in children are positively associated with the quality of family life, the relationship quality between parents and children, as well as their social-emotional development and psychological well-being (Chen et al., 2016). Conversely, elevated levels of AFP in children are often linked to tension in parent–child relationships and are positively associated with psychological distress and problematic behaviors, such as depression, anxiety, and aggressive and deviant behaviors (see Olwen & Yeh, 2019; Tsao & Yeh, 2019). However, when both are elevated, RFP has the capacity to mitigate or even transform the negative effects of AFP into positive outcomes.

The attributes of RFP align with the co-experienced positive affects in the Positivity Resonance Theory (Fredrickson, 2016). This theory suggests that interpersonal connection characterized by shared positivity, mutual care and concern, and behavioral and biological synchrony—referred to as perceived positivity resonance—is strongly correlated with the well-being of individuals (Major et al., 2018; Zhou et al., 2022).

These previous findings implied that relationship quality or relationship integration between parents and children should be the key factor leading to the adaptive development and well-being of the children. As for what kind of parenting style or practices can improve the children's filial beliefs or the quality of the parent–child relationship, an empirical study (Yeh & Cheng, 2005) indicated that children who perceive their parents adopting the authoritative parenting style tend to develop both reciprocal and authoritarian filial beliefs. Conversely, those who perceive their parents as employing the authoritarian parenting style experience a notable positive impact on the development of their authoritarian filial beliefs. In contrast, the influence on the development of both filial beliefs is low for children who perceive their parents as adopting the indulgent parenting style. Those who perceive their parents adopting the neglectful parenting style, however, tend to experience a negative impact on the development of both reciprocal and authoritarian filial beliefs. Another empirical study (Huang & Yeh, 2013) further demonstrated that the impact of perceived parental authoritative parenting style on children's reciprocal filial beliefs is primarily mediated by children's feelings of gratitude toward their parents. In contrast, the influence of perceived parental authoritative parenting style on children's authoritarian filial beliefs is predominantly mediated by children's feelings of committed compliance to their parents, that is, children obey their parents wholeheartedly, feel a real sense of commitment to what their parents ask for, and can identify with their parents' requirements. In other words, the study illustrates that when children perceive a parental authoritative parenting style, the rules established by parents are more profoundly internalized or integrated into children's values and behaviors. Significantly, the impact of perceived parental authoritarian parenting style on children's authoritarian filial beliefs may be mediated by children's feelings of situational compliance. This compliance lacks intrinsic commitment or personal identification, being mainly superficial and influenced by the awareness of potential consequences, especially in public situations. Notably, this dynamic is observed more distinctly to the father as the target, rather than the mother.

In short, the previous empirical evidence implied that the authoritative parenting style is a highly recognized good parenting style because it is closely related to the reciprocal filial piety of children and is also closely integrated with a good parent–child relationship; while the authoritarian parenting style is disapproving in nature, as it is closely linked to the development of authoritarian filial piety in children. This association tends to result in heightened tension in parent–child relationships, along with increased psychological distress and problematic behaviors in children. However, many scholars (Arendell, 1997; Doepke & Zilibotti, 2019; Lan, 2019) believe that the so-called good or bad upbringing style for children is not only determined by the parenting style itself. A large determinant of "appropriateness" comes from the judgment of good or bad in the social and cultural context at that time. Some scholar (Chao, 1994) even argued that parenting concepts, such as "authoritarian" and "restrictive" are not very relevant for Chinese parents, especially in the domains of children's school learning and academic performance or for fostering family harmony.

The Evolution of Taiwan's Dominant Parenting Styles

How to be a competent or good parent in a challenging globalizing world not only is an individual's own choice but also involves the family's expectations and society's norms on the role of parents (Lan, 2019). Parents usually understand their children's behavior based on the beliefs accumulated in their own growth experiences, view their children's development and form expectations for their children based on these experiences, and adopt these beliefs as the core basis for their parenting behavior (Lin, 2003). But, in addition to what parents want their children to be, based upon the filial norm in Chinese society, children shoulder the responsibility of carrying on the family line and displaying the family's reputation. Therefore, family members other than parents will also hold parents accountable for their children's achievement performance, thereby affecting parents' parenting behavior (Yeh & Yang, 1997). More importantly, the so-called competent parenting concepts or practical strategies are originally the result of social construction and requirements. The social construction of a good parent and a mature child through formal educational institutions affects parents' role identity. Parents are given the responsibility to raise children to meet society's expectations. Therefore, how to raise children is also governed by social norms and ethos. Many Taiwanese parents' parenting anxiety today actually often comes from conflicts between the above three sources (personal choice, family expectations, and parents' role and responsibilities in society). Furthermore, global economic trends have presented challenges to the skills and characteristics essential for the talent competition of the next generation. This, in turn, has heightened parenting anxiety and uneasiness among Taiwanese parents (Lan, 2019).

As Taiwanese parents today, how should they face the ongoing pressure of raising new generation children? Perhaps we can review and examine the evolution of Taiwanese filial piety concepts and family values under the impact of modernization and globalization in the past six decades, and how the adjustments they brought about affect the concepts of parent–child interaction and parenting styles. When understanding the possible underlying mechanisms of these changes, parents may be able to figure out how to cultivate children with life adaptability and talent competitiveness for the future artificial intelligence generation.

Many scholars have used Western modernization theory to explain the changing trends in family structure and values in Taiwan (e.g., Chu, 1986; Lee et al., 1994; Lin et al., 2003). This approach is problematic for three reasons: (1) the modernization process itself is diverse. It has different developmental processes and results across the social and cultural contexts. Taiwanese family structure and value change need to be understood through the historical, cultural, and political context of Taiwan's modernization; (2) the modernization process is not the only factor that affects family structure and values change. When discussing family structure and values change, it is necessary to take into account both Taiwan's domestic policy and global trends; and (3) Western modernization theory often uses the traditional/modern dichotomy to define the possible connotations of and forms of change. It also focuses on the increase and decrease of specific values. These analyses constrain proper interpretations of the features and implications of family structure and values transitions.

1965–85 in Taiwan

The Kuomintang (KMT) government moved to and ruled Taiwan and declared martial law in 1949. Martial law refers to emergency measures taken by the government during special periods such as foreign wars and internal rebellions that seriously endanger social security and political stability. When martial law is imposed, judicial and administrative powers are partially or fully taken over by the military. The key transformation of Taiwan's industrial structure began in 1965 (Hsiao, 1995). Meanwhile, post-war baby boomers made Taiwan's population grow sharply, and the KMT government began to implement a family planning policy in 1970. After 1980, the average number of children in Taiwanese families gradually declined. This family planning policy created an external condition for the change in family structure.

From 1965 to 1985 modernization in Taiwan was most evident in terms of economic development and industrial transformation. However, the effects of other aspects of modernization were constrained to a relaxing of traditional norms. After withdrawing from the United Nations and breaking with the United States in the 1970s, the KMT government began partial democratization to maintain the legitimacy of its rule. However, the main goal of the government's strategic policy was to buffer against protests from outside the party, so it had little impact on social and family values. For example, the KMT began to promote the "Chinese Culture Renaissance Movement" in the late 1960s and invited scholars from various fields to explore the possible development and application of traditional or Confucian values in the new era. In 1977, as part of the Chinese Cultural Renaissance Movement, some scholars proposed a call for "new filial piety," emphasizing that filial piety should be a personal expression, rather than simply a role demanding for children (Yang, 1985). However, this new filial piety emphasizing reform resulted in only a slight relaxing of children's roles and the nature of the parent–child relationship. There was no deeper transformation of family values in the society. The government continued to incorporate traditional family values in the school curricula as standard subjects (citizen ethics and life ethics in primary and secondary schools). These materials were closely integrated with the KMT's national ideology emphasizing the inheritance of Chinese culture (Chen, 2006). The goal was always to shape the KMT as the defender of the Chinese orthodoxy culture, not to promote social modernization.

On the whole, the period from 1965 to 1985 was a critical period for Taiwan's transformation from a traditional society to a modern society. However, martial law was still enforced in Taiwan, and the basic operation of the social system was still closely integrated with the authority of the ruling party. With the transformation of population and family structure and the superficial democratization, the power of parental authority was still emphasized, and the nature of parent–child relationship was also tilted towards parents. Therefore, the authoritarian or parent-centered parenting style was more common than other parenting styles in Taiwan during this period. The authoritarian parenting style is one in which parents require obedience and strict control from their children (Baumrind, 1968). Authoritarian parents attempt to shape, control, and evaluate their children's behavior according to a set of behavioral standards, which are often absolute standards driven and established by a higher authority. It was not uncommon for Taiwanese parents at the time to physically punish their children or use the strategy that inflicted shame sense on their children when they committed transgressions (Fung, 1999; Ho, 1981; Wu, 1981).

In other words, although the new social thinking emphasized the removal of existing restraints and an increase in social mobility, the result was only superficial openness. The function and role of the family and parents in Taiwanese society remained similar to those of traditional society.

The family and parents are responsible for educating children to master social norms and etiquette. Thus, parental control and authority are the necessary ways to maintain societal norms and values (Mead, 1978). Appropriately depicting the characteristics of Taiwanese parenting during this period reflects the transformation of the orthodox values advocated by the KMT government into acceptable forms based on the revival of Chinese cultural traditions.

However, for Chinese or Taiwanese, parental control and restriction may not always manifest parental hostility and mistrust or involve "domination" of children per se, but may be equated with parental concern, caring, or involvement during this period (Chao, 1994). From the perspective of Chinese culture, "chiao-shun" or "guan" in Chinese or "child training" may be a proper term for understanding Chinese or Taiwanese parenting. Most Chinese or Taiwanese parents believe that when children reach school age, they have the ability to "understand things" and should be trained to be self-disciplined, diligent, and responsible for their own behaviors (Shek & Chan, 1999). "Chiao-shun" or "guan" contains the ideas of training children in the appropriate or expected behavior, but also involves an immense devotion and sacrifice on the part of the parents. Additionally, the "training" also emphasizes the importance of "family-based" control to maintain family harmony and the integrity of the family unit by instilling children's hard work, self-discipline, and obedience. It frequently occurs in the context of parental support, high involvement, and physical contact with the child, which differ from the implications of authoritarian parenting rooted in European culture (Chao, 1994, 1996).

Therefore, even if the authoritarian parenting style is used here to describe the way most Taiwanese parents raised their children during this period, it does not imply that this parenting style always has a negative impact on the children. A few studies (Blair & Qian, 1998; Leung et al., 1998; Steinberg et al., 1994) found that authoritarian parenting style had a positive relationship with school performance of Chinese adolescents or Asian American youth. A prominent example is Amy Chua's controversial book "Battle Hymn of the Tiger Mother," which noted that although she was strict and demanding, she spent "approximately ten times as much time per day engaged in academic activities with her children as Western parents," which is why following these "Chinese values" is more conducive to raising successful Chinese children. In other words, it's not that Taiwanese parents do not care about their children in this period, but it is hidden in their authority and discipline, which is quite subtle and may not be noticed by their children (Li, 1998). I would like to call the Taiwanese parenting style of this period a hybrid style of authoritarian and authoritative parenting styles as defined by Baumrind. However, regardless of how we define the way Taiwanese parents raise their children or evaluate the impact of authoritarian parenting style on their children, we can expect that the parent–child relationship and parenting trend in Taiwanese society have been gradually opened up with subsequent reforms in political and educational systems.

1986–2008 in Taiwan

Taiwan implemented educational reforms in 1986, and in 1987 it lifted the martial law which had been in effect for 38 years. With the lifting of martial law, a series of important political and educational system reforms were completed. These have brought unprecedented changes to Taiwanese society. Among them, democratic social movements were surging and civil rights becoming increasingly powerful. Taiwan has taken the step of democratic constitutional reform, moving from an authoritarian to a democratic and free country, laying the foundation for the subsequent development of equality and freedom. In terms of politics, in 1987, the establishment of new or opposing political parties, freedom of speech, and the establishment of private media were allowed; in 1991, the temporary regulations on counter-insurgency mobilization were abolished and full direct elections of Congress were implemented; in 1996, the direct election of the national president was implemented; in the 2000 presidential election, the Democratic Progressive Party (DPP) won and became the ruling party, while the KMT lost the election and became the opposition party overseeing the government. In terms of education, the Executive Yuan Education Reform Review Committee was formally established in 1994; in 1999, the Basic Education Law was promulgated, which stipulates that the people are the main body of education, the power of education was devolved from the central government to local governments, and school textbooks could be compiled by the private sectors to reduce the constraints of a single standard and improve the quality of textbooks through free market competition. Since 2000 Taiwanese society entered the post-modernization era, and social changes have focused on the in-depth transformation of social norms and values.

In this period, as we could see, in addition to a new emphasis on the individuality and uniqueness of students in teaching practices, there were a series of reforms in the national curriculum to advocate for autonomy and equality in Taiwan (Wu, 2016). For example, in 2001, the civic and life ethics courses were abolished, meaning that several traditional cultural norms were no longer propagated through the formal education system. Social transformation had an obvious impact in the form of equalizing various interpersonal relationships. Taiwan middle-class parents became more open to Western-style education and parenting conceptions, emphasizing love and two-way communication rather than authority and obedience to cultivate children's autonomy and individuality. They gained a new awareness of practices supporting a new form of parent–child relationship that did not rely so heavily on parental control or power. A study investigating the shifts in the concept of filial piety among Taiwanese individuals (Yeh, 1997) analyzed data from the Taiwan Social Change Survey—a nationwide survey. The findings revealed that Taiwanese people placed greater emphasis on and held stronger beliefs in RFP compared with AFP during this period.

During the period 1986–2008, middle-class parents in Taiwan especially liked to follow Western trends. Therefore, they endorsed reciprocal filial belief more than authoritarian filial belief. They spent more time paying attention to and learning how to raise their children than their parents. The main learning channels were through parenting-related books or attending parenting lectures to obtain professional information about parenting (Liou, 2001). The authoritative parenting style was the much-respected way among middle-class parents in Taiwan at this time when raising their children (Lin, 2008; Wei, 2002). Authoritative parents, like authoritarian parents, want to influence their children's behavior and choices. However, they do not achieve their goals through command and discipline, but through reasoning (Baumrind, 1968). Authoritative parents attempt to direct their children's activities in a rational, problem-oriented manner. Autonomous self-will and disciplined obedience are valued simultaneously. They share the rationale behind the policy with children and solicit children's objections when they refuse to comply. Therefore, this kind of parenting style controls the points of disagreement between parents and children but does not strictly require children's absolute obedience and allows children to put forward their own opinions. Although parents insist on their own opinions, they also admit that their children have personal interests and specific ways. Authoritative parents affirm their children's current qualities but also set standards for future behavior. They use reason, power, regime shaping, and reinforcement to achieve their goals rather than making decisions based on the individual child's desires.

The authoritative parenting style had become the prototype of appropriate parenting in Western societies at that time and was also highly supported by middle-class parents in Taiwan, but like the aforementioned authoritarian parenting style, there has been controversy over whether this parenting style has the same positive impact on Chinese children (Chao, 2001). In a notable study, the authoritative parenting style consistently demonstrated a positive correlation with the academic performance of European American students; however, this relationship was not evident among Asian American students (Dornbusch et al., 2016). Another investigation by Steinberg et al. (1994) revealed that authoritative parenting had positive impacts on the school performance of both European and Asian American adolescents. However, the influence was found to be comparatively less advantageous for Asian American youth than their European American counterparts. Conversely, authoritarian parenting was observed to be relatively more beneficial for Asian American youth. These ethnic variations in parenting effects may stem from differing conceptualizations of parenting approaches (Chao, 2000).

Besides, some Taiwanese parents would like their children to live a happy life without too much stress, so they would adopt a child-centered or more laissez-faire approach to raising their children and let children make their own choices (Chao, 2011). Taiwanese permissive parents attempt to behave in a non-punitive, acceptant, and affirmative manner toward their children's impulses, desires, and actions, but they also hope that their children's future life will be better than their own current life. Academic performance is perceived to a great extent as relating to personal future achievement and career development in Taiwan. As a result, parents usually regulate their children's efforts to do well academically, but they do not want to be too strict when the child fails to meet the demands (Wei, 2002). Therefore, I call this parenting style a hybrid style of authoritative and permissive parenting styles as defined by Baumrind. However, when the social environment changes too fast, making people full of uncertainty about the future world, it is natural for parents to feel anxious and uneasy about how to raise their children to adapt to the future world. And this is exactly the portrayal of Taiwanese society in the following period.

Taiwan since 2009

The global financial tsunami occurred in 2008, which severely impacted Taiwan's economy and society too. Taiwan's economic growth rate dropped to 0.73 percent that year, and even negative economic growth appeared in the following year, reaching –1.81 percent. This not only resulted in a decline in investment and the closure of many companies, but also aggravated the gap between the rich and the poor (expanded to 6.34 times) and the unemployment issue. During this period, Taiwan witnessed two more political parties taking turns in power again: the KMT assuming power in 2008, followed by the DPP taking the helm in 2016. Additionally, the Sunflower Student Movement, also known as the Occupy Congress incident, unfolded as a collaborative social movement initiated by university students and citizen groups in Taiwan from March 18 to April 10, 2014. This movement, led by protesting students, involved the occupation of the Legislative Yuan (i.e., the Legislature) and attempts to occupy the adjacent

Executive Yuan (i.e., the Cabinet in the United States) in Taipei City. The gravity of these political and social dynamics was further compounded by the global impact of the COVID-19 pandemic, spanning from late 2019 to early 2023. All these occurrences had a noticeable impact on the ideological perspectives of Taiwanese parents regarding parenting and child healthcare.

Since 2011 Taiwan's total fertility rate has been one of the lowest in the world. In a society with a declining birthrate, children become more valuable assets, especially for families with only one child, which calls on parents to invest more effort in raising their children. This is why the "intensive parenting style" is more popular in Taiwan at this time (Wu, 2016), especially for middle-class parents. Sharon Hays (1996) in her book, *The Cultural Contradictions of Motherhood*, postulated that "intensive mothering" is the ideology that now governs mothering within the United States, and serves as the ideal form of parenting that differentiates "good" and "bad" mothers. She advises mothers to expend a tremendous amount of time, energy, and money in raising their children, even those who lack the resources to enact this form of motherhood. In contemporary Taiwan, middle-class parents—particularly mothers, who bear the primary responsibility for child-rearing—adhere to a similar philosophy of intensive mothering. This approach is characterized by the following key aspects (Lan, 2019): firstly, mothers prioritize being child-centered, maintaining constant attention to their children, and considering an understanding of children's needs as paramount; Secondly, the mothering has evolved into a more labor-intensive endeavor, demanding both physical and emotional investments at a high level; Thirdly, the notion of "proper parenting" aligns with expert advice, emphasizing the importance of following guidance from professionals (Hung, 2015); Lastly, the financial costs associated with raising children are on the rise, with a notable increase in expenditures for various extracurricular activities. This type of parent–child relationship provides parents with significant emotional comfort and a profound sense of meaning. However, it also leads to a notable exhaustion among contemporary Taiwanese parents as they navigate the complexities of raising their children. This delicate balance can be aptly described as "all joy and no fun," as highlighted by Senior (2014).

In addition to the prevailing intensive parenting ideology inducing anxiety and unease among today's Taiwanese middle-class parents regarding their parenting strategies, society itself is rife with contradictions in various parenting-related perspectives, amplifying parental apprehension. These contradictions surface in the logical discourse surrounding intergenerational relationships, incongruities in the objectives of parenting appeals, and inconsistencies in parenting implementation (Lan, 2019). Firstly, the contradiction in the discourse logic of intergenerational relationships in contemporary Taiwan is as follows: On one hand, society emphasizes the democratic nature of intimate relationships, advocating for equality and independence in parent–child relationships. However, on the other hand, traditional Chinese filial piety concepts and hierarchical authority resurge during periods of social turmoil, placing the responsibility for the future achievement of children squarely on the shoulders of parents. Secondly, the contradiction in parenting appeals' objectives is as follows: While Taiwanese society persists in gauging the success of parenting using the yardstick of "instrumental rationality," considering parenting as a means to attain children's success in academics and the workplace, there is a growing emphasis on "value rationality" as well. The emphasis values the emotional intimacy between parents and children and the inherent joy of a child's growth as the purpose of parenting. Finally, the contradiction in parenting implementation is as follows: On one hand, parenting has become increasingly financially intensive, necessitating parents to invest significant time in the workplace to earn sufficient economic resources to cover parenting expenses. On the other hand, parenting also demands more time and labor intensity, expecting parents to allocate extended periods of companionship and emotional attention to their children.

As Taiwanese parents grapple with the complexities of these conflicting parenting cultures, they are left trying to find their paths and find a way to settle down. The kind of adaptation is to respond to the opportunities and constraints brought by the institutional structure and the external environment, and to try to master and alleviate the challenges brought by the contradictions. Among them, parents with more favorable economic conditions have the ability to actively assemble diverse educational resources for their children. During their children's formative years, these parents may opt to send them abroad for education or enroll them in domestically private schools. Despite the associated expenses, these institutions emphasize the cultivation of an elite habitus. The primary goal is to pave the way for their children's future global competitiveness. Parents with moderate economic means, adhering to Taiwan's 12-year compulsory education policy, guide their children through the educational system progressively. Additionally, they make endeavors to enroll their children in various private talent training courses and extracurricular classes, aiming for their children to surpass their peers, smoothly enter a top national university, and graduate to secure higher-paying job opportunities. Conversely, those in the lower economic strata, such as working-class parents, are preoccupied with earning a livelihood to cover family expenses. They lack the surplus mental energy or time to invest in their children. Consequently, these parents rely on their children to be self-reliant and strive for upward mobility; otherwise, their children's future prospects may be confined to the ongoing struggle for survival in the working class.

From a psychological perspective, the core elements of parenting are inevitably related to love and affection. However, when it comes to the expectations of investment and returns in parenting, parents will naturally tailor their efforts based on the resources and conditions available to them, as well as their expectations for the future living of their children. At this point, it becomes necessary to delve into a deep analysis of the family's socio-economic status and the educational resources that society can provide, involving both sociological and economic perspectives. In other words, stratification is a core issue in parenting research (Lareau, 2018). The substantial disparities in social class structures have significantly predetermined the potential parenting approaches of Taiwanese parents, not leaving much room for individual choices in the implementation of parenting ways. Economists (Doepke & Zilibotti, 2019) have also issued a cautionary note about the global trend emphasizing "competitiveness" in parenting, warning against the emergence of a phenomenon known as the "parenting gap trap." This phenomenon occurs when contemporary middle-class parents heavily invest in maintaining their socioeconomic status through higher education, resulting in the escalating cost of quality education and imposing a burden on parents in lower socioeconomic strata who struggle to keep up. Perhaps this prevailing state of social inequality is the fundamental source of parenting anxiety among contemporary Taiwanese parents. Here inevitably prompts the question of whether "parenting" is a costly commodity requiring financial purchase or if it should be regarded as a basic choice for every parent.

The Roles of Future Parents

Predicting the exact future of parenting in Taiwan is challenging, but we can anticipate some trends and potential changes based on current societal shifts. First, Digital Parenting: As technology continues to evolve, parents are likely facing new challenges in managing their children's screen time, online interactions, and exposure to digital content. Parents may need to stay informed about the latest technologies and social media platforms to guide their children effectively (Modecki et al., 2022). Second, Emphasis on Mental Health: There is a rising recognition of the significance of mental health, leading parents to prioritize the promotion of emotional well-being in their children. This is particularly evident through the influence of neurodevelopment (Bush et al., 2020) and the adoption of techniques like mindfulness and stress management (Khng, 2023), which may increasingly become integral components of parenting strategies. Third, Flexible

Education Models: The traditional education system may see changes, with an increasing emphasis on personalized and flexible learning options. Parents may need to explore various educational approaches, including online learning, homeschooling, and alternative education models (Li, 2023). Fourth, Environmental Consciousness: With the growing concern for the environment, parents may incorporate eco-friendly practices into their parenting, such as promoting sustainable habits and teaching children about environmental responsibility (Güven & Yılmaz, 2017). Fifth, Cultural Competence: In an increasingly globalized world, parents may focus on raising culturally competent children who appreciate diversity and possess intercultural skills. Exposure to different cultures and languages may be integrated into parenting practices (Coakley & Buehler, 2008). Sixth, Financial Literacy: Teaching children about financial literacy may become increasingly important as economic landscapes change. Parents may focus on instilling money management skills and a strong work ethic (Serido & Deenanath, 2016).

It's important to note that these trends are speculative, and the actual parenting landscape in the coming years in Taiwan will be influenced by various factors, including cultural shifts, technological advancements, and societal changes. Flexibility, adaptability, and open communication with children will likely remain key aspects of effective parenting in the future.

Conclusion

In conclusion, the ever-evolving world continually shapes Taiwanese society, impacting the beliefs and practices of parents in their crucial role as educators. Parenting, however, is not a value-neutral endeavor; rather, it mirrors societal values and standards, influencing the upbringing of children (LeVine, 2003). Historically, Taiwan's authoritarian era profoundly influenced parent–child relationships, centering discussions on children's learning around the concept of "authority." The contemporary shift emphasizes understanding children's needs, desires, and unique personalities, aligning with the Chinese slogan "teaching a child in accordance with his/her aptitude." Maintaining a positive relationship with the child becomes a prominent element within this shift. These suggestions collectively encourage parents to adapt their interactions accordingly and transcend rigid parenting ideologies. As societal changes accelerate, fostering uncertainty about the future, parents grapple with the challenge of preparing their children for an evolving world. This uncertainty contributes to parental anxiety, highlighting the absence of a definitive or universally successful parenting approach. Instead, it underscores the necessity for patience and the refinement of parenting strategies over time.

In the pursuit of ensuring their children's happiness and success, contemporary advice for Taiwanese parents emphasizes positive strategies. This involves actively praising desired behaviors and engaging in enjoyable activities with children, fostering a relationship grounded in positivity and equality. In contrast, negative strategies, particularly concerning young children, caution against excessive instructions and criticism, acknowledging the challenges in processing criticism during early development. Essentially, the advocated positive strategies, centered on praise and attentiveness, align with the understanding that parenting style reflects the type of relationships parents cultivate with their children. Recognizing parenting style as a global construct reflecting the overall emotional tone of the parent–child relationship, it becomes crucial to avoid excessive criticism and directives, emphasizing the paramount importance of cultivating a healthy and positive parent–child relationship.

References

Arendell, T. (1997). A social constructionist approach to parenting. In T. Arendell (Ed.). Contemporary parenting: Challenges and issues (pp. 1–44). Thousand Oaks, CA: Sage Publications.

Baumrind, D. (1968). Authoritarian vs. authoritative parental control. *Adolescence, 3*(11), 255–272.

Bedford, O. & Yeh, K.-H. (2019). The history and the future of the psychology of filial piety: Chinese norms to contextualized personality construct. *Frontiers in Psychology, 10*, 100. https://doi.org/10.3389/fpsyg.2019.00100.

Blair, S. L. & Qian, Z. (1998). Family and Asian students' educational performance. *Journal of Family Issues, 19*, 355–374. https://doi.org/10.1177/019251398019004001.

Bush, N. R., Wakschlag, L. S., LeWinn, K. Z., Hertz-Picciotto, I., Nozadi, S. S., Pieper, S.,... & Posner, J. (2020). Family environment, neurodevelopmental risk, and the environmental influences on child health outcomes (ECHO) initiative: looking back and moving forward. *Frontiers in psychiatry, 11*, 547. https://doi.org/10.3389/fpsyt.2020.00547.

Chao, H.-L. (2011). The "New Good Father" revealed in the press and the politics of fatherhood in Taiwan. *Journal of General Education, 16*, 73–106. https://doi.org/10.7107/JGED.201106.0073.

Chao, R. K. (1994). Beyond parental control and authoritarian parenting style: Understanding Chinese parenting through the cultural notion of training. *Child development, 65*(4), 1111–1119. https://doi.org/10.1111/j.1467-8624.1994.tb00806.x.

Chao, R. K. (1996). Chinese and European American mothers' beliefs about the role of parenting in children's school success. *Journal of cross-cultural psychology, 27*(4), 403–423. https://doi.org/10.1177/0022022196274002.

Chao, R. K. (2000). The parenting of immigrant Chinese and European American mothers: Relations between parenting styles, socialization goals, and parental practices. *Journal of Applied Developmental Psychology, 21*(2), 233–248. https://doi.org/10.1016/S0193-3973(99)00037-4.

Chao, R. K. (2001). Extending research on the consequences of parenting style for Chinese Americans and European Americans. *Child development, 72*(6), 1832–1843. https://doi.org/10.1111/1467-8624.00381.

Chen, C.-Y. (2006). The nation-building in Taiwan primary school textbooks after World War II (1968–1989). Unpublished master thesis. National Hsinchu University of Education, Hsinchu, Taiwan.

Chen, W.-W., Wu, C.-W., & Yeh, K.-H. (2016). How parenting and filial piety influence happiness, parent–child relationships, and quality of family life in Taiwanese adult children. *Journal of Family Studies, 22*(1), 80–96. https://doi.org/10.1080/13229400.2015.1027154.

Chu, R.-L. (1986). Parental parenting styles as perceived by adolescents. In Hei-Yuan Chiu & Ying-Hwa Chang (Eds), *Social and cultural change in Taiwan, volume 2* (pp. 617–654). Taipei: Institute of Ethnology, Academia Sinica.

Coakley, T. M. & Buehler, C. (2008). Toward a theory of cultural competence in transcultural parenting: The role of cultural receptivity. *Journal of Public Child Welfare, 2*(4), 401–425. https://doi.org/10.1080/15548730802523174.

Doepke, M. & Zilibotti, F. (2019). *Love, money, and parenting: How economics explains the way we raise our kids*. Princeton University Press.

Dornbusch, S. M., Ritter, P. L., Leiderman, P. H., Roberts, D. F., & Fraleigh, M. J. (2016). The relation of parenting style to adolescent school performance. In *Cognitive and Moral Development, Academic Achievement in Adolescence* (pp. 276–289). Routledge.

Fredrickson, B. L. (2016). Love: Positivity resonance as a fresh, evidence-based perspective on an age-old topic. In L. F. Barrett & J. M. Haviland (Eds), *Handbook of emotions*, 4th ed. (pp. 847–858). New York: Guilford Press.

Fung, H. (1999). Becoming a moral child: The socialization of shame among young Chinese children. *Ethos, 27*(2), 180–209.

Güven, S. & Yılmaz, N. (2017). Role and importance of family at preschool children environmental education. *European Journal of Sustainable Development, 6*(4), 105–114. https://doi.org/10.14207/ejsd.2017.v6n4p105.

Hays, S. (1996). *The cultural contradictions of motherhood.* Yale University Press.

Ho, D. Y. F. (1981). Traditional patterns of socialization in Chinese society. *Acta Psychologica Taiwanica, 23,* 81–95.

Ho, D. Y. F. (1994). Filial piety, authoritarian moralism, and cognitive conservatism in Chinese societies. *Genetic, Social and General Psychology Monographs, 120,* 349–365.

Ho, D. Y. F. (1996). Filial piety and its psychological consequences. In M. H. Bond (Ed.), *The handbook of Chinese psychology.* New York: Oxford University Press.

Huang, K. J. & Chen, J. H. (2024). Filial piety and the development of independence and interdependence during emerging adulthood: A longitudinal study of Taiwanese adolescents. *Journal of Youth and Adolescence, 53,* 1232–1243. https://doi.org/10.1007/s10964-023-01929-w.

Huang, L.-L. & Chu, R.-L. (2012). Is it the wind shearing or the tide going in and out? Searching for core values and its changing trend in Taiwan. *The Journal of Kaohsiung Behavior Sciences, 3,* 60–90.

Huang, S.-J. & Yeh, K.-H. (2013). The effect of perceived parenting styles on adolescents' dual filial belief: A mediational analysis. *Indigenous Psychological Research in Chinese Societies, 39*, 119–164.

Hung, H.-F. (2015). The situation and the challenges of new-generation mothers in Taiwan: The cultural contradiction of employed mothers as caregiver and worker. *Taiwanese Journal of Social Welfare, 13*(1), 87–149. https://doi.org/10.6265/TJSW.2015.13(1)3.

Hsiao, H.-H. (1995). The social consciousness and soc al participation of the X-generation. *Journal of Labors' Friends, 535*, 6–9.

Khng, K. H. (2023). Deep breathing and mindfulness: Simple techniques to promote students' self-regulation and well-being from the inside out. In Positive psychology and positive education in Asia: Understanding and fostering well-being in schools (pp. 311–325). Singapore: Springer Nature Singapore.

Lan, P.-C. (2014). Compressed modernity and global entanglement: The contested transformation of parenting discourses in postwar Taiwan. *Current Sociology, 62*(4), 531–549. https://doi.org/10.1177/0011392114524509.

Lan, P.-C. (2019). *Struggling to raise children: Globalization, parental anxieties and unequal childhoods*. Taipei: Spring-Hill Publishing.

Lareau, A. (2018). *Unequal childhoods: Class, race, and family life*. In Inequality in the 21st Century (pp. 444–451). Routledge.

Lee, Y. J., Parish, W. L., & Willis, R. J. (1994). Sons, daughters, and intergenerational support in Taiwan. *American Journal of Sociology, 99*(4), 1010–1041. https://doi.org/10.1086/230370.

Leung, K., Lau, S., & Lam, W. L. (1998). Parenting styles and achievement: A cross-cultural study. *Merrill-Palmer Quarterly, 44*, 157–172. www.jstor.org/stable/23093664.

LeVine, R. A. (2003). *Childhood socialization: Comparative studies of parenting, learning, and educational change*. Hong Kong: University of Hong Kong.

Li, M. (2023). Home Education as an Effective Educational Method: A Study. *Research and Advances in Education, 2*(5), 27–34. www.paradigmpress.org/rae/article/view/610.

Li, M.-C. (1998). The connotation and function of Chinese parent–child relationship: Taking college students as an example. *Indigenous Psychological Research in Chinese Societies, 9*, 3–52.

Lin, H.-Y. (2008). Latent class analyses of maternal beliefs, childrearing goals, and parenting practices: Associations with children's academic performance. *Research in Applied Psychology, 37*, 181–213. www.airitilibrary.com/Article/Detail?DocID=15609251-200803-x-37-181-213-a.

Lin, I.-F., Goldman, N., Weinstein, M., Lin, Y.-H., Gorrindo, T., & Seeman, T. (2003). Gender differences in adult children's support of their parents in Taiwan. *Journal of Marriage and Family, 65*(1), 184–200.

Lin, W.-Y. (2003). The influence of parents' theories of human nature on parenting belief: The case of theories of intelligence. *Indigenous Psychological Research in Chinese Societies, 20*, 253–293. https://doi.org/10.6254/2003.20.253.

Liou, T.-H. (2001). The parenting belief of modern mothers of young children - taking those who with college educational degrees as an example. *Journal of National Hsin-Chu Teachers College, 14*, 355–405.

Major, B. C., Le Nguyen, K. D., Lundberg, K. B., & Fredrickson, B. L. (2018). Well-being correlates of perceived positivity resonance: Evidence from trait and episode-level assessments. *Personality and Social Psychology Bulletin, 44*(12), 1631–1647. https://doi.org/10.1177/0146167218771324.

Mead, M. (1978). *Culture and commitment: The new relationships between the generations in the 1970s*. New York: Columbia University Press.

Modecki, K. L., Goldberg, R. E., Wisniewski, P., & Orben, A. (2022). What is digital parenting? A systematic review of past measurement and blueprint for the future. *Perspectives on Psychological Science, 17*(6), 1673–1691. https://doi.org/10.1177/17456916211072458.

Serido, J. & Deenanath, V. (2016). Financial parenting: Promoting financial self-reliance of young consumers. In J. Xiao (Ed.), *Handbook of consumer finance research* (pp. 291300). Cham: Springer. https://doi.org/10.1007/978-3-319-28887-1_24.

Senior, J. (2014). *All joy and no fun: The paradox of modern parenthood*. New York: Harper Collins.

Shek, D. T. & Chan, L. K. (1999). Hong Kong Chinese parents' perceptions of the ideal child. *The Journal of psychology, 133*(3), 291–302. https://doi.org/10.1080/00223989909599742

Steinberg, L., Lamborn, S. D., Darling, N., Mounts, N. S., & Dornbusch, S. M. (1994). Over-time changes in adjustment and competence among adolescents from authoritative, authoritarian, indulgent, and neglectful families. *Child Development, 65*, 754–770. https://doi.org/10.1111/j.1467-8624.1994.tb00781.x.

Tsao, W.-C. & Yeh, K.-H. (2019). Indigenous implications and global applications of the Dual Filial Piety Model: A psychological re-conceptualization of 'Xiao'. In: K. H. Yeh (Ed.), Asian indigenous psychologies in the global context (pp. 195–219). Palgrave Studies in Indigenous Psychology. Palgrave Macmillan, Cham. https://doi.org/10.1007/978-3-319-96232-0_9.

Wei, S.-T. (2002). Assessing parenting styles in Chinese culture. *Journal of Ilan Institute of Technology, 9*, 341–369. https://doi:10.6179/nit.lam.2002.09.32.

Wu, C.-W. & Yeh, K.-H. (2021). Self-sacrifice is not the only way to practice filial piety for Chinese adolescents in conflict with their parents. *Frontiers in Psychology, 12*, 661335. https://doi.org/10.3389/fpsyg.2021.661335.

Wu, D. Y. (1981). Child abuse in Taiwan. In J. E. Korbin (Ed.), *Child abuse and neglect: Cross-cultural perspectives* (pp. 139–165). Berkeley, CA: University of California Press.

Wu, M.-Y. (2016). Parenting dilemma: Sociological analysis of parenting teenagers in Taiwan. Taipei: Wu-nan Publications Corporation.

Yang, K.-S. (1985). New filial piety in modern Chinese societies. *Renaissance of Chinese Culture Monthly, 19*(1), 51–67.

Yeh, K.-H. (1997). Changes in the Taiwanese people's concept of filial piety. In L.-Y. Chang, Y.-H. Lu, & F.-C. Wang (Eds), *Taiwanese Society in 1990s* (pp. 171–214). Taipei: The Preparatory Office of the Institute of Sociology, Academia Sinica.

Yeh, K.-H. (2003). The beneficial and harmful effects of filial piety: An integrative analysis. In K.-S. Yang, K.-K. Hwang, P. B. Pederson, & I. Daibo (Eds), *Progress in Asian social psychology: Conceptual and empirical contributions* (pp. 67–82). Westport, CT: Praeger.

Yeh, K.-H. & Bedford, O. (2003). A test of the dual filial piety model. *Asian Journal of Social Psychology, 6*, 215–228. https://doi.org/10.1046/j.1467-839X.2003.00122.x.
Yeh, K.-H. & Cheng, S.-P. (2005). Parenting, children's empathy and compliance, and filial types. Paper presented at the 113th Annual Convention of the American Psychological Association (APA), Washington, DC, USA.
Yeh, K.-H., Yi, C.-C., Tsao, W.-C., & Wan, P.-S. (2013). Filial piety in contemporary Chinese societies: A comparative study of Taiwan, Hong Kong and China. *International Sociology, 28*(3), 277–296. https://doi.org/10.1177/0268580913484345.
Yeh, M.-H. & Yang, K.-S. (1997). Chinese familism: Conceptual analysis and empirical assessment. *Bulletin of the Institute of Ethnology, Academia Sinica, 83*, 169–225.
Zhou, J., Prinzing, M. M., Le Nguyen, K. D., West, T. N., & Fredrickson, B. L. (2022). The goods in everyday love: Positivity resonance builds prosociality. *Emotion, 22*(1), 30–45. https://doi.org/10.1037/emo0001035.

14

CHANGES AND PRESERVATION OF TRADITION IN ASIAN PARENTING

Comparisons of Family Process among South Korean, Korean American, and Korean Chinese Families

Yoonsun Choi, Michael Park, Yishan Shen, and Kihyun Kim

Culture fundamentally shapes the family process, including childrearing goals and values, parenting behaviors, and parent–child relationships, which, in turn, influence child development (Harkness & Super, 2002). During the last century, global migrations have occurred in large volumes, along with rapid industrialization and Westernization, disproportionately affecting non-Western populations. Koreans are one of the examples, with significant sizes of diasporic communities both near (e.g., China and Japan) and far (e.g., the United States and Brazil) from the Korean Peninsula. Cultural characteristics of Korean parenting might have been inevitably complicated, particularly among migrants who settled in various sociopolitical contexts as racial/ethnic and cultural minorities. However, it remains unclear how the families have modified or preserved their culture while juggling minority status and reinventing the family process.

Several critical questions emerge. For example, does traditional Korean parenting change more when Koreans migrate to Western societies like the U.S., compared with those who settle in other Asian countries? Despite cultural proximity and similar phenotypes, Korean Chinese, who settled in Manchuria in the early 1900s, remain a distinct ethnic minority group in China where Han Chinese is the dominant group. Reasons and pathways for migrations significantly vary, resulting in distinctive demographics of migrants in each context, e.g., Korean Americans, relatively newer immigrants post the Immigration Act of 1965, are predominantly urban middle class (Min, 2010). Korean American family process may primarily be a product of a middle-class background. Socioeconomic class plays a significant role in shaping parenting, likely above and beyond the impact of

DOI: 10.4324/9781003383949-14

heritage culture (Zhang et al., 2023). Conversely, have Koreans maintained their traditional parenting? Is preservation of the tradition good for child development? Empirical data to document how heritage culture perseveres or changes in family processes in variant contexts remains seriously limited, while cultural traits of parenting are reduced to stereotypes and misperceptions (e.g., "tiger parenting"). Filling this gap, this study compares the patterns of Korean parenting reported by three groups of Korean adolescents, i.e., in Seoul, South Korea, the Midwest in the U.S., and Yanbian, China, and how they are associated with youth adjustments.

Asian Parenting and Youth Adjustments

Bestsellers of parenting [e.g., *Battle Hymn of the Tiger Mother* (Chua, 2011); *Bringing Up Bébé* (Druckerman, 2014)] capitalize on parent anxiety to seek parenting practices that are effective in fostering desired characters in children. In this quest for "good" parenting, Asian parenting has been a subject of attention in Western literature as a reason for Asian American children's stronger academic performance and positive adjustments. However, adjustments among Asian Americans are complex. Although young Asian Americans seemingly conform to the "model minority" myth because they, as an aggregate, perform better academically and have fewer externalizing problems (e.g., substance use, violence), they have more serious internalizing problems (e.g., depression, suicidality) than youth in other racial/ethnic groups (Choi et al., 2022). Korean American youth squarely fit this idiosyncratic pattern of adjustments, a co-existence of favorable external behaviors and serious mental health struggles, coined as the Asian American Paradox (Choi et al., 2020). Interestingly, South Korean youth show a similar pattern of adjustment, i.e., outstanding academic performance in international assessments (e.g., PISA, TIMSS: OECD, 2023) but alarmingly poor mental health with suicide as the leading cause of death among adolescents (Ryou et al., 2019). Although there is a dearth of data on Korean Chinese, emerging evidence suggests that Korean Chinese similarly show a paradoxical pattern, i.e., the "model minority" who perform well at school, but with a serious level of mental distress (Zhang et al., 2023). Before we would even ask whether a certain "cultural" parenting style, e.g., Korean or Asian parenting, can produce math whiz and music protégé as the stereotype dictates or blame such parenting for mental distress and suicidality, it is imperative to consider what Korean parenting is and how it may be practiced differently in various sociocultural settings.

The etiology of the mixed adjustments is likely to vary across different contexts. For example, racial discrimination is a notable stressor among Korean Americans, which is unlikely applicable to South Koreans who are the dominant group. Meanwhile, for Korean Chinese youth, perceived discrimination perpetrated by co-ethnic individuals in South Korea—their ancestral homeland—can be even more salient and harmful than ethnic discrimination from Han Chinese (Zhao et al., 2024). Additionally, being left behind by parents who have migrated for jobs (often to South Korea) can be a unique stressor for Korean Chinese youth (Cui et al., 2014). Academic pressure in South Korea tends to be relentless, unimaginable in the U.S., and often blamed for the disturbing rate of mental distress (Soenens et al., 2012). A more refined understanding of family processes among Korean families across various contexts can help identify traits of Korean parenting that are beneficial or harmful and address the pernicious combination of externalized and internalized behaviors. Likewise, comparative analyses across countries would elucidate how culture, race/ethnicity, and class intersect to shape parenting in different geopolitical contexts and inform the development of parenting interventions appropriate to each context.

Asian vs. Western Parenting

Traditional Asian families are culturally collectivistic, emphasizing interdependence, conformity, emotional self-control, and humility (Kurasaki et al., 2002). Asian cultural values produce deeply ingrained family values, such as a strong sense of family obligation and obedience to parents (Chao & Tseng, 2002). In stark contrast, desired traits in Western cultures are independence, individualism, assertiveness, and confidence (Chao, 1995). Regarded as the most ideal, *authoritative* parenting style that establishes firm rules, employs inductive reasoning and expressive warmth, and allows autonomy is thought to build close parent–child relations and yield positive youth outcomes. When assessed by conventional Western measures, Asian parenting is often depicted as controlling, strict, and emotionally distant (i.e., *authoritarian*) (Kagitçibasi, 2007) and its associations with child adjustments are inconsistent and can even be confusing (e.g., corporal punishment may not be significantly and negatively associated with parent–child conflict (Deater-Deckard et al., 2005)).

In recent decades, our understanding of Asian parenting has been enhanced and we know that assessing Asian parenting through the Western perspective can produce misleading knowledge. For example, a more nuanced conceptualization sees Asian parental control as *order-keeping* rather than *dominating* (Jose et al., 2000; Kagitçibasi, 1996). Dominating control is coercive, punitive, and emotionally distant. Order-keeping control is more directive and restrictive than authoritative parenting but is practiced with reasoning, praise, and warmth. Parental restrictions are often motivated by the strong emphasis on education and are accompanied by persistent teaching of education's value (Louie, 2004). Corporal punishment also appears different from harsh parenting (Kim & Hong, 2007). Thus, more restrictive Asian parenting may not damage parent–child relations and in fact, prevent externalizing problems by reducing opportunities for risks.

Asian parents may also express warmth differently from Western parents. A traditional Asian parenting virtue is sternness, with fewer overt expressions of love (Kim, 2006), thus warmth, identified as *qin* (親), is often expressed nonverbally and indirectly and through instrumental support, parental devotion and sacrifice, and support for education (Wu & Chao, 2011). The same is found among Korean Americans (Choi et al., 2013). Similarly, while existing Western theories operationalize a child's bonding to parents as sharing feelings and thoughts with parents, and feeling very close to them (Choi et al., 2005), in Asian families, there may be other critical indicators of close parent–child relations, such as a sense of obligation to family or to care for aging parents (Fuligni et al., 2002) and, like parent's indirect expression of warmth to a child, youth may also express their bonding to parents more indirectly (Choi & Kim, 2010).

Chinese *guan* (管) parenting (Chao, 1995) is a prime example of Asian parenting and practiced among Chinese American families. *Guan* ("to govern and love") practices directive control and close monitoring of child behaviors while building close parent–child relationships. Korean family process *ga-jung-kyo-yuk* (가정교육) (Choi et al., 2013) is another example. Korean parents, along with other East Asian parents who are influenced by Confucian teachings, may exert strict discipline and training so that their children can learn to control personal desires, conform to authority, and behave well in society. The literal translation of *ga-jung-kyo-yuk* is "home education" and is best translated into the Western concept of family socialization or parenting. Its core values include family hierarchy, demonstration of respect for the elderly via appropriate etiquette, and family obligations. *Ga-jung-kyo-yuk* also governs childrearing practices (e.g., strict parenting styles) and, as the word *kyo-yuk* (i.e., education) connotes, emphasizes teaching in the family. Empirical data corroborates that both *guan* and *ga-jung-kyo-yuk* are neither authoritative nor authoritarian but are a distinct combination of authoritarian and authoritative parenting styles.

Koreans in South Korea, China, and the United States

Korea is a traditionally collectivistic, agrarian society profoundly influenced by Confucianism, Taoism, Mahayana Buddhism, and shamanism, and post the Korean War (1950–53), South Korea underwent massive industrialization and urbanization. Although ethnic/racial diversity is on the rise with a growing number of migrant workers and international marriages (predominantly East and Southeast Asian women who immigrated to marry South Korean men), it remains largely homogenous with the national pride in homogeneity of the people. China also is a traditionally collectivistic, agrarian society with a historical influence of Confucianism and has experienced rapid economic development and social changes since the 1980s.

Korean Chinese have settled in China more than three generations ago. Major migrations of Koreans to China started in the early 1900s through the last years of declining *Chosun*, the last dynasty of Korea, and the Japanese occupation between 1910 and 1945 (Choi, 2001). Reasons for migrations varied—to flee from the Imperial Japanese atrocity, to organize efforts for independence, and to seek economic opportunities. With the division of Korea into South and North and the subsequent Korean War, Korean Chinese did not have contact with South Korea until the late 1990s when they started migrating to South Korea for job opportunities. In 2019, more than 1.8 million Korean Chinese were in China, largely in the Northeast regions. Yanbian Korean autonomous prefecture of Jilin province has the largest concentration of Korean Chinese, who make up nearly 36 percent of the local population (Yanbian Bureau of Statistics, 2020). The most recent Chinese census (National Bureau of Statistics of China, 2020) show that 11.9 percent of Korean Chinese had a bachelor's or higher degree, higher than the national average (7.7 percent). Although Korean Chinese are phenotypically indistinguishable from the majority group Han Chinese and are considered the "model minority" because of their higher education level and contributions to the economic development of Northeast China (Choi, 2001), they continue to face discrimination (e.g., difficulty in employment) because of their Korean heritage (Lee et al., 2007).

Korean Americans, the fifth-largest Asian American subgroup, are a visible (i.e., non-White) ethnic/racial minority. In 2019, more than 1.9 million Korean Americans were living in the U.S., concentrated in metropolitan areas such as Los Angeles, New York, Washington, D.C., and Chicago (Budiman, 2021). They are mostly from educated, urban, and middle-class families. In 2019, 57 percent of Korean Americans above age 25 had a bachelor's or higher degree, above the national average (33 percent; Budiman, 2021). Although they, like many other groups of Asian Americans, are referred to as the "model minority," they are subject to racial discrimination (Park, Choi, Yasui, et al., 2021) and are often ostracized as "perpetual foreigners," struggling to be fully accepted in American society (Park, Choi, Yoo, et al., 2021).

Acculturation and Enculturation

Culture constantly evolves, and the cultural characteristics of family process are not static. People of non-Western nations have been swiftly Westernized during the last few decades and the effects have permeated the family process. For example, modern-day Asian families place great importance on independence and autonomy—virtues valued in modern and industrialized society. Education continues to be critical, not only because it has been traditionally valued, but also because it is in high demand in the industrialized economy. Contemporary parenting scholars in Korea, for instance, encourage Korean parents to practice more "democratic" parenting, such as giving praise and granting autonomy, similar to Western authoritative parenting.

Im/migrant families also partially or fully alter the family process in response to the social and cultural expectations of mainstream culture (Booth et al., 1997). For example, Asian immigrant parents in the U.S. largely preserve their traditional core parenting values (Kibria, 2002; Louie, 2004). In resistance to assimilative pressure, im/migrants may adhere to their culture even more than their counterparts do in their country of origin (Rosenthal & Feldman, 1992). Nonetheless, acculturative pressures are inevitable and they are modifying parenting, creating a cultural hybrid of Asian American parenting that is different from Asian or Western parenting (Choi et al., 2017). The gist of integration policies in China is to grant respective ethnic groups to keep their language and cultural traditions. Ethnic groups have mainly resided in autonomous districts until recently. The geographical isolation has enabled the preservation of ethnic culture but also resulted in limited integration of ethnic groups. Despite very different goals of the two countries, Koreans as a minority in both the U.S. and China have voluntarily or involuntarily preserved their distinct heritage culture.

A minority status in a society may have unique implications for parenting, beyond the impacts of culture (Garcia Coll & Pachter, 2002). Minority families face specific stressors from their marginalized position (e.g., discrimination), which are key to understanding minority youth development and parenting (Garcia Coll et al., 1996). For example, ethnic/racial minority parents may use their cultural model (e.g., emphasis on education) as an adaptation strategy for coping with the potential barriers associated with their minority status (Xie & Goyette, 1997). Indeed, Korean ethnic minority parents in China and the U.S. reported higher levels of academic socialization than Korean parents in South Korea (Zhang et al., 2023). Asian American parents intentionally work to retain their heritage culture and strengthen child's sense of ethnic/racial pride to prepare their children to navigate racialized society (Juang et al., 2018). Thus, minority status may facilitate the preservation of traditional culture in the family.

Current Study

This study compared family processes across Korean youth living in South Korea, China, and the U.S. who share the same heritage culture but live in distinct cultural, socioeconomic, and political contexts. We organized the family process as (1) traditional family values (e.g., parental emphasis on traditional manners and etiquettes that symbolize age veneration and relational hierarchy, and youth endorsement of core values such as respect for adults, and harmony and sacrifice for the greater good at the expense of individual desires); (2) traditional parenting behaviors (e.g., parental behaviors that promote ideal cultural values, commitment to education, gendered norms, pressure to succeed, implicit affection, academic-oriented parental control, and *qin*); (3) Western parenting behaviors (e.g., granting autonomy, authoritarian and authoritative parenting styles, parental acceptance, rejection, rules and regulations, and monitoring behavior); and (4) parent–child relations (e.g., intergenerational cultural conflict, parent–child communication, bonding, and conflict). We examined the associations among these variables and with youth adjustments including mental health (e.g., depressive symptoms and suicidality), academic performance (e.g., GPA), and antisocial behaviors. Comparisons of means/proportions and bivariate correlations were used to document how family processes, especially its traditional traits, are similar across three contexts and related to youth outcomes. Significant differences across the groups would then reflect the intersection of culture, acculturation and enculturation, racial/ethnic minority vs. majority status, and class and their collective influence on the family process among Korean families in three different countries.

Comparative Data

Survey of Korean Youth in Three Countries

Data were from three interrelated studies of Korean youth in South Korea, China, and the U.S. In 2014, a total of 408 Korean American youth (M_{age}=14.76 [SD=1.91]; 47.3 percent female) in the greater Chicago area were surveyed, which was the first wave of the Midwest Longitudinal Study of Asian American Families (MLSAAF) that follows Filipino American and Korean American families. In 2017, a total of 524 Korean youth (M_{age}=14.98 [SD=1.45]; 50.1 percent female) from socioeconomically diverse families in Seoul were surveyed. In 2019, a total of 267 Korean Chinese youth (M_{age}=15.24 [SD=1.66]; 58.9 percent female) were recruited from the Yanbian Korean Autonomous Prefecture of China.

Of the participating families, 61 percent Korean American parents, and 42 percent of the Korean Chinese mothers had a college or associate degree. This information was not collected in the South Korean survey, but the sampling strategy was intentional to sample family socioeconomic status (SES) evenly by recruiting youth from schools in high, middle, and low-income neighborhoods. Nevertheless, 90 percent of the youth sample in South Korea, as well as 94 percent in China, and 81 percent in the U.S., self-rated their families as middle or higher class. Of the participating students, 16 percent in South Korea and 26 percent in the U.S. were provided with free lunches at school. Korean youth in China and the U.S. reported speaking more Korean than the society's dominant language at home.

Korean American youth were recruited from the greater Chicago area via multiple sources, including school rosters, phonebooks, and ethnic community organizations. Parental consent and adolescent assent were obtained. The survey was available both in English and Korean languages and 85 percent used the English version. South Korean youth were recruited from middle and high schools in the *Eunpyeong-Gu* School District, Seoul, including three schools in high-income (31 percent), four in middle-income (42 percent), and two in low-income (27 percent) neighborhoods. Passive parental consent and adolescent assent were obtained. Youth filled out a paper-pencil survey. Korean Chinese youth were recruited from grades 7 and 8 in one dual-language middle school and grades 10 and 11 in one dual-language high school in Yanbian, China. Passive parental consent and adolescent assent were obtained. Participating youth completed a paper-pencil questionnaire in Korean. Approvals were obtained from the Institutional Review Board of the respective universities of the Investigators.

Measures

Measures of *ga-jung-kyo-yuk* were first developed by the Korean American Families Project and expanded in the MLSAAF. They were included in surveys in South Korea and China. Details of how the measures were developed and tested for psychometric properties are available elsewhere (e.g., Choi et al., 2017). Unless noted, response options were a five-point Likert scale (e.g., 1 = *not at all* to 5 = *very well*), and scores were averaged across the items of a scale.

Traditional Family Values: *Traditional Manners and Etiquette* (a four-item scale) assesses how much parents emphasize practicing a set of traditional manners and etiquettes that symbolize respect for elders, e.g., to greet adults by bowing and saying appropriate greeting words (e.g., "*an-nyung-ha-se-yo*"). *Respect for Adults* (three-item) assesses youth endorsement of the importance of obedience to and respect for adults. *Harmony and Sacrifice* (three-item) measures youth endorsement of needing to make sacrifices for the family or others.

Traditional Parenting Behaviors: *Parental Behaviors Promoting Ideal Cultural Traits* (eight-item) assesses the level of parent efforts to reinforce traits idealized in Asian culture, such as humility, suppression of negative emotions, and compliance, e.g., "My parents discourage me from confronting adults." *Commitment to Child's Education* (two-item) (Wu & Chao, 2011) measures parental support for a child's education, e.g., "My parents do everything for my education and make any sacrifice." *Gendered Norms* (seven-item) asks gendered expectations, e.g., "My parents think that girls should not date while in high school." *Pressure to Succeed* (ten-item) assesses parental pressure to excel, e.g., "My mother pressures me to go to a top college." *Parental Implicit Affection* (two-item) measures the indirect expression of parental love, i.e., my mom "will put my needs before her own needs." *Academically Orientated Parental Control* (seven-item) (Chao & Wu, 2001) assesses parental control specific to a child's schoolwork such as limiting social activities. *Qin* (nine-item) (Wu & Chao, 2011) measures the indirect expression of parent–child closeness, e.g., "My parents understand my difficulties even though they don't say anything."

Western Parenting Behaviors: The selected measures were *Granting Autonomy* (Grolnick et al., 1991; Silk et al., 2003) (eight-item, e.g., "Whenever possible, my mom allows me to choose my own directions in life."), *Authoritarian Parenting Style* (four-item, e.g., "My mom does not allow me to question any decision she makes.") *Authoritative Parenting Style* (two-item, e.g., "My mom consistently gives me direction and guidance in rational and objective ways." (Buri, 1991), *Parental Acceptance* (nine-item) and *Rejection* (15-item) from PARQ, *Parental Rules and Restrictions* (response options were "Yes" and "No"), and a single-item *Parental Monitoring* (Eddy et al., 2000), e.g., parental knowledge of a child's whereabouts when not home.

Parent–child Relationship: *Intergenerational Cultural Conflict* (ICC) used the Asian American Family Conflicts Scale (nine-item) (Lee et al., 2000) to measure generational conflict, e.g., "Your parents want you to sacrifice personal interests for the sake of the family, but you feel this is unfair." *Parent–child Communications* (Eddy et al., 2000) used four items (e.g., "I talk with my parents about what is going on in my life."), *Parent–child Bonding five-items* (e.g., "How close do you feel to your mom?") from Add Health, and *Parent–child Conflict* four-item from Prinz (1977) about parents and children getting angry at each other.

Youth Adjustments: *Depressive Symptoms* used the 14 items from the Children's Depression Inventory (Angold et al., 1995) and the Seattle Personality Questionnaire for Children (Kusche et al., 1988). *Suicidal Ideation* was measured by having suicidal thoughts in the months prior to the survey ("Yes" or "No"). GPA was estimated on the core subjects in each country (Zhang et al., 2023). Finally, nineteen items of antisocial behaviors, originally from DSM-V but considered antisocial in all countries, were selected (such as fighting and stealing).

Results

Rate Differences

Unadjusted means and standard deviations for continuous variables and proportions for dichotomous variables are summarized by each group in Table 14.1. Overall, traditional family values were statistically higher among immigrant and racial/ethnic minority groups (i.e., Korean Chinese [KC] and Korean Americans [KA]). Youth endorsement of traditional values (e.g., *Respect* and *Harmony*) was highest among KA. Similarly, traditional parenting behaviors were also higher among KC and KA, and particularly, academic-related constructs (including *Education*, *Pressure,* and *Academic Control*), *Ideal Traits,* and *Qin* were highest among KA, with *Pressure* and *Qin* equally high in KC. Notably, *Gendered* was highest among KC. When assessed by the Western parenting behavior measures, except for *Authoritative* for which KC reported the highest, KA reported the highest levels in *Autonomy*, *Authoritarian*, *Acceptance*, *Rules*, and *Monitoring*. *Acceptance* was lowest among SK, whereas *Rejection* was lowest among KA. *Rules* was high among KC. Parent–child relations were somewhat mixed. Rather counterintuitively, *ICC* was higher among SK and KC than KA, but *Communication* was highest among SK. *Bonding* was higher among KA than the other two groups. Interestingly, *Conflict* was not significantly different across the three groups. Lastly, mental health outcomes were significantly worse among KC, especially *Suicidal* was nearly two to three times higher than the other two groups (i.e., 26.55 percent vs. 14.29 percent SK or 9.48 percent KA). In terms of *GPA* and *Antisocial*, SK fared worst, whereas KA reported the best adjustment.

Bivariate Correlations

Bivariate correlations among the variables are summarized in Table 14.2. We report only notable patterns in the text, both similarities and/or differences. First, across all three groups, *Ideal Traits* was significantly and positively associated with parenting behaviors generally perceived as negative, such as *Gendered*, *Pressure*, *Academic Control*, *Authoritarian*, and *Rejection* and negative parent–child relationships such as *ICC* and *Conflict*. However, for KA, *Ideal Traits* seemed to carry fewer relational and developmental costs as compared with the other two groups (i.e., nonsignificant correlations with *Communication* and *Bonding*; not significantly correlated with mental distress and *Antisocial*). In some cases, *Ideal Traits* even carried relational and developmental benefits in KA, e.g., a positive correlation with *Authoritative*, whereas such a correlation was absent in the other two groups.

TABLE 14.1 Descriptive Statistics

Measures	*South Korean (SK)*	*Korean Chinese (KC)*	*Korean American (KA)*	*Differences* $(p < .05)$
	N (%) or M (SD)			
Traditional family values				
Traditional Manners	3.97 (0.85)	4.22 (0.76)	4.32 (0.74)	SK<KC, SK<KA
Respect for Adults	2.77 (0.87)	3.12 (0.87)	3.85 (0.73)	SK<KC<KA
Harmony & Sacrifice	3.1 (0.9)	3.34 (0.86)	3.81 (0.63)	SK<KC<KA
Traditional parenting				
Promoting Ideal Traits	3.15 (0.69)	3.17 (0.71)	3.43 (0.67)	SK<KA, KC<KA
Commitment to Education	3.91 (0.87)	4.36 (0.85)	4.55 (0.6)	SK<KC<KA
Gendered Norms	2.29 (0.81)	3.25 (0.8)	2.65 (0.76)	SK<KA<KC
Pressured to Succeed	2.21 (0.91)	2.34 (0.89)	2.44 (0.79)	SK<KC, SK<KA
Implicit Affection	3.77 (0.91)	4.25 (0.78)	4.27 (0.68)	SK<KC, SK<KA
Academic Control	2.51 (0.71)	2.63 (0.89)	2.9 (0.77)	SK<KC<KA
Qin	3.34 (0.76)	3.85 (0.81)	3.89 (0.62)	SK<KC, SK<KA
"Western" parenting				
Granting Autonomy	3.29 (0.69)	3.5 (0.74)	3.67 (0.56)	SK<KC<KA
Authoritarian	2.37 (0.99)	2.51 (1)	2.95 (0.84)	SK<KC<KA
Authoritative	3.35 (0.88)	3.66 (0.95)	3.29 (0.82)	SK<KC, KA<KC
Acceptance	3.6 (0.84)	3.75 (0.79)	3.76 (0.78)	SK<KC, SK<KA
Rejection	1.91 (0.69)	1.89 (0.74)	1.58 (0.45)	KA<SK, KA<KC
Rules	1.85 (1.76)	2.66 (1.88)	2.81 (1.73)	SK<KC, SK<KA
Monitoring	3.62 (0.95)	3.69 (0.98)	4.37 (0.76)	SK<KA, KC<KA
Parent–child relationship				
Intergenerational Conflict	2.6 (0.97)	2.7 (0.92)	2.39 (0.78)	KA<SK, KA<KC
Parent–child Communication	3.86 (0.96)	3.68 (0.94)	3.58 (0.83)	KA<SK, KC<SK
Parent–child Bonding	3.79 (0.95)	3.78 (0.91)	4.01 (0.7)	SK<KA, KC<KA
Parent–child Conflict	2.22 (0.9)	2.31 (0.78)	2.22 (0.79)	n.s.
Youth adjustments				
Depressive Symptoms	1.86 (0.79)	2.12 (0.78)	1.81 (0.73)	SK<KC, KA<KC
Suicidal Ideation	14.29%	26.55%	9.48%	KA<SK<KC
GPA	1.63 (1.24)	2.9 (0.85)	3.54 (0.54)	SK<KC<KA
Antisocial Behaviors	1.51 (1.93)	1.12 (1.68)	0.77 (1.41)	KA<KC<SK

Relatedly, only among KA, *Authoritative*, viewed as ideal in Western literature, was positively associated with rather negative family processes including *Gendered* ($r=.22$, $p<.001$), *Pressure* ($r=.19$, $p<.001$), *Authoritarian* ($r=.30$, $p<.001$), *Rules* ($r=.22$, $p<.001$), *ICC* ($r=.16$, $p<.01$), *Rejection* ($r=.11$, $p<.05$), and *Conflict* ($r=.12$, $p<.01$). Its nonsignificant association with youth outcomes among KA was also notable because it was indeed associated with youth outcomes in expected directions among SK and KC.

TABLE 14.2 Bivariate Correlations

	1	*2*	*3*	*4*	*5*	*6*	*7*	*8*	*9*	*10*	*11*	*12*	*13*
1. Manners	—												
	—												
	—												
2. Respect	0.30***	—											
	0.29***	—											
	0.27***	—											
3. Harmony	0.17***	0.45***	—										
	0.29***	0.48***	—										
	0.16**	0.39***	—										
4. Ideal Traits	0.18***	0.19***	0.24***	—									
	0.15*	−0.00	0.16*	—									
	0.35***	0.31***	0.29***	—									
5. Education	0.24***	0.21***	0.22***	−0.01	—								
	0.27***	0.19**	0.17**	0.15*	—								
	0.20***	0.27***	0.26***	0.22***	—								
6. Gendered	−0.08	0.02	0.00	0.33***	−0.18***	—							
	0.17**	0.28***	0.29***	0.39***	0.15*	—							
	0.21***	0.21***	0.08	0.43***	0.01	—							
7. Pressured	−0.08	−0.07	−0.06	0.27***	−0.19***	0.42***	—						
	−0.16*	−0.08	−0.05	0.33***	−0.11	0.25***	—						
	0.04	0.09	−0.05	0.25***	0.04	0.36***	—						

(Continued)

TABLE 14.2 (Continued)

	1	2	3	4	5	6	7	8	9	10	11	12	13
8. Implicit	0.19***	0.13**	0.24***	0.01	0.49***	−0.17***	−0.32***	—					
	0.44***	0.28***	0.24***	−0.02	0.37***	0.17**	−0.26***	—					
	0.22***	0.20***	0.28***	0.08	0.35***	−0.11*	−0.17***	—					
9. Academic Con.	0.08	0.03	0.05	0.15***	0.12**	0.14**	0.35***	0.10*	—				
	0.10	0.17**	0.19**	0.22***	0.04	0.34***	0.41***	0.03	—				
	0.18***	0.30***	0.13*	0.31***	0.28***	0.26***	0.38***	0.07	—				
10. Qin	0.27***	0.24***	0.28***	0.12**	0.60***	−0.16***	−0.23***	0.63***	0.21***	—			
	0.42***	0.23***	0.23***	0.05	0.40***	0.31***	−0.20***	0.65***	0.11	—			
	0.24***	0.37***	0.39***	0.31***	0.57***	0.06	−0.03	0.54***	0.33***	—			
11. Autonomy	0.23***	0.22***	0.24***	−0.06	0.41***	−0.27***	−0.36***	0.42***	0.04	0.53***	—		
	0.32***	0.17**	0.18**	0.00	0.30***	0.09	−0.22***	0.35***	0.06	0.43***	—		
	0.23***	0.13**	0.26***	0.03	0.25***	−0.21***	−0.29***	0.37***	−0.05	0.38***	—		
12. Authoritarian	−0.08	−0.07	0.01	0.41***	−0.23***	0.42***	0.56***	−0.31***	0.19***	−0.21***	−0.36***	—	
	−0.12	0.04	0.13*	0.34***	−0.10	0.33***	0.46***	−0.17**	0.30***	−0.18**	−0.11	—	
	0.09	0.17***	0.08	0.42***	0.07	0.42***	0.57***	−0.09	0.31***	0.06	−0.26***	—	
13. Authoritative	0.28***	0.24***	0.27***	0.04	0.42***	−0.16***	−0.20***	0.45***	0.17***	0.56***	0.51***	−0.26***	—
	0.29***	0.15*	0.20**	−0.09	0.24***	0.04	−0.30***	0.32***	0.03	0.39***	0.51***	−0.07	—
	0.16**	0.16**	0.21***	0.32***	0.20***	0.22***	0.19***	0.13**	0.24***	0.43***	0.16**	0.30***	—

	14	15	16	17	18	19	20	21	22	23	24	25
14. Acceptance	—											
	—											
	—											
15. Rejection	−0.53***	—										
	−0.49***	—										
	−0.52***	—										
16. Rules	0.00	0.19***	—									
	−0.06	0.20**	—									
	0.02	0.11*	—									
17. Monitoring	0.39***	−0.25***	0.18***	—								
	0.41***	−0.15*	−0.01	—								
	0.29***	−0.11*	0.05	—								
18. ICC	−0.39***	0.61***	0.26***	−0.19***	—							
	−0.23***	0.54***	0.28***	0.03	—							
	−0.43***	0.57***	0.27***	−0.17***	—							
19. Communication	0.59***	−0.58***	−0.06	0.33***	−0.49***	—						
	0.53***	−0.52***	−0.15*	0.26***	−0.44***	—						
	0.61***	−0.51***	−0.02	0.24***	−0.49***	—						
20. Bonding	0.76***	−0.65***	−0.03	0.34***	−0.46***	0.68***	—					
	0.70***	0.47***	−0.06	0.43***	−0.29***	0.62***	—					
	0.69***	−0.48***	0.09	0.28***	−0.39***	0.70***	—					
21. Conflict	−0.47***	0.71***	0.24***	−0.17***	0.56***	−0.46***	−0.53***	—				
	−0.40***	0.54***	0.20***	−0.18**	0.42***	−0.32***	−0.45***	—				
	−0.38***	0.60***	0.13**	−0.08	0.52***	−0.46***	−0.44***	—				

(Continued)

TABLE 14.2 (Continued)

	14	15	16	17	18	19	20	21	22	23	24	25
22. Depressive	−0.26***	0.41***	0.08	−0.07	0.28***	−0.30***	−0.33***	0.31***	—			
	−0.24***	0.34***	0.16**	−0.12	0.32***	−0.29***	−0.28***	0.38***	—			
	−0.23***	0.38***	−0.02	−0.01	0.29***	−0.34***	−0.24***	0.36***	—			
23. Suicidal	−0.22***	0.29***	0.12**	0.00	0.21***	−0.29***	−0.28***	0.25***	0.48***	—		
	−0.17**	0.18**	0.17**	−0.12	0.22***	−0.22***	−0.22***	0.23***	0.43***	—		
	−0.07	0.13**	−0.01	−0.02	0.18***	−0.18***	−0.13**	0.18***	0.38***	—		
24. GPA	0.14**	−0.11*	−0.01	0.18***	0.01	0.10*	0.06	−0.11*	−0.14**	−0.10*	—	
	0.20***	−0.04	0.17**	0.16*	0.07	0.13*	0.20***	−0.04	−0.12	−0.11	—	
	0.04	−0.11*	−0.00	0.15**	−0.14**	0.11*	0.05	−0.03	−0.14**	−0.03	—	
25. Antisocial	−0.16***	0.32***	0.11*	−0.21***	0.24***	−0.26***	−0.21***	0.30***	0.27***	0.13**	−0.11*	—
	−0.20***	0.35***	0.14*	−0.23***	0.21***	−0.20***	−0.21***	0.23***	0.27***	0.33***	−0.05	—
	−0.20***	0.28***	0.02	−0.27***	0.17***	−0.26***	−0.28***	0.31***	0.17***	0.14**	−0.22***	—

Notes.

Manners = Traditional Manners; Respect = Respect for Adults; Harmony = Harmony & Sacrifice; Ideal Traits = Promoting Ideal Traits; Education = Commitment to Education; Gendered = Gendered Norms; Pressured = Pressured to Succeed; Implicit = Implicit Affection; Academic Con. = Academic Control; Autonomy = Granting Autonomy; ICC = intergenerational cultural conflict; Communication = Parent–child Communication; Bonding = Parent–child Bonding; Conflict = Parent–child Conflict; Depressive = Depressive Symptoms; Suicidal = Suicidal Ideation; Antisocial = Antisocial Behaviors.

Within each variable, the first, second, and third rows represent the correlation for Koreans, Korean Chinese, and Korean Americans, respectively. For example, the correlation between traditional manners and respect for adults is.30 for Koreans,.29 for Korean Chinese, and.27 for Korean Americans.

$^{***}p < .001$. $^{**}p < .01$. $^{*}p < .05$.

Gendered was positively associated with traditional values and traditional parenting behaviors mainly among KC who reported the highest rate among the three groups. It was associated with negative family processes, particularly among SK (e.g., less *Autonomy*, *Acceptance*, *Monitoring*, and *Bonding*; more *Rejection* and *Conflict*; and more mental distress and *Antisocial*). On the contrary, these associations were generally not significant among KC. Its associations with youth outcomes were not statistically significant among KA either.

Traditional values were significantly associated with youth adjustments but somewhat inconsistently across the three groups. We found that youth endorsement of *Respect* was negatively associated with *Depressive* among KC (r=-.19, p<.01) and KA (r=-.17, p<.001) but not SK, also negatively with *Suicidal* among SK (r=-.10, p<.05) and KC (r=-.14, p<.05) but not among KA, and significantly and positively associated with GPA only among KC (r=.15, p<.05). It was however negatively associated with *Antisocial* in all three groups (respectively, r=-.12, r=-.19 and r=-.13, p<.01). *Harmony* was significantly associated with *Depressive* (r=-.15, p<.05), *GPA* (r=.16, p<.01) and *Antisocial* (r=-.13, p<.05) among KC, but not in the other groups and with *Suicidal* among SK (r=-.10, p<.05) but not the other groups.

In addition, *Autonomy* was overall positively associated with all three traditional family values and other family processes that can be construed as positive, such as more *Education*, *Implicit*, *Qin*, *Authoritative*, *Monitoring*, *Communication*, *Bonding* and less *Pressure*, *Authoritarian*, *ICC*, and importantly, less *Depressive*. These patterns were largely consistent and significant across all three groups. It was also significantly associated with less *Suicidal* among SK (r=-.21, p<.001) and less *Antisocial* among KC (r=-.20, p<.001).

Discussion

Rapid globalization and massive migration have brought about serious challenges as well as new opportunities for both the U.S. and global citizens. Among the challenges are the acculturation and enculturation processes among migrant families and their children. Asian youth in the U.S. and abroad comprise a silent minority in many ways; their positive externalized behaviors garner attention while their undetected negative internalized behaviors make them vulnerable to preventable self-harming injury and even death. Recent research suggests that intervening during the critical acculturation and enculturation processes both in and outside of the U.S. can help youth realize their full potential (Choi et al., 2013). Yet, to do so, an enhanced understanding of whether and how indigenous and Western parenting shapes youth outcomes is needed. A richer understanding of this process can also add to the knowledge base on child development in a multicultural, globalizing, and dynamic world.

The comparative analyses in this study found that Korean Americans have maintained their heritage in the family more so than Korean Chinese and South Koreans. The pattern was found in both parenting behaviors and youth endorsement of traditional values. Diaspora communities who have migrated or immigrated to a different cultural or socioeconomic country and often as a racial/ethnic minority may deliberately preserve their heritage and tradition as a way to buffer the negative impact of minority status. The results of this study illustrate that it is not an imagination that immigrant communities such as Korean Americans may indeed adhere to their tradition, more so than those in the country of origin or who have migrated to a context with cultural and racial similarity. In frequent interviews with Korean American community leaders and families, we have often heard that their family process feels "antique." It is possible that given their distinct minority status and the significant cultural distance from the Western mainstream, Korean Americans have reactively and deliberately held on to their tradition, while South Korean and Korean Chinese families have westernized themselves more readily in the process of rapid industrialization.

In addition, socioeconomic class may not have been adequately accounted for in understanding the impact of culture on family processes. For example, although the Asian culture is generally believed to put a strong emphasis on children's education, such a belief may be an overgeneralization, as our data (e.g., Zhang et al., 2023) have revealed how parenting behaviors focused on the promotion of academic achievement may vary across ethnic Korean families from different communities. Korean Americans, as compared with South Koreans and Korean Chinese, generally reported higher levels of academically oriented parenting, which may be explained by their recent immigrant status (i.e., first- and second-generation), reasons for immigration (i.e., primarily driven by economic and educational motivations), and SES (i.e., mostly middle and upper-middle class). Similarly, SES also may explain significantly higher problem behaviors among South Koreans (i.e., a larger variability) and higher mental distress in South Koreans and Korean Chinese who may be less resourced than Korean Americans on average.

Our data further suggest that ICC—a phenomenon that is believed to be particularly relevant to immigrant families, as a result of the parents and the child acculturating to the mainstream Western culture at different paces—may be more prominent in the Majority World. As parts of the Majority World (e.g., China, Korea) have gone through rapid social and economic development in the past few decades, parent–child acculturation discrepancy may well present itself in Asian families, whether or not they have an immigrant/migrant background. Relatedly, even though acculturation is mainly discussed in the literature involving immigrants, it can occur in any context where two or more streams of cultures meet (Berry & Sam., 2016). Indeed, our data suggest that parents in the Majority World may have selectively acculturated to the mainstream Western culture in their parenting, whereby some aspects of their parenting are more traditional while others are more Western (e.g., highest *Gendered Norms* AND highest *Authoritative Parenting* in Korean Chinese families; lowest *Autonomy Support* AND lowest *Gendered Norms* in South Korean families). In addition, SES may play a role in non-significant differences in ICC. That is, a lower SES is associated with higher parent–child conflict and the middle-class background of Korean Americans may help keep the level of ICC similar to other groups despite significant intergenerational cultural differences.

The distinctive ways in which traditional elements of the family process among Korean Americans are maintained (i.e., in a cultural hybrid) and, further, how they are related to youth adjustments (i.e., mixed impact) are intriguing. Those family processes typically regarded as negative (i.e., parental efforts to preserve traditional values, authoritarian style, and gendered norms) may not be as harmful among Korean American families as in other groups. Combined with Korean Americans maintaining the core heritage culture more so than the other groups, the findings of this study demonstrate a complex intersection of culture, class, and racial/minority status in the family process. Active cultural socialization is pervasive among non-White, immigrant families in the U.S. It is plausible that parental adherence to their tradition is seen as an extension of enculturation efforts to strengthen racial/ethnic pride as a buffer against the negativity of racial/ethnic minority status. Consequently, Korean American youth may be less influenced by some of the negativity derived from traditional values or parenting behaviors, and in fact, their cultural understanding may help parent–child relationships and improve adjustment. In other words, upholding one's heritage and tradition may have a unique benefit among the racialized and/or culturally marginalized families.

Limitations and Future Directions

The three samples in the current study were regionally and strategically recruited and are not nationally representative of the ethnic Korean populations in the three societies, which warrants caution in the cross-cultural interpretations of the results. For example, all three samples were recruited from urban contexts, and rural adolescents' experiences are not represented in the data. The sole recruitment of Korean Chinese youth who attend Korean ethnic schools limits the representativeness of the sample further, as the Korean-learning Korean Chinese youth population is rapidly shrinking. The experiences of the more assimilated Korean Chinese youth remain unknown. However, the three study sites used the same measures to assess family processes across groups of Korean heritage in different sociopolitical contexts—this is rare, if not the first study to do so. The data were collected at different times, another limitation, but they were still close to one another within a few years during which the family process would unlikely shift significantly. Cultural changes tend to take a long time.

Despite these limitations, this study offers several important insights on how culture, class, and race/ethnicity may collectively shape family process and implications for practice and future directions. First, a unique cultural hybrid of heritage and Western parenting among Korean groups in variant contexts shows that modern Korean parenting (and a cautious extension to Asian parenting), regardless of its geographical and sociopolitical location, is quite flexible and far different from the narrow definition of "traditional" Korean (or Asian) parenting that is stereotyped to be harsh and controlling. Instead, Korean families have found a balance between Western and heritage parenting that would be appropriate and adaptive in respective contexts. Moreover, what is conventionally considered "Western" may also be part of the parenting practices of a large group of Asian families.

Additional analyses are warranted to examine why and how the idiosyncratic combination of positive external adjustment and negative internal struggle is shared across the three groups. The optimal balance of cultures that produces positive adjustment might look slightly different depending on which context they live in (e.g., more academic control in China and the U.S.). In future analyses, SES and other crucial related matters should be directly accounted for to discern the impact of class, and the experiences of being a minority and growing up without parents (e.g., the proportion of left-behind children was prominent in Korean Chinese). In all contexts, Korean families are flexible and adapt quickly to the rapidly changing economic/social context, and parenting that is associated with ideal adjustments will illustrate how to strike a balance between "new" and "old" cultural practices in parenting.

References

Angold, A. C., Costello, E. J., Messer, S. C., & Pickles, A. (1995). Development of a short questionnaire for use in epidemiological studies of depression in children and adolescents. *International Journal of Methods in Psychiatric Research*, *5*(4), 237–249.

Berry, J. W. & Sam., D. (2016). Theoretical perspectives. In D. Sam & J. W. Berry (Eds), *The Cambridge Handbook of Acculturation Psychology* (pp. 11–29). Cambridge University Press.

Booth, A., Crouter, A. C., & Landale, N. S. (Eds). (1997). *Immigration and the family: research and policy on U.S. immigrations*. Lawrence Erlbaum Associates.

Budiman, A. (2021). *Koreans in the U.S. Fact Sheet*. Pew Research Center. www.pewresearch.org/social-trends/factsheet/asian-americans-koreans-in-the-u-s.

Buri, J. R. (1991). Parental Authority Questionnaire. *Journal of personality assessment, 57*(1), 110–119.

Chao, R. K. (1995). Chinese and European American cultural models of the self reflected in mother's childrearing beliefs. *Ethos, 23*(3), 328–354.

Chao, R. K. & Tseng, V. (2002). Parenting of Asians. In M. H. Bornstein (Ed.), *Handbook of Parenting* (Vol. 4, pp. 59–93). Lawrence Erlbaum Associates.

Chao, R. K. & Wu, C. (2001). *Guan parenting behaviors*. University of California at Riverside.

Choi, W.-G. (2001). The Korean minority in China: The change of its identity. *Development and Society, 30*(1), 119–141.

Choi, Y., Harachi, T. W., Gillmore, M. R., & Catalano, R. F. (2005). Applicability of the social development model to urban ethnic minority youth: Examining the relationship between external constraints, family socialization and problem behaviors. *Journal of Research on Adolescence, 15*(4), 505–534.

Choi, Y., Jeong, E., & Park, M. (2022). Asian Americans' parent–child conflict and racial discrimination may explain mental distress. *Policy Insights from Behavioral and Brain Sciences* 9(1), 377–392.

Choi, Y. & Kim, Y. S. (2010). Acculturation and enculturation: Core vs. peripheral changes in the family socialization among Korean Americans. *Korean Journal of Studies of Koreans Abroad, 21*, 135–190.

Choi, Y., Kim, Y. S., Pekelnicky, D. D., & Kim, H. (2013). Preservation and Modification of Culture in Family Socialization: Development of Parenting Measures for Korean Immigrant Families. *Asian American Journal of Psychology, 4*(2), 143–154.

Choi, Y., Park, M., Lee, J. P., Kim, T. Y., & Tan, K. P. H. (2017). Culture and family process: Examination of culture specific family process via development of new parenting measures among Filipino and Korean American families with adolescents. In Y. Choi & H. C. Hahm (Eds), *Asian American Parenting: Family Process and Intervention* (pp. 37–68). Springer.

Choi, Y., Park, M., Lee, J. P., & Lee, M. (2020). Explaining the Asian American youth paradox: Universal factors vs. Asian American family process among Filipino and Korean American youth. *Family Process, 59*(4), 1818–1836.

Chua, A. (2011). *Battle hymn of the tiger mother*. Bloomsbury Publishing.

Cui, W., Gu, Y., Shi, S., Zhang, M., & Wang, Y. (2014). Relationship among Korean-Chinese left-behind adolescents' life events, resilience and prospective adaptation. *Chinese Journal of School Health, 35*(1), 69–72. https://doi.org/http://dx.doi.org/10.16835/j.cnki.1000-9817.2014.01.026.

Deater-Deckard, K., Dodge, K. A., & Sorbring, E. (2005). Cultural differences in the effects of physical punishment. In M. Rutter (Ed.), *Ethnicity and causal mechanisms* (pp. 204–226). Cambridge University Press.

Druckerman, P. (2014). *Bringing up Bébé: One American mother discovers the wisdom of French parenting*. Penguin Press.

Eddy, J. M., Reid, J. B., & Fetrow, R. A. (2000). An Elementary School-Based Prevention Program Targeting Modifiable Antecedents of Youth Delinquency

and Violence: Linking the Interests of Families and Teachers (LIFT). *Journal of Emotional and Behavioral Disorders, 8*(3), 165–176.
Fuligni, A. J., Yip, T., & Tseng, V. (2002). The impact of family obligation on the daily activities and psychosocial well-being of Chinese American adolescents. *Child Development, 73*(1), 302–314.
Garcia Coll, C., Lamberty, G., Jenkins, R., McAdoo, H. P., Crnic, K., Wasik, B. H., & Garcia, H. V. (1996). An integrative model for the study of developmental competencies in minority children. *Child Development, 67*, 1891–1914.
Garcia Coll, C. & Pachter, L. M. (2002). Ethnic and Minority Parenting. In M. H. Bornstein (Ed.), *Handbook of Parenting* (Vol. 4, pp. 1–20). Lawrence Erlbaum Associates.
Grolnick, W. S., Ryan, R. M., & Deci, E. L. (1991). Inner Resources for School Achievement: Motivational Mediators of Children's Perceptions. *Journal of Educational Psychology, 83*(4), 508–517.
Harkness, S. & Super, C. M. (2002). Culture and parenting. In M. H. Bornstein (Ed.), *Handbook of parenting* (Vol. 2, pp. 253–280). Lawrence Erlbaum Associates.
Jose, P. E., Huntsinger, C. S., Huntsinger, P. R., & Liaw, F.-R. (2000). Parental values and practices relevant to young children's social development in Taiwan and the United States. *Journal of Cross Cultural Psychology, 31*(6), 677–702.
Juang, L. P., Park, I. J. K., Kim, S. Y., Lee, R. M., Qin, D. B., Okazaki, S., Swartz, T. T., & Lau, A. (2018). Reactive and proactive ethnic–racial socialization practices of second-generation Asian American parents. *Asian American Journal of Psychology, 9*(1), 4.
Kagitçibasi, Ç. (1996). *Family and human development across cultures*. Lawrence Erlbaum Associates.
Kagitçibasi, Ç. (2007). *Family, self, and human development across cultures: Theory and applications*, 2nd edition. Lawrence Erlbaum.
Kibria, N. (2002). *Becoming Asian American: Second generation Chinese and Korean American identities*. Johns Hopkins University.
Kim, E. & Hong, S. (2007). First-generation Korean-American parents' perception of discipline. *Journal of Professional Nursing, 23*(1), 60–68.
Kim, K. (2006). Hyo and parenting in Korea. In H. R. Kenneth & O. B. Chung (Eds), *Parenting beliefs, behaviors, and parent–child relations: A cross-cultural perspective* (pp. 207–222). Pschology Press.
Kurasaki, K. S., Okazaki, S., & Sue, S. (Eds). (2002). *Asian American Mental Health: Assessment theories and methods*. Kluwer Academic/Plenum Publishers.
Kusche, C., Greenberg, M., & Beilke, R. (1988). Seattle personality questionnaire for young school-aged children. Unpublished manuscript. University of Washington, Seattle.
Lee, R. M., Choe, J., Kim, G., & Ngo, V. (2000). Construction of the Asian American Family Conflicts Scale. *Journal of Counseling Psychology, 47*(2), 211–222.
Lee, R. M., Noh, C.-Y., Yoo, H. C., & Doh, H.-S. (2007). The psychology of diaspora experiences: Intergroup contact, perceived discrimination, and the ethnic identity of Koreans in China. *Cultural Diversity and Ethnic Minority Psychology, 13*(2), 115–124.
Louie, V. S. (2004). *Compelled to excel: Immigration, education, and opportunity among Chinese Americans*. Stanford University Press.

Min, P. G. (2010). *Preserving ethnicity through religion in America: Korean protestants and Indian Hindus across generations*. New York University.

National Bureau of Statistics of China (2020). *Tabulation on the 2010 population census of the People's Republic of China [Data set]*. www.stats.gov.cn/sj/pcsj/rkpc/6rp/indexch.htm.

OECD (2023). *Education GPS*. Retrieved October 18, 2023 from https://doi.org/10.1007/s10964-023-01845-z.

Park, M., Choi, Y., Yasui, M., & Hedeker, D. (2021). Racial discrimination and the moderating effects of racial and ethnic socialization on mental health of Asian American youth. *Child Development, 92*(6), 2284–2298.

Park, M., Choi, Y., Yoo, H. C., Yasui, M., & Takeuchi, D. (2021). Racial stereotypes and Asian American youth paradox. *Journal of youth and adolescence*, (50), 2374–2393. https://doi.org/10.1007/s10964-021-01519-8.

Prinz, R. (1977). *The Assessment of Parent-Adolescent Relations: Discriminating Distressed and Non-distressed Dyads [doctoral dissertation]*. Stony Brook: State University of New York.

Rosenthal, D. A. & Feldman, S. S. (1992). The nature and stability of ethnic identity in Chinese youth: Effects of length of residence in two cultural contexts. *Journal of Cross-Cultural Psychology, 23*(2), 214–227.

Ryou, B., Choi, Y., Hong, J. S., & Kim, K. (2019). Cultural Orientations and psychosocial adjustments among immigrant adolescents in South Korea. *Journal of Immigrant and Minority Health, 21*, 767–777.

Silk, J. S., Morris, A. S., Kanaya, T., & Steinberg, L. (2003). Psychological Control and Autonomy Granting: Opposite Ends of a Continuum or Distinct Constructs? *Journal of Research on Adolescence, 13*(1), 113–128.

Soenens, B., Park, S.-Y., Vansteenkiste, M., & Mouratidis, A. (2012). Perceived parental psychological control and adolescent depressive experiences: A cross-cultural study with Belgian and South-Korean adolescents. *Journal of Adolescence, 35*(2), 261–272.

Wu, C. & Chao, R. K. (2011). Intergenerational cultural dissonance in parent-adolescent relationships among Chinese and European Americans. *Developmental Psychology, 47*(2), 493–508.

Xie, Y. & Goyette, K. (1997). The racial identification of biracial children with one Asian parent: Evidence from the 1990 census. *Social Forces. 76*, 547–570.

Yanbian Bureau of Statistics (2020). *Statistical communiqué of Yanbian Korean autonomous prefecture on the 2019 national economic and social development*. http://www.yanbian.gov.cn/sj/tjgb/202006/t20200604_152275.html.

Zhang, M., Shen, Y., Choi, Y., & Kim, K. (2023). Parental academic socialization and youth's adjustments: A comparisons of Korean youth in South Korea, China, and the United States. *Journal of youth and adolescence, 52*, 2526–2544. https://doi.org/https://doi.org/10.1007/s10964-023-01845-z.

Zhao, Z., Shen, Y., & Wang, J. (2024). Profiles of identity and discrimination and the psychological, health, and academic outcomes of Korean ethnic minority youth in China. *Journal of Research on Adolescence. 34*(2), 313-326.

15

PARENTING IN MAJORITY WORLD ASIAN COUNTRIES

W. Andrew Rothenberg, Florrie Fei-Yin Ng, and Marc H. Bornstein

Introduction

In 2015 the United Nations adopted the Sustainable Development Goals (SDGs), a set of actions for the world to become more peaceful and prosperous by 2030 (UNICEF, 2017). SDG 4 endeavors to "Ensure inclusive and equitable quality education and promote lifelong learning opportunities for all," and indicators of this goal include identifying the extent to which children under the age of five receive stimulating caregiving in their home environments. To accomplish SDG 4, attention needs to be paid to caregiver provision of stimulating caregiving in majority world countries, which are still underrepresented in the developmental science literature, despite the advocacy of numerous scientists over many years (e.g., Sun et al., 2016; Tomlinson et al., 2014).

This chapter focuses on caregivers' provision of stimulating caregiving in majority world countries in Asia. Although Asia is home to approximately 60 percent of the world's population, Asian parenting is vastly understudied and, when studied, is usually cast in comparison to parenting and child development in minority world countries (Ng & Wang, 2019; Raval, 2023). The focus of this chapter on stimulating caregiving can shed light on cultural caregiving strengths in majority world Asian countries as well as advance understanding of how caregiving to young children may be viewed as an adaptation to social and cultural ecologies (Bornstein et al., 2022a). Indeed, developmental scholars have identified that core values of many Asian cultures, such as interdependence, duty to family, and achievement as a family endeavor, serve to place caregiving and family strengthening

DOI: 10.4324/9781003383949-15

at the center of life in many Asian societies (Joseph, 2018; Ng & Li, 2024; Roche, 2017). Unfortunately, many majority world Asian countries have been subject to centuries of colonization and oppression that have made it more likely for families to be exposed to adverse contexts, such as high poverty, that undermine the provision of stimulating caregiving (McCoy et al., 2022; Raval, 2023). Yet, the first decades of the 21st century have witnessed burgeoning initiatives for early childhood interventions across majority world countries in Asia (UNESCO, 2010; 2023). For example, Bangladesh and Vietnam are two majority world countries that UNICEF highlights as nations that have invested in effective early intervention programs to promote child development (Aboud & Akhter, 2011).

This chapter attempts to understand how parents in majority world Asian countries provide caregiving to their young children by examining four issues associated with their cognitive and socioemotional caregiving practices through UNICEF's nationally representative, internationally comparable Multiple Indicator Cluster Surveys (MICS; UNICEF, 2017). The data set includes 53,044 families with children 36–59 months old in 12 majority world Asian countries. Examining these caregiving practices is vital to better understanding the nature of stimulating caregiving in these majority world countries and furthering world progress toward SDG 4. First, the chapter recounts the importance of studying cognitive and socioemotional caregiving and reviews perspectives on four issues, *viz.* differences in mothers', fathers', and other caregivers' cognitive and socioemotional caregiving in these Asian countries, associations between cognitive and socioemotional caregiving practices among mothers, fathers, and other caregivers, associations between caregivers' cognitive and socioemotional caregiving practices and child gender, and how caregivers' cognitive or socioemotional caregiving practices are associated with early childhood development. Next, the chapter reviews the methods, procedures, sampling, and statistical techniques used to examine these issues. Results for each of the four issues of caregiver differences, associations among caregivers, associations between caregivers' caregiving practices and child gender, and associations of caregiving with early childhood development are then reported. The meaning of these results for each issue is discussed, and before concluding, the chapter reviews limitations, strengths, and future directions of the current work.

Families in Majority World Asian Countries

Parents' cognitive and socioemotional caregiving practices do not exist in a vacuum. To understand these caregiving practices in majority world Asian countries, it is necessary to consider the sociocultural context in which these practices occur. The 12 Asian countries in the UNICEF Multiple

Indicator Cluster Surveys (MICS) studied here span a large geographic area: Mongolia is in East Asia; Laos, Thailand, and Vietnam are in Southeast Asia; Bangladesh, Bhutan, and Nepal are in South Asia; Iraq and the State of Palestine are in West Asia; and Kazakhstan, Kyrgyzstan, and Turkmenistan are in Central Asia. Although these Asian countries differ in ways that reflect regional variations in dimensions such as religion and gender roles (Ng & Li, 2024), they share some cultural values and practices that similarly structure family life and govern interpersonal dynamics among family members.

All 12 of these Asian countries are collectivistic in that they emphasize the group over the individual and the family is considered as the basic unit of the society (Ng & Li, 2024). Large households with six or more members—many of which are multigenerational—are more common in countries in West Asia (e.g., 49 percent in the State of Palestine) and South Asia (e.g., 31 percent in Bhutan) than in Southeast Asia (e.g., 9 percent in Thailand), with countries in Central Asia (e.g., 25 percent in Kyrgyzstan) and East Asia (24 percent in Mongolia) falling in between (United Nations, 2019). Regardless of their residential arrangement, parents and young children frequently interact with extended family members, who are often actively involved in childcare (Ng & Wang, 2019). In most majority world Asian countries, household hierarchy is based on age and gender, with older (vs. younger) and male (vs. female) family members enjoying higher statuses. However, majority world Asian countries vary in the extent to which they are patriarchal: Countries in West and South Asia rank among the lowest in the world in terms of gender parity, but countries in Southeast Asia rank high, especially regarding women's economic participation and opportunity (World Economic Forum, 2023). Indeed, in contrast to other regions of Asia in which women tend to shoulder most, if not all, caregiving responsibilities in the family, males and females in Southeast Asia have traditionally shared such responsibilities (Ng & Li, 2024).

The Importance of Studying Cognitive and Socioemotional Caregiving

Scholars of Asian parenting were among the first to identify that stimulating caregiving practices in UNICEF's MICS dataset could be theoretically and empirically disaggregated into cognitive caregiving (i.e., stimulating children to engage and understand the environment by describing, demonstrating, and providing opportunities to learn) and socioemotional caregiving (i.e., stimulating children to engage in interpersonal interactions; Bornstein & Putnick, 2012; Sun et al., 2016). We adopted this conceptualization and believe that it is especially informative to distinguish cognitive and socioemotional caregiving in majority world Asian countries for several reasons. First, prior research suggests that cognitive caregiving might be especially important for child development in Asian contexts because many Asian parents are invested in educating their children on account of the emphasis on education in traditional and religious teaching and the positive implications of educational achievement for upward mobility and family honor (Ng & Wang, 2019; Roche, 2017). Second, with respect to socioemotional caregiving, in traditionally interdependent societies, such as is true in Asia, socialization of interpersonal sensitivity and group harmony is promoted and esteemed (Chen, 2023; Ng & Li, 2024).

Differences in Mothers', Fathers', and Other Caregivers' Cognitive and Socioemotional Caregiving in Majority World Asian Countries

One fundamental question to explore in investigating cognitive and socioemotional caregiving is to understand who in the family is providing such caregiving. This question is especially intriguing to investigate in the context of majority world Asian countries, in which there are often multiple caregivers in the household and the nature of modern caregiving has been changing with socioeconomic development (Joseph, 2018; Ng & Li, 2024; Roche, 2017). On the one hand, scholars investigating Asian parenting have noted that traditional divisions of childcare and household responsibilities are similar across regions in Asia (Ng & Wang, 2019; Shwalb et al., 2014). In this traditional family structure, fathers oversee discipline and make major family decisions, while mothers play more nurturing roles with children, spend more time actually parenting children, and feel more efficacious in childrearing (Ng & Wang, 2019; Shwalb et al., 2014). Mothers are often joined in this caregiving role by other female members of the household, such as grandmothers and aunts (Mehta & Thang, 2012; Ng & Wang, 2019). The provision of care by these "other" caregivers is common in these Asian countries because Asian households are more likely to have multiple generations of a family living together, compared with the "nuclear" family structure common in Western societies (Joseph, 2018; Ng & Li, 2024). This traditional division of gender roles suggests that mothers and other caregivers might engage in more cognitive and socioemotional caregiving than fathers, and caregiving data from majority world Asian countries supports this inference. UNICEF data collected in majority world countries between 2005 and 2010 revealed that mothers engaged in more cognitive and socioemotional caregiving than fathers in all Asian nations examined (Sun et al., 2016), and UNICEF data collected between 2009 and 2017 revealed that in majority world countries mothers engaged in higher levels of stimulating caregiving than fathers or other caregivers, and other caregivers engaged in higher levels of stimulating caregiving than fathers (Cuartas et al., 2018; McCoy et al., 2022).

On the other hand, there are limitations to the aforementioned studies. Older evaluations which focused specifically on Asian nations relied on data collected between 2005 and 2010 (Bornstein & Putnick, 2012). Since that time parenting in Asian nations has changed with fathers becoming more involved in parenting and mothers joining the workforce at higher rates, suggesting that the gap between father and mother/other caregiver caregiving may be closing (Lansford et al., 2021; Ng & Wang, 2019). Given these competing influences of traditional family structure and contemporary trends in parenting, it is especially important to examine the contemporary state of mothers', fathers', and other caregivers' cognitive and socioemotional caregiving in majority world Asian countries.

Associations between Cognitive and Socioemotional Caregiving Practices Among Mothers, Fathers, and Other Caregivers in Majority World Asian Countries

In addition to knowing the sheer number of cognitive and socioemotional caregiving activities mothers, fathers, and other caregivers engage in, it is useful to understand the extent to which one caregiver's cognitive and socioemotional caregiving practices correspond with those of children's other caregivers in the same household. Knowing how correlated multiple caregivers' actions are provides insight into the likelihood that increasing cognitive or socioemotional caregiving practices in one caregiver might "spread" or "spill over" to the caregiving practices of other caregivers (Maital & Bornstein, 2003, 2022; Rothenberg, 2019). Again, traditional family structures in Asian societies and contemporary parenting influences in Asian societies provide competing explanations for the extents to which caregivers' cognitive and socioemotional caregiving practices correspond to one another.

On the one hand, traditional family structures in many Asian societies sanction female caregivers to wield considerable power when it comes to dictating how to provide caregiving (Ng & Wang, 2019; Roche, 2017). Caregiving responsibilities are often shared among mothers and other female members of the family, like grandmothers and aunts (Ng & Wang, 2019; Tapanya, 2011). In such households, the hierarchy is generational, and deference and obedience to senior members of the household are emphasized, such that there may be high correspondence in caregiving practices among female caregivers within the household (Ng & Li, 2024). Moreover, if mothers and other older female relatives dictate caregiving patterns in the household, and men take their cues from these caregivers, then high correspondence in cognitive and socioemotional caregiving among all caregivers in the household would be expected.

On the other hand, as consequence of contemporary urbanization, mothers and fathers in majority world Asian countries are increasingly working outside the home (Lansford et al., 2021; Ng & Wang, 2019; Yotanyamaneewong et al., 2021). This trend suggests that mothers' and fathers' caregiving will correspond more highly with each other than with other caregivers' caregiving behaviors because other caregivers will often engage in caregiving when mothers and fathers are at work. Given these competing traditional and contemporary influences, the present study investigates how highly mothers, fathers, and children's other caregivers' caregiving behaviors are correlated in these Asian countries.

Associations Between Cognitive and Socioemotional Caregiving Practices and Child Gender in Majority World Asian Countries

Child gender might influence the extent to which caregivers engage in cognitive and socioemotional caregiving with children (Bornstein & Putnick, 2016). This gender differentiation might be especially true in Asian nations, where the traditionally patriarchal nature of many societies leads to a parental preference for sons (Ng & Wang, 2019; Shwalb et al., 2014). This preference has been driven by pragmatic concerns about socioeconomic conditions; in most majority world Asian countries, parents' old-age support was for many centuries reliant on having a male heir (although this reliance is waning as parents increasingly rely on their daughters and their own financial resources for support; Ng & Li, 2024; Ng & Wang, 2019). Because of son preference, there is some evidence of gender bias in parents' resource allocation, with sons often benefiting from lower mortality rates, more attention, nutrition, and medical treatment (Attane & Guilmoto, 2007). This differential resource allocation is especially likely in poverty-stricken families, and poverty is more prevalent in majority world countries (Bornstein & Rothenberg, 2021; Guilmoto & Jones, 2016). It stands to reason that this traditional preference for greater parental resource allocation for sons in majority world Asian countries may be reflected in caregiving, with sons receiving more cognitive and socioemotional caregiving than daughters. Yet, work that examines majority world countries worldwide—many of which are patriarchal with son preference—finds that cognitive and socioemotional caregiving practices do not differ based on child gender (Bornstein & Putnick, 2016; Bornstein et al., 2022a). Therefore, traditional cultural preferences for sons in Asia and evidence from majority world countries worldwide contrast in predicting whether caregiver caregiving differs based on child gender. This study investigates these competing hypotheses by examining whether mother, father, and other caregiver caregiving practices vary based on child gender.

Which Caregivers' Cognitive and Socioemotional Caregiving Practices are Most Powerfully Associated with Early Childhood Development in Majority World Asian Countries

Examining whether mothers, fathers, or other caregivers engage in the most cognitive or socioemotional caregiving practices is not the same as investigating which of these caregivers' parenting practices might be most influential in promoting early childhood development. For instance, even though fathers typically engage in less caregiving than mothers in majority world countries, mothers' and fathers' stimulating caregiving activities are each uniquely associated with better child development (Jeong et al., 2016, 2017). However, no work has directly compared associations between mothers', fathers', and other caregivers' cognitive and socioemotional caregiving in particular (as opposed to stimulating behaviors in general) with early childhood development in any majority world countries.

Examining unique associations of cognitive and socioemotional caregiving is especially important in the Asian context. As described, caregivers in Asian nations often place importance on parenting children in ways that promote achievement and learning (Ng & Wang, 2019). Consequently, Asian parents believe that learning should begin early in life (Ng & Wang, 2019). Emphasis on cognitive caregiving practices, including joint book reading, counting, and story-telling, is associated with high achievement in Asian children (Lau et al., 2011; Ng & Wang, 2019; Rafiq et al., 2013). Although cognitive caregiving might be an especially powerful predictor of child development outcomes across majority world Asian countries, it remains unclear who among mothers, fathers, and other caregivers might exert the most influence over early childhood development.

Given the more central role that mothers play in childrearing across many Asian nations (Ng & Wang, 2019), it is possible that when directly compared, associations between maternal caregiving and child development might be larger than those of paternal caregiving. No literature examines how other caregivers' caregiving practices might be uniquely associated with child development after considering effects of mother and father practices. Answering this question is important in Asian contexts, where other caregivers often live in the same household as children, provide caregiving to those children, and are richly involved in young children's lives (Cuartas et al., 2020; Ng & Wang, 2019). The current study examines the extent to which mothers', fathers', and other caregivers' caregiving practices are associated with early childhood development, even after accounting for one another's caregiving.

The Importance of Accounting for Variability in Caregiving Across Majority World Asian Countries

Although general cultural patterns are shared across many Asian countries, helping to explain caregiving patterns and correlates, Asian countries are not a monolith; each nation may have distinct cultural strengths and ways of caregiving (Ng & Wang, 2019). Indeed, the 12 majority world countries investigated here vary widely in the number of children who experience early stimulation at home (from 44 percent–92 percent; UNICEF, 2023) and in the number of children whom UNICEF deems developmentally "on-track" (from 65 percent–95 percent; UNICEF, 2023). Moreover, within any particular country, there can be significant variability in cognitive and socioemotional caregiving depending on a number of family characteristics (e.g., socioeconomic status, family structure, etc.; Ng & Wang, 2019). Although the present study attempts to identify patterns across 12 majority world Asian countries, it also attempts to account for differences in caregiving within and across those countries analytically.

The Current Study

This study examines cognitive and socioemotional caregiving practices of mothers, fathers, and children's other caregivers in 12 Majority world Asian countries. Specifically, it examines (1) how many out of three basic cognitive and three basic socioemotional caregiving practices mothers, fathers, and other caregivers reportedly engage in; (2) how these different reports of caregivers' cognitive and socioemotional caregiving practices are associated with one another; (3) how these reports of cognitive and socioemotional caregiving practices differ depending on the gender of the child they are being provided to; and (4) how strongly reports of each of these caregivers' cognitive and socioemotional caregiving practices are associated with early childhood development. Attention is given to variations in the patterns within and across the 12 Asian countries.

Methods Used to Address The Four Issues

Participants

A total of 53,044 families with children ages three to four years from 12 majority world Asian countries provided the MICS4 and MICS5 data examined here. Each country selected a representative probability sample, national in coverage (Bornstein et al., 2022a; UNICEF, 2009). Children were, on average, 47.33 months old (*SD*=6.91), and the sample was evenly divided with 48.93 percent girls and 51.07 percent boys. On average, 3.09 children under the age of 18 years (*SD*=1.85) lived in each household. To obviate within-family or within-household variance, one child between 36 and 59 months was randomly selected from families with more than one child in the target age range for the current analyses. The mother in each family reported on mother, father, and other caregiver caregiving practices and child development. Mothers were on average 31.35 years old (*SD*=7.85) and 21.16 percent reported receiving no formal education, 29.75 percent primary, 35.39 percent secondary, and 13.70 percent higher education.

Procedures and Measures

MICS4 and MICS5. Each country followed the same MICS4/MICS5 implementation procedures to ensure standardization and cultural/linguistic equivalences across nations. Participating governments forward- and backward-translated all measures into local languages (UNICEF, 2009; UNICEF, 2013). Field teams were recruited and trained in interview techniques, contents of the questionnaires, field procedures, and use of equipment. These field teams then interviewed participants in their homes. All data were entered twice into standard databases and centrally archived. The questions and measures used in this study were unchanged across the MICS4/5.

Cognitive and Socioemotional Caregiving Practices. The MICS4 and MICS5 asked mothers whether the mother, father, or any other caregiver in the household over 15 years of age engaged in each of three different cognitive and socioemotional caregiving practices over the past three days. The three cognitive caregiving practices were: (1) read books or looked at picture books with the child; (2) told stories to the child; and (3) named, counted, or drew with the child. The three socioemotional practices were: (1) sang songs to or with the child, including lullabies; (2) took the child outside the home, compound, yard, or enclosure; and (3) played with the child. These items were selected for inclusion in the MICS via a three-stage process that included several pilot studies and reaching consensus on appropriate items among two panels of experts worldwide. All items demonstrate measurement invariance and psychometric soundness across cultural contexts (Kariger et al., 2012). In this study, separate scores were calculated for each caregiver: mothers, fathers, and other caregivers. Aligning with previous work (Bornstein & Putnick, 2012), the items were summed to form cognitive and socioemotional caregiving indices for each caregiver wherein 0=*the caregiver engaged in no activities in the last three days* to 3=*the caregiver engaged in all three activities in the last three days*.

Early Childhood Development Index. The Early Childhood Development Index (ECDI; UNICEF, 2017) consists of ten questions that measure four domains of early childhood development in children ages 36–59 months, including literacy/numeracy development (e.g., knowing and using numbers/letters/words), socioemotional development (e.g., recognizing and expressing thoughts/feelings), physical health (e.g., developing gross and fine motor abilities), and approaches to learning (e.g., following directions and independently completing tasks). These items were selected for inclusion in the MICS via a four-stage process that included identification of items by an expert panel and field-testing items to examine their psychometric soundness, clarity, relevance, measurement invariance, and validity (UNICEF, 2017). To complete the ECDI, the mother of the child was asked whether the child displayed a particular behavior related to child development. Following UNICEF (2017) guidelines, answers that indicated positive child development were then summed to compute a total Early Childhood Development Index Score (0–10 scale; higher scores indicated more advanced child development). Across the 12 majority world Asian countries, the ECDI mean was 6.10 (SD=1.77). See Table 15.1 for ECDI scores in each participating LMIC.

Child and Caregiver Sociodemographic Characteristics. Child age in months and gender (0=female, 1=male) and mother age in years and education (0=no education to 3=higher education) were controlled in analyses.

Other Caregivers Resided in the Home. Whether other caregivers resided with children was controlled in all analyses. Other caregivers resided in 56.60 percent of homes in the 12 Asian countries.

Overall Quality of the Physical Home Environment. To account for effects of household wealth and physical assets in the home, a composite measure that captured the overall quality of the physical home environment (called the Overall Quality of the Physical Home Environment, or OQPHEI; Bradley et al., 2022) was used. The OQPHEI was created by standardizing scores of each of the Quality Housing Index (a sum score capturing eight aspects of the home environment including source of water, toileting facility, house construction materials, and cooking fuel used), Household Wired Appliances Index (a sum score capturing which of five different types of wired appliances are present in the home), Family Amenities Index (a sum score that indicates which of seven transportation and communication items a family owns), and Learning Materials Index (a sum score that indicates which of five different types of learning materials are available in the home) and then summing those standardized scores. The resulting OQPHEI had a mean of 0 with higher scores indicating better overall quality of the physical home environment.

The Human Development Index. Given the focus on majority world countries, we used the United Nations' Human Development Index (HDI; UN Development Programme, 2014) to control for the effects of nations' human development conditions. The HDI measures the conditions countries provide to promote the development of people and their capabilities (UN Development Programme, 2014). The HDI has three major components: (1) life expectancy (years); (2) education (the adult literacy rate and combined gross enrollment in primary, secondary, and tertiary school); and (3) gross domestic product (GDP). The HDI varies from 0 (low) to 1 (high). The average household HDI score across this entire Asian sample was 0.66 (SD=0.07), indicating that, on average, households are living in nations at the "medium" human development level.

Results for the Four Issues

Differences in Cognitive and Socioemotional Caregiving Provided by Mothers, Fathers, and Other Caregivers in Majority World Asian Countries

Significant differences emerged for reports of mothers', fathers', and other caregivers' cognitive (Table 15.1) and socioemotional (Table 15.2) caregiving practices. Specifically, across the entire sample, mothers engaged in an average of 1.19 cognitive and 1.19 socioemotional caregiving practices in the past three days, compared with 0.48 cognitive and 0.74 socioemotional practices for fathers, and 0.75 cognitive and 1.13 socioemotional practices and for other caregivers. Moreover, 40.26 percent of mothers, 70.20 percent of fathers, and 59.58 percent of other caregivers participated in no cognitive caregiving practices, and 34.93 percent of mothers, 51.87 percent of fathers, and 38.68 percent of other caregivers participated in no socioemotional caregiving practices. Each of these differences among caregivers is small-to-medium in effect size (Table 15.1 cognitive caregiving practices, SMD_{range}=0.23–0.48 for whole sample; Table 15.2 socioemotional practices, SMD_{range}=0.05–0.41 for whole sample) even after accounting for nesting of caregivers within families and countries and controlling for covariates. Overall, in these 12 Asian countries, mothers engaged in the most reported cognitive and socioemotional caregiving practices, followed by other caregivers in the home, followed by fathers; this pattern was replicated in most individual nations (Tables 15.1 and 15.2).

Correlations in Cognitive and Socioemotional Caregiving Practices Among Mothers, Fathers, and Other Caregivers in Majority World Asian Countries

Partial correlations, controlling for the effects of family and country membership as well as the other covariates, revealed that reports of mother and father cognitive caregiving scores ($r(53036)=.16$, $p<.01$) and socioemotional caregiving scores ($r(53034)=.26$, $p<.01$) were positively associated, and these associations were small-to-medium in magnitude (Cohen, 1988). In contrast, reports of mother and other caregiver cognitive ($r(53036)=-.17$, $p<.01$) and

TABLE 15.1 Mother, Father, and Other Caregiver Cognitive Caregiving, Differences Between Caregivers, and Early Childhood Development Index by Country

Country	*N*	*Mother Cognitive Caregiving M (SD) (0–3 Scale)*	*Father Cognitive Caregiving M (SD) (0–3 Scale)*	*Other Caregiver Cognitive Caregiving M (SD) (0–3 Scale)*	*Mother-Father Standardized Mean Difference*	*Mother-Other Caregiver Standardized Mean Difference*	*Other Caregiver-Father Standardized Mean Difference*	*ECDI M (SD) (0–10 Scale)*
Whole sample	53044	1.19 (1.17)	0.48 (0.85)	0.75 (1.05)	0.48***	0.30***	0.23***	6.10 (1.77)
Bangladesh	8767	1.71 (1.17)	0.53 (0.90)	0.86 (1.08)	0.77***	0.55***	0.31***	5.62 (1.70)
Bhutan	2403	0.56 (0.87)	0.45 (0.82)	0.59 (0.90)	0.13***	-0.03	0.15***	5.94 (1.66)
Iraq	13960	0.86 (1.01)	0.37 (0.73)	0.43 (0.78)	0.37***	0.33***	0.07***	5.59 (1.78)
Kazakhstan	4200	1.83 (1.16)	0.39 (0.78)	1.03 (1.18)	0.81***	0.45***	0.48***	6.81 (1.47)
Kyrgyzstan	1778	1.35 (1.15)	0.28 (0.60)	0.78 (1.06)	0.65***	0.35***	0.40***	5.74 (1.33)
Laos	4472	0.73 (0.98)	0.62 (0.93)	0.89 (1.09)	0.09***	-0.12***	0.19***	6.28 (1.59)
Mongolia	3672	0.97 (1.09)	0.42 (0.80)	0.63 (1.03)	0.43***	0.26***	0.21***	6.49 (1.32)
Nepal	2241	1.06 (1.17)	0.60 (0.94)	0.92 (1.12)	0.31***	0.09***	0.23***	5.55 (1.89)
State of Palestine	3217	1.69 (1.05)	0.56 (0.83)	0.57 (0.91)	0.71***	0.71***	0.01	5.84 (1.70)
Thailand	4214	0.67 (1.06)	0.62 (1.06)	1.46 (1.32)	0.06*	-0.85***	0.61***	7.74 (1.56)
Turkmenistan	1492	2.49 (0.85)	0.69 (0.94)	0.45 (0.83)	0.92***	1.04***	-0.29***	6.84 (1.10)
Vietnam	2628	1.37 (1.16)	0.59 (0.89)	0.71 (0.99)	0.43***	0.37***	0.09***	6.65 (1.70)

Note. All standardized mean difference scores can be interpreted as if the second caregiver listed is the caregiver score that is being compared with, and these differences emerged after controlling for the nested structure of the data and covariates as reported in the Analytic Plan. $^*p < .05$, $^{**}p < .01$, $^{***}p < .001$

TABLE 15.2 Mother, Father, and Other Caregiver Socioemotional Caregiving and Differences Between Caregivers by Country

Country	*N*	*Mother Socioemotional Caregiving M (SD) (0–3 Scale)*	*Father Socioemotional Caregiving M (SD) (0–3 Scale)*	*Other Caregiver Socioemotional Caregiving M (SD) (0–3 Scale)*	*Mother-Father Standardized Mean Difference*	*Mother-Other Caregiver Standardized Mean Difference*	*Other Caregiver-Father Standardized Mean Difference*
Whole sample	53044	1.19 (1.09)	0.74 (0.91)	1.13 (1.09)	0.41***	0.05***	0.38***
Bangladesh	8767	1.06 (0.98)	0.67 (0.77)	1.39 (0.97)	0.39***	-0.34***	0.64***
Bhutan	2403	1.22 (0.99)	0.68 (0.95)	1.06 (1.02)	0.55***	0.16***	0.42***
Iraq	13960	0.98 (0.97)	0.73 (0.86)	0.90 (0.92)	0.21***	0.07***	0.15***
Kazakhstan	4200	1.71 (1.11)	0.79 (0.93)	1.26 (1.17)	0.62***	0.30***	0.37***
Kyrgyzstan	1778	0.97 (1.03)	0.48 (0.79)	1.04 (1.14)	0.39***	-0.06	0.44***
Laos	4472	1.09 (1.07)	0.72 (0.97)	1.40 (1.17)	0.24***	-0.21***	0.40***
Mongolia	3672	1.14 (1.08)	0.60 (0.89)	0.67 (1.00)	0.48***	0.42***	0.07**
Nepal	2241	1.17 (1.11)	0.59 (0.88)	1.32 (1.12)	0.43***	-0.11***	0.51***
State of Palestine	3217	1.95 (1.01)	1.06 (0.95)	0.82 (1.02)	0.58***	0.73***	-0.23***
Thailand	4214	0.46 (0.89)	0.67 (1.07)	1.75 (1.26)	-0.30***	-1.84***	0.79***
Turkmenistan	1492	2.35 (0.83)	1.12 (0.87)	0.59 (0.86)	0.70***	1.00***	-0.60***
Vietnam	2628	1.78 (1.12)	1.02 (1.02)	1.16 (1.17)	0.51***	0.41***	0.12***

Note. ECDI = Early Childhood Development Index. All standardized mean difference scores can be interpreted as if the second caregiver listed is the caregiver score that is being compared with, and these differences emerged after controlling for the nested structure of the data and covariates as reported in the Analytic Plan. *$p < .05$, ** $p < .01$, ***$p < .001$.

socioemotional ($r(53036)=-.21$, $p<.01$) caregiving, and father and other caregiver cognitive ($r(53036)=-.08$, $p<.01$) and socioemotional ($r(53036)=-.17$, $p=.01$) caregiving were both negatively associated and between small and medium in magnitude (Cohen, 1988). This same pattern of correlations was replicated in most nations in the sample (results available from first author). These results indicate that, according to mothers, the more that mothers engaged in cognitive and socioemotional caregiving practices, the more fathers engaged in those practices as well. In contrast, the more mothers and fathers engaged in cognitive and socioemotional caregiving practices, the less other caregivers in the home engaged in these practices.

Cognitive and Socioemotional Caregiving Practices Provided by Mothers, Fathers, and Other Caregivers by Child Gender in Majority World Asian Countries

After accounting for nesting of caregivers within families and countries and controlling for other covariates, mothers ($M_{Girls}=1.20$, $M_{Boys}=1.19$; $SMD=-0.01$, $p>.05$) and other caregivers ($M_{Girls}=0.75$, $M_{Boys}=0.74$; $SMD=-0.01$, $p>.05$) engaged in equal amounts of cognitive caregiving activities with girls and boys, whereas fathers reportedly engaged in slightly more cognitive caregiving activities with boys than girls ($M_{Girls}=0.47$, $M_{Boys}=0.50$; $SMD=0.09$, $p<.05$). For socioemotional caregiving, mothers reportedly engaged in slightly more socioemotional ($M_{Girls}=1.21$, $M_{Boys}=1.16$; $SMD=-0.05$, $p<.05$) caregiving with girls than boys, whereas fathers reportedly engaged in slightly more socioemotional caregiving activities with boys than girls ($M_{Girls}=0.71$, $M_{Boys}=0.77$; $SMD=0.08$, $p<.05$). Other caregivers reportedly engaged in equal amounts of socioemotional caregiving activities with girls and boys ($M_{Girls}=1.14$, $M_{Boys}=1.13$; $SMD=-0.01$, $p>.05$). However, the sizes of all these differences were not of practical significance (i.e., all were under the $SMD=0.2$; Cohen, 1988), indicating that girls and boys experienced equivalent levels of reported caregiving regardless of whether that caregiving was delivered by mothers, fathers, or other caregivers in the home. Notably, however, small effect sizes early in life can aggregate to large effects later in life, and small effect sizes at the population level may be meaningful.

Mother, Father, and Other Caregiver Cognitive and Socioemotional Caregiving Practices in Association with Early Childhood Development in Majority World Asian Countries

At the between-country level, neither the two types of caregiving nor country HDI predicted differences between countries in child ECDI scores (Table 15.3). This means that country-level differences in average levels of

TABLE 15.3 Multilevel Models Comparing the Simultaneous Associations of Cognitive and Socioemotional Caregiving and Demographic Characteristics with the Early Childhood Development Index

	B *[95 percent Confidence Interval]*	*p*	*Significant after Bonferroni Correction?*
Between-Country Associations with Early Childhood Development Index			
Mothers' Cognitive Caregiving Practices	-0.34 [-1.21, 13.95]	.33	No
Fathers' Cognitive Caregiving Practices	6.19 [-1.56, 13.95]	.09	No
Other Caregivers' Cognitive Caregiving Practices	-2.64 [-9.58, 4.30]	.35	No
Mothers' Socioemotional Caregiving Practices	0.57 [-1.21, 2.32]	.43	No
Fathers' Socioemotional Caregiving Practices	-3.43 [-10.78, 3.92]	.26	No
Other Caregivers' Socioemotional Caregiving Practices	2.07 [-2.83, 6.97]	.31	No
Human Development Index	11.55 [-3.64, 26.75]	.10	No
Within-Country Associations with Early Childhood Development Index			
Mothers' Cognitive Caregiving Practices	0.19 [0.18, 0.21]	<.001	Yes
Fathers' Cognitive Caregiving Practices	0.15 [0.13, 0.17]	<.001	Yes
Other Caregivers' Cognitive Caregiving Practices	0.17 [0.15, 0.18]	<.001	Yes
Mothers' Socioemotional Caregiving Practices	-0.03 [-0.05, -0.02]	<.001	Yes
Fathers' Socioemotional Caregiving Practices	-0.03 [-0.05, -0.01]	<.001	Yes
Other Caregivers' Socioemotional Caregiving Practices	-0.03 [-0.05, -0.01]	<.001	Yes
Child Gender (0 = Female, 1 = Male)	-0.19 [-.21, -0.16]	<.001	Yes
Child Age (Months)	0.04 [0.04, 0.04]	<.001	Yes
Mother Age (Years)	0.01 [0.00, 0.01]	<.001	Yes
Mother Education (0–3 Range)	0.19 [0.17, 0.21]	<.001	Yes
Other Caregiver in the Home Environment (0 = No, 1 = Yes)	-0.07 [-0.11, -0.03]	<.001	Yes
Overall Quality of the Physical Home Environment (Range: -7.17, 8.44)	0.10 [0.09, 0.11]	<.001	Yes

Note. Bonferroni-corrected critical p-value was p =.003.

mother, father, and other caregiver cognitive and socioemotional differences did not predict differences in child ECDI scores. Put another way, differences across these 12 Asian countries in average levels of caregiving were not significant predictors of child development scores.

However, at the within-country level, mothers, fathers, and other caregivers who reportedly engaged in larger numbers of cognitive caregiving practices than is typical in their country had young children who demonstrated more advanced development (Table 15.3). All three caregivers' caregiving were similarly associated with early childhood development (as demonstrated by the overlapping 95 percent confidence intervals); the only difference was that fathers' cognitive caregiving was slightly less strongly associated with early childhood development than was mothers' cognitive caregiving (as demonstrated by the barely non-overlapping 95 percent confidence intervals). Collectively, mothers', fathers', and other caregivers' cognitive caregiving accounted for 1.9 percent of unique within-country variance in early childhood development scores separate and apart from all other variables, all small effects (Cohen, 1988). However, these small effects are still notable, given that they persisted in the face of universal developmental effects (i.e., children aging) and other protective factors (e.g., mother education) that have demonstrated substantial power in predicting child outcomes (Bornstein et al., 2022b).

When cognitive caregiving scores were removed from the model, mothers, fathers, and other caregivers who used a larger number of socioemotional caregiving practices had young children who demonstrated more advanced development (results available from the first author). However, when included in the model with cognitive caregiving, socioemotional caregiving strategies collectively accounted for only 0.7 percent of unique within-country variance in the ECDI scores in this model, which is considered not practically meaningful (Cohen, 1988).

Collectively, these within-country results highlight the universally promotive effect of cognitive caregiving strategies on early childhood development. Even when comparing caregivers who share the same cultural context, mothers, fathers, and other caregivers who engage in more cognitive caregiving practices have children with higher ECDI scores.

The Meaning of the Four Findings for Parenting and Early Childhood Development in Majority World Asian Countries

The United Nations has long advocated for majority world countries to invest in the provision of responsive, stimulating caregiving for young children given its implications for children's physical, cognitive, emotional, and social development (UNESCO, 2010, 2023). In majority world Asian countries, a number of intervention programs have been developed to support caregivers in this regard (e.g., Aboud & Akhter, 2011). Nevertheless, empirical evidence on caregivers' provision of stimulating caregivers and relations of stimulating caregiving to early childhood development in majority world countries in Asia, especially Central and West Asia, remains scarce. Focusing on 12 majority world countries across different regions of Asia, the current study examined mothers', fathers', and children's other caregivers' cognitive and socioemotional caregiving as well as associations of those practices with early childhood development. Among the three types of caregivers, mothers appear to provide cognitive and socioemotional caregiving the most, although fathers and other caregivers are also actively engaged in both sorts of caregiving. The results also indicate that all three types of caregivers may play major roles in supporting young children's development, with their cognitive caregiving practices being more important compared with their socioemotional caregiving practices.

Differences in Cognitive and Socioemotional Caregiving Provided by Different Caregivers in Majority World Asian Countries

On average mothers reportedly engaged in the most cognitive and socioemotional caregiving practices, followed by other caregivers in the home, and last fathers. That mothers in these Asian countries reportedly engage in more cognitive and socioemotional caregiving activities than fathers aligns with existing literature on broader patterns of caregiving in majority world countries (Bornstein & Putnick, 2016; Cuartas et al., 2020). In these Asian countries, this finding may be accounted for by the traditional division of childcare roles where mothers assume larger caregiving responsibilities (Ng & Wang, 2019).

However, the current study builds on the existing literature by revealing that children's other caregivers participated in more caregiving practices than fathers in this sample (Cuartas et al., 2018; McCoy et al., 2022). We attribute this finding to the multigenerational structure of most majority world Asian countries households; in this sample, other caregivers resided in 56.60 percent of homes. Although the MICS do not reveal the identity of those other caregivers, in most Asian multigenerational households they are women, often grandmothers or aunts, who spend substantial amounts of time with children and hold considerable power in modeling and shaping caregiving interactions (Ng & Wang, 2019). Therefore, it is not surprising that other caregivers were reported to engage in more cognitive and socioemotional caregiving practices than were fathers in this sample.

Correlations in Caregiving Practices Among Different Caregivers in Majority World Asian Countries

Based on mothers' reports, the more mothers engaged in cognitive and socioemotional caregiving practices, the more fathers did: however, the more mothers and fathers engaged in cognitive and socioemotional caregiving practices, the less children's other caregivers did. We interpret these differences in light of contemporary trends in family life in Asian countries. If current trends toward urbanization force mothers and fathers outside the home more frequently, and consequently force other caregivers to serve as substitutes for working parents, negative correlations between mother/father caregiving and other caregiver caregiving would be expected (Lansford et al., 2021; Ng & Wang, 2019; Meng et al., 2023; Yotanyamaneewong et al., 2021). The data appear to support this second, "contemporary economic trends" explanation.

Additionally, the positive correlation between reports of mothers' caregiving practices and fathers' caregiving practices builds on existing MICS literature in terms of positive correlations in cognitive and socioemotional parenting practices among mothers and fathers living in majority world countries between 2005 and 2009 (Bornstein & Putnick, 2016; Sun et al., 2016). The current data extend this finding to 2009–2017 and replicate it in majority world Asian countries. The strong positive association between mother and father caregiving practices may reflect assortative mating before or mutual modeling or decision making in childrearing after the birth of a child. Encouragingly, it may also mean that, if cognitive or socioemotional caregiving practices can be increased for one caregiver, they might also increase in the other (Rothenberg, 2023). This result might be an especially important consideration for the design of interventions to promote cognitive and socioemotional caregiving in parents, as intervening with one parent might "spill over" to increase the number of caregiving behaviors in the other parent. Importantly, the negative correlations between mothers and children's other caregivers, and fathers and children's other caregivers, mean that when parents choose other caregivers to care for their children they cannot be guaranteed that those other caregivers will behave with their children the way parents themselves behave.

Cognitive and Socioemotional Caregiving Practices in Majority World Asian Countries and Child Gender

Girls and boys in majority world Asian countries experienced roughly equivalent levels of caregiving regardless of whether their caregiving was reportedly provided by mothers, fathers, or their other caregivers. These results align with previous MICS work in other countries around the world that found that reported caregiver use of several different caregiving practices did not differ based on their child's gender (Bornstein & Putnick, 2016; Bornstein et al., 2022b). It is encouraging that, at least according to the measures used in the MICS, Asian parents do not seem to favor boys or girls in their early caregiving practices. Sometimes, owing to the traditionally patriarchal nature of many Asian societies, sons are preferred to daughters and family resources are unequally distributed towards sons (Ng & Wang, 2019; Guilmoto & Jones, 2016). However, as Asian nations become wealthier and more industrialized over time, treatment for boys and girls appears to become more equal (Ng & Wang, 2019; Roche, 2017; Rosenzweig & Zhang, 2014). It could be that, with improving economic conditions and increased female workforce participation, parents rely less on their sons and more on their daughters or themselves to secure their financial future and therefore invest their caregiving in a similar way in their boys and girls. Of course, these data apply to the three- to four-year-olds, and gender differences in socialization could emerge later in children's development.

How Caregivers' Caregiving is Associated with Early Childhood Development in Majority World Asian Countries

Mother, father, and other caregiver cognitive and socioemotional caregiving practices in the 12 majority world Asian countries examined here appear to be differentially associated with early childhood development. Although differences between countries did not predict ECDI scores, at the within-country level mothers, fathers, and other caregivers who engaged in more cognitive caregiving practices compared with their same-country peers had children who demonstrated more advanced development on the ECDI. The lack of between-country associations between caregiving and ECDI highlights the myriad cultural practices, strengths, traditions, and ways of caregiving that exist across Asia (Ng & Wang, 2019). Because societies are so heterogeneous and therefore specific in the ways that they impact child development, it may be less likely that any single uniform measure of caregiving predicts child development between these contexts (Bornstein, 2019; Ng & Wang, 2019). Additionally, it may be that the number of majority world Asian countries included in this analysis (i.e., 12) is too small, or that there was little between-country variability in ECDI scores, and consequently between-country cross-cultural analyses are simply underpowered to expose significant effects. Moreover, the within-cultural effects found in the current analyses reinforce calls from researchers of Asian parenting that emphasize heterogeneity in caregiving across Asian cultures (e.g., Ng & Wang, 2019; Raval, 2023).

The within-culture findings align with our hypothesis that cognitive caregiving practices might more powerfully predict early childhood development in majority world Asian countries compared with socioemotional caregiving practices. These results are consistent with the values of many Asian parents, who prioritize parenting in ways that foster learning and achievement to promote upward economic mobility and family honor (Ng & Wang, 2019). Parents in Asia have been documented to use all three of the cognitive caregiving behaviors examined here (reading to, counting/naming/drawing with, and storytelling to their children) to promote child achievement from an early age (Lau et al., 2011; Ng & Wang, 2019; Rafiq et al., 2013), so it comes as little surprise that those same behaviors promote early childhood development. It is also notable that, although caregivers' cognitive caregiving predicts more advanced child development around the world, the collective impact of caregivers' cognitive caregiving on child development in these majority world Asian countries is almost double that of majority world countries in general (i.e., 1.9 percent of within-country variance in ECDI scores predicted in majority world Asian countries versus 1.0 percent of variance in ECDI scores predicted in majority world countries in general; Bornstein et al., 2022b). This evidence supports the inference that many Asian cultures' emphasis on promoting cognitive caregiving practices may "pay off" in advancing child development.

It is also notable that, at the within-culture level, fathers' cognitive caregiving practices were only slightly less powerful predictors of early childhood development than were mothers' or other caregivers' cognitive caregiving practices. One might expect such differences to be larger given the more central caregiving role mothers and other caregivers play in caregiving in many Asian Majority world countries (Ng & Wang, 2019). However, these results accord with other investigations of MICS data in many Majority world countries worldwide that find mother and father stimulating parenting both matter in predicting early childhood development and are close to equal in magnitude (e.g., Jeong et al., 2016, 2017). These results underscore that the caregiving of all three caregivers "matter" to child development and that having at least one engaged caregiver, no matter who that caregiver is, promotes child development (Jeong et al., 2016). Nevertheless, mother cognitive caregiving practices are still stronger correlates of more advanced early childhood development scores than father cognitive caregiving practices, probably owing to mothers' more central role in caregiving in contemporary Asian Majority world countries (Ng & Wang, 2019).

Caregiving in Majority World Asian Countries: Blending Traditional and Contemporary Trends?

Taken together, our findings suggest an interplay in majority world Asian countries between traditional values and caregiving roles on the one hand

and contemporary trends associated with socioeconomic development on the other. On the one hand, families' retention of traditional caregiving roles and multigenerational family structures, and retention of traditional values that emphasize cognitive caregiving to promote early learning, might account for disparities in cognitive and socioemotional caregiving across caregivers. On the other hand, contemporary trends towards parents working outside the home might drive patterns of correspondence in caregiving across caregivers, and contemporary economic trends and the de-emphasis on son preference might drive equitable caregiving across child gender. Our results suggest that, even as caregivers in Majority world Asian countries retain many aspects of traditional family structure and caregiving values, they adapt those structures and values to the changing world around them to promote child flourishing (Ng & Wang, 2019).

Limitations and Future Directions, Strengths, and Conclusions

This study has several limitations that are important to note. First, mothers reported on the caregiving practices of all three types of caregivers in a household and also reported on child development outcomes. These methods introduced the threat of shared source variance that might have inflated associations between caregiving practices and child outcomes and failed to capture the full range of caregiving behaviors undertaken by all caregivers. Future work should capture multiple caregivers' perspectives on their caregiving. Second, the MICS measure of cognitive and socioemotional caregiving has only six items which do not nearly encompass the full range of caregiving practices. Future work that captures a broader range of caregiving practices would enrich the existing literature. Third, caregiving practices and child development were measured contemporaneously, so the direction of effects cannot be determined. It could very well be that children who are developing better evoke more caregiving practices from their caregivers. Examining longitudinal trends in both caregiving and its associations with child development is an essential next step. Fourth, unfortunately MICS data do not allow us to identify the specific "other caregivers," so the "other caregiver" category could include teenage siblings, grandparents, other relatives, and unrelated household members. Future work examining the prevalence of, and differences in, caregiving engagement among these heterogeneous subsamples is needed.

That said, the current study has several notable strengths, including the use of a nationally representative and internationally comparable data set that examined more than 50,000 families in 12 under-researched majority world Asian countries. It also examined and compared caregiving practices of mothers, fathers, and other caregivers to address multiple gaps in the developmental science literature in understanding the roles of different agents in children's lives.

Collectively, these findings provide a new perspective into what caregiving looks like and how it operates in majority world Asian countries. Our results highlight the greater role other caregivers play in providing caregiving in majority world Asian countries than is typically seen in more commonly studied minority world countries. Attesting to the cultural strengths of majority world Asian countries, the multigenerational structure and collective commitment to the welfare of the family in their cultures mean that Asian parents could harness the help of other caregivers as they adjust their caregiving in adaptation to the changing environments of Asia. Encouragingly, and in contrast with older literature, this study finds that caregivers report providing similar amounts of cognitive and socioemotional caregiving regardless of whether they have sons or daughters. Finally, this study reveals that cognitive caregiving is more strongly associated with child development compared with socioemotional caregiving and that each caregiver's cognitive caregiving practices matter in child development. These findings suggest that providing caregivers the opportunities and supports necessary to enact more cognitive caregiving activities could help parents overcome the systematic barriers faced in many majority world countries and draw on unique strengths of Asian family structures and values to promote child development.

References

Aboud, F. E. & Akhter, S. (2011). A cluster-randomized evaluation of a responsive stimulation and feeding intervention in Bangladesh. *Pediatrics, 127*(5), e1191–e1197. https://doi-org.proxy.lib.duke.edu/10.1542/peds.2010-2160.

Attane, I. & Guilmoto, C. Z. (Eds) (2007). *Watering the neighbor's garden: The growing demographic female deficit in Asia*. Paris, France: Committee for International Cooperation in National Research in Demography.

Bornstein, M. H. (2019). "It's about time!" Ecological systems, transaction, and specificity as key developmental principles in children's changing worlds. In R. D. Parke & G. H. Elder (Eds), *Children in changing worlds: Sociocultural and Temporal Perspectives* (pp. 277–286). Cambridge University Press. https://doi.org/10.1017/9781108264846.010.

Bornstein, M. H. & Putnick, D. L. (2012). Cognitive and socioemotional caregiving in developing countries. *Child Development, 83*(1), 46–61. https://doi.org/10.1111/j.1467-8624.2011.01673.x.

Bornstein, M. H. & Putnick, D. L. (2016). Gender in low- and middle-income countries: IV Mothers' and fathers' parenting practices with their daughters and sons in low- and middle-income countries. *Monographs of the Society for Research in Child Development, 81*(1), 60–77. https://doi.org/10.1111/mono.12226.

Bornstein, M. H., Rothenberg, W. A., Bizzego, A., Bradley, R. H., Deater-Deckard, K., Esposito, G., Lansford, J. E., Putnick, D. L., & Zietz, S (2022a). Introduction and general methods: Parenting, national development, and early childhood development in 51 low- and middle-income countries. In M. H. Bornstein, W. A. Rothenberg, A. Bizzego, R. H. Bradley, K. Deater-Deckard, G. Esposito, J. E. Lansford, & S. Zietz (Eds), *Parenting and child development in low- and middle-income countries* (pp. 1–51). Routledge.

Bornstein, M. H., Rothenberg, W. A., Lansford, J. E., Bradley, R. H., Deater-Deckard, K, Bizzego, A., & Esposito, G. (2021). Child development in low- and middle-income countries. *Pediatrics, 148*(5), e2021053180. https://doi.org/10.1542/peds.2021-053180.

Bornstein, M. H., Rothenberg, W. A., & Putnick, D. L. (2022b). Socioemotional and socioemotional caregiving, national development, and early childhood development in 51 low- and middle-income countries. In M. H. Bornstein, W. A. Rothenberg, A. Bizzego, R. H. Bradley, K. Deater-Deckard, G. Esposito, J. E. Lansford, & S. Zietz (Eds), *Parenting and child development in low- and middle-income countries* (pp. 79–127). Routledge.

Bradley, R. H. & Rothenberg, W. A. (2022). Children's physical home environment, national development, and early childhood development in 51 low- and middle-income countries. In M. H. Bornstein, W. A. Rothenberg, A. Bizzego, R. H. Bradley, K. Deater-Deckard, G. Esposito, J. E. Lansford, & S. Zietz (Eds), *Parenting and child development in low- and middle-income countries* (pp. 160–209). Routledge.

Chen, X. (2023). *Socialization and socioemotional development in Chinese children*. In M. H. Bornstein (Series Editor), *Cambridge elements in child development*. Cambridge University Press. doi:10.1017/9781009072380.

Cohen, J. (1988). *Statistical power analysis for the behavioral sciences* (2nd ed.). Lawrence Erlbaum Associates.

Cuartas, J., Jeong, J., Rey-Guerra, C., McCoy, D. C., & Yoshikawa, H. (2020). Maternal, paternal, and other caregivers' stimulation in low-and-middle-income countries. *PLoS One, 15*(7), e0236107. https://doi.org/10.1371/journal.pone.0236107.

Guilmoto, C. Z. & Jones, G. W. (Eds). (2016). Forty percent of the world. In Y. Charbit and I. Pool (Series Eds), *Demographic transformation and socio-economic development: Vol. 5. Contemporary demographic transformations in China, India, and Indonesia*. Springer International.

Jeong, J., McCoy, D. C., & Fink, G. (2017). Pathways between paternal and maternal education, caregivers' support for learning, and early child development in 44 low-and middle-income countries. *Early Childhood Research Quarterly, 41*, 136–148. https://doi.org/10.1016/j.ecresq.2017.07.001.

Jeong, J., McCoy, D. C., Yousafzai, A. K., Salhi, C., & Fink, G. (2016). Paternal stimulation and early child development in low- and middle-income countries. *Pediatrics, 138*(4), e20161357. https://doi.org/10.1542/peds.2016-1357.

Joseph, S. (Ed.). (2018). *Arab family studies*. Syracuse University Press. https://press.syr.edu/supressbooks/189/arab-family-studies.

Kariger, P., Frongillo, E. A., Engle, P., Britto, P. M., Sywulka, S. M., & Menon, P. (2012). Indicators of family care for development for use in multicountry surveys. *Journal of Health, Population, and Nutrition, 30*(4), 472–486. https://doi.org/10.3329/jhpn.v30i4.13417.

Lansford, J. E., Rothenberg, W. A., & Bornstein, M. H. (Eds). (2021). *Parenting across cultures across development: Parenting from childhood to adolescence in nine countries.* Routledge.

Lau, E.Y.H., Li, H., & Rao, N. (2011). Parental involvement and children's readiness for school in China. *Educational Research, 53*, 95–113.

Maital, S. L. & Bornstein, M. H. (2003). The ecology of collaborative childrearing: A systems approach to child care on the kibbutz. *Ethos, 31*, 274–306. https://doi.org/10.1525/eth.2003.31.2.274.

Maital, S. L. & Bornstein, M. H. (2022). Israel: Parenting infants in the city and on kibbutz In M. H. Bornstein, *Parenting, infancy, culture: Specificity and commonality in Argentina, Belgium, Israel, Italy, and the United States* (pp. 213–280). Routledge.

McCoy, D. C., Seiden, J., Cuartas, J., Pisani, L., & Waldman. M. (2022). Estimates of a multidimensional index of nurturing care in the next 1000 days of life for children in low-income and middle-income countries: a modelling study. *The Lancet Child & Adolescent Health*, 6(5), 324–334. https://doi.org/10.1016/S2352-4642(22)00076-1.

Mehta, K. K. & Thang, L. L. (Eds). (2012). *Social indicators research series: Vol. 47. Experiencing grandparenthood: An Asian perspective.* Springer.

Meng, C., Gustafsson, B., & Knight, J. (2023). *Economic Transformation and Income Distribution in China over Three Decades* (Elements in Development Economics). Cambridge: Cambridge University Press. doi:10.1017/9781009357616.

Ng, F. F. & Li. Y. (2024). Parenting goals and values in Asian cultures. In. X. Chen (Ed.) *Asian Parenting: Meanings, characteristics, and implications* (pp. xxx–xxx). Routledge.

Ng, F. F. & Wang, Q. (2019). Asian and Asian American parenting. In M.H. Bornstein (Ed.) *Handbook of Parenting* (3rd ed., Vol. 4, pp. 108–169). Routledge.

Rafiq, H.M.W., Fatima, T., Sohail, M. M., Saleem, M., & Khan, M. A. (2013). Parental involvement and academic achievement: A study on secondary school students of Lahore, Pakistan. *International Journal of Humanities and Social Science, 3*, 209–223.

Raval, V. V. (2023). From the margins to the center: Advancing research on caregiver socialization of emotion in Asia. *Child Development Perspectives*. https://doi-org.proxy.lib.duke.edu/10.1111/cdep.12487.

Roche, S. (Ed.). (2017). *The family in central Asia: New perspectives.* De Gruyter. https://www.degruyter.com/document/doi/10.1515/9783112209271.

Rosenzweig, M. R. & Zhang, J. (2014). *Co-residence, life-cycle savings and inter-generational support in urban China*. Center Discussion Paper (No. 1039). Economic Growth Center and Yale University Press. www.nber.org/papers/w20057?.

Rothenberg, W. A. (2019). Intergenerational continuity in parenting: A review and theoretical integration. *Marriage & Family Review, 55*(8), 701–736. https://doi.org/10.1080/01494929.2019.1589618.

Rothenberg, W.A. & Bornstein, M.H. (2023). Cognitive and Socioemotional Caregiving in Mothers, Fathers, and Children's Other Caregivers from 51 Low and Middle-Income Countries. *Parenting: Science and Practice, 23*(3–4), 197–218. doi:10.1080/15295192.2023.2250827.

Shwalb, D. W., Shwalb, B. J., Nakazawa, J., Hyun, J. H., Le, H. V., & Satiadarma, M. P. (2014). East and Southeast Asia: Japan, South Korea, Vietnam, and Indonesia. In M. H. Bornstein (Ed.) *Handbook of Cultural Developmental Science* (pp. 445–464. Psychology Press.

Sun, J., Liu, Y., Chen, E. E., Rao, N., & Liu, H. (2016). Factors related to parents' engagement in cognitive and socio-emotional caregiving in developing countries: Results from Multiple Indicator Cluster Survey 3. *Early Childhood Research Quarterly, 36,* 21–31. https://doi.org/10.1016/j.ecresq.2015.12.003.

Tapanya, S. (2011). Attributions and attitudes of mothers and fathers in Thailand. *Parenting: Science and Practice, 11,* 190–198.

Tomlinson, M., Bornstein, M. H., Marlow, M., & Swartz, L. (2014). Imbalances in the knowledge about infant mental health in rich and poor countries: Too little progress in bridging the gap. *Infant Mental Health Journal, 35,* 624–629. https://doi.org/10.1002/imhj.21462.

UN Development Programme (2014). *Human development report 2014: Sustaining human progress: Reducing vulnerabilities and building resilience.* http://hdr.undp.org/sites/default/files/hdr14-report-en-1.pdf.

UNESCO (2010). *Early childhood care and education in the Asia Pacific region: Moving towards Goal 1.* Retrieved from https://unesdoc.unesco.org/ark:/48223/pf0000190526.

UNESCO (2023). *Region report for Arab states: Education starts early: Progress, challenges, and opportunities.* Retrieved from https://unesdoc.unesco.org/ark:/48223/pf0000385580.

UNICEF (2009). *Multiple Indicator Cluster Surveys 4 Manual.* https://mics.unicef.org/tools?round=mics4.

UNICEF (2013). *Multiple Indicator Cluster Surveys 5 Manual.* https://mics.unicef.org/tools?round=mics5.

UNICEF (2017). *Development of the Early Childhood Development Index in MICS surveys.* http://mics.unicef.org/files?job=W1siZilsIjIwMTcvMDkvMTUvMjEvMTUvNDMvMzc4L01JQ1NfTWV0aG9kb2xvZ2ljYWxfUGFwZXJfNi5wZGYiXV0&sha=85c096f0b2c5b0c8.

UNICEF (2023, November). *Country Profiles (2023).* Nurturing Care for Early Childhood Development. https://nurturing-care.org/resources/country-profiles.

United Nations (2019). *Patterns and trends in household size and composition: Evidence from a United Nations dataset.* www.un.org/en/development/desa/population/publications/pdf/ageing/household_size_and_composition_technical_report.pdf.

World Economic Forum (2023). *Global gender gap report 2023.* www.weforum.org/publications/global-gender-gap-report-2023.

Yotanyamaneewong, S., Rothenberg, W. A., & Tapanya, S. (2021). Four domains of parenting in Thailand. In J. E. Lansford, W. A. Rothenberg, & M. H. Bornstein (Eds), *Parenting across cultures across development: Parenting from childhood to adolescence in nine countries* (pp. 172–192). Routledge.

INDEX

Note: **Bold** page numbers refer to tables; *italic* page numbers refer to figures and ***bold italic*** page numbers refer to boxes.